Baillière's Study Skills for Nurses and Midwives

D0702193

Senior Commissioning Editor: Ninette Premdas
Development Editor: Sally Davies
Project Manager: Frances Affleck
Designer: Kirsteen Wright
Illustration Manager: Gillian Richards
Illustrator: Oxford Illustrators; David Banks

Baillière's Study Skills for Nurses and Midwives

FOURTH EDITION

EDITED BY

Sian Maslin-Prothero RN RM DIPN(LOND) CERT ED

Dean of the Graduate School and Professor of Nursing, Keele University, Keele, UK

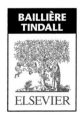

BAILLIÈRE
TINDALL

ELSEVIER

Edinburgh London New York Oxford Philadelphia St Louis Sydney Toronto 2010

BAILLIÈRE
TINDALL
ELSEVIER

First edition © Baillière Tindall 1997
Second edition © Harcourt Publishers Limited 2001, © Elsevier Science Limited 2002
Third edition © Elsevier Science Limited 2005
Fourth edition © 2010, Elsevier Limited. All rights reserved.

ISBN 978-0-7020-3142-7

British Library Cataloguing in Publication Data
A catalogue record for this book is available from the British Library

Library of Congress Cataloging in Publication Data
A catalog record for this book is available from the Library of Congress

Notice
Neither the Publisher nor the Editor assume any responsibility for any loss or injury and/or damage to persons or property arising out of or related to any use of the material contained in this book. It is the responsibility of the treating practitioner, relying on independent expertise and knowledge of the patient, to determine the best treatment and method of application for the patient.

The Publisher

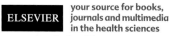

ELSEVIER   your source for books,
journals and multimedia
in the health sciences
www.elsevierhealth.com

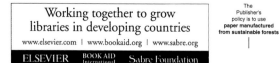

Working together to grow
libraries in developing countries
www.elsevier.com | www.bookaid.org | www.sabre.org

ELSEVIER   BOOK AID   Sabre Foundation
International

The Publisher's policy is to use paper manufactured from sustainable forests

Printed in China

CONTENTS

Contents

CONTRIBUTORS

Denis Anthony BA(Hons) MSc PhD RMN SRN RN(Canada)
Professor of Nursing, School of Nursing and Midwifery, De Montfort University, Leicester, UK

Sue Brain BA(Hons) PGCE DipLib MCLIP
Library Manager, NHS Direct, Southampton, UK

Lisa Common BA(Hons) RM
Community Midwife, CitiHealth Nottingham City, Nottingham, UK

Andrew Finney BSc(Hons) RN PGCHE
Clinical Skills Lecturer, School of Nursing and Midwifery, Keele University, Staffordshire, UK

Elizabeth A Rosser (née Girot) DPhil MN DipNEd DipRM RN RM
Professor/Associate Dean (Nursing), Bournemouth University, School of Health and Social Care, Bournemouth, UK

Neil Gopee BA(Hons) MEd PhD RN CertEd
Senior Lecturer, Faculty of Health and Life Sciences, Coventry University, Coventry, UK

Rebecca Hoskins BSc(Hons) MA FFEN RGN RN
Consultant Nurse and Senior Lecturer in Emergency Care, School of Health and Social Care, University of the West of England, Bristol, UK

Netta Lloyd-Jones MN DipN CMS RGN CertEd
Head of Practice Education, School of Health and Social Care, Oxford Brookes University, Oxford, UK

Kym Martindale BA(Hons) MA PhD
Senior Lecturer in English with Media Studies, University College Falmouth, Penryn, Cornwall, UK

Sian Maslin-Prothero RN RM DipN(Lond) CertEd
Dean of the Graduate School and Professor of Nursing, Keele University, Keele, Staffordshire, UK

Abigail Masterson BSc MPA MN RN PGCEA FRSA
Director, Abi Masterson Consulting Ltd, London, UK

Jenny Spouse MSc PhD RGN SCM RCNT DipN RNT
Formerly Associate Dean for Practice Education, St Bartholomew School of Nursing and Midwifery, City University London, UK; Consultant in practice education

Heather J Wharrad BSc PhD
Reader and Associate Professor in Education and Health Informatics, School of Nursing, Midwifery and Physiotherapy, University of Nottingham Medical School, Nottingham, UK

INTRODUCTION

From personal experience I know how important it is to have strategies that can help you to be a successful learner – even if you have been a successful learner in the past. We work in a climate of rapid change in which, as health professionals, we are expected to be creative, critical thinkers who can respond to the dynamic health and social-care environment in order to meet the needs and requirements of our clients and their carers.

In the UK, we are required by our regulatory body – the Nursing and Midwifery Council – to demonstrate our competency to practise. Regardless of where you are – an Access course college student, a pre-qualifying midwifery or nursing student, or an experienced post-qualifying student – this book aims to develop skills for life-long learning; all the skills essential for you to become an independent learner.

How to use this book

I have listened to the feedback from reviewers of the previous edition, and made changes in light of this. The book is divided into two sections; Section 1 focuses on developing initial study skills, and Section 2 explores skills needed to learn from practice.

The aim of the book is to be interactive, and the structure of the chapters is devised so that – at a glance – you see what the key issues are, followed by an introduction. Within each chapter there are: tips and hints, reflection points, activities, case studies, references, websites and further reading. You can decide whether the chapter has what you need – the order in which you access the chapters is up to you.

Reflection points

 These will raise issues that allow you a few moments to reflect on what you are learning and how you might learn from your experiences.

Activities

 These invite you as the reader to consider issues which require you to move beyond reflection. They may require you to note down some of your ideas or to carry out some more research into a given topic. You may wish to come back to these after you finish reading the chapter.

Tips/Hints

 Useful tips have been indicated and highlighted for quick reference. These are often based on the writer's own experiences and we hope they will help you avoid some of the common pitfalls.

ACKNOWLEDGEMENTS

I would like to thank the current and previous contributors to the book, who have made this a different study skills text that continues to be of value to learners.

This book is dedicated to Jack, Charlotte and Paul.

SECTION 1
DEVELOPING YOUR STUDY SKILLS

SECTION CONTENTS

1 Getting ready to study

Lisa Common and Sian Maslin-Prothero

KEY ISSUES

- Preparation
- Setting realistic goals
- Making a timetable
- Making plans
- Defining priorities
- Thinking strategically
- Creating a suitable environment
- Developing networks for support

Introduction

If you have recently started or are just about to start a course of study, you are also likely to have a high degree of motivation to succeed. One of the things you will realize is that studying is a serious and time-consuming activity and not something to be done as and when you feel like it. You have committed yourself to this course and you should aim to maintain your current drive and enthusiasm. Don't forget to look back on your progress from time to time to see what you have achieved; this will motivate you to continue.

This first chapter looks at how you can approach studying to make the best use of your time and resources. It considers timetabling and time management as measures for improving the quality of study time, and as strategies for completing important tasks. The final sections discuss where you study and provide some resources that you might find useful.

Take a look at yourself – what impact is this course going to have on your life for the foreseeable future? There is no such thing as a 'typical student' and your circumstances will be different to those of your fellow students.

Preparing for your course

The phrases 'adult learner' and 'life-long learning' crop up everywhere in healthcare education. Essentially, they mean that you – yes, *you* – are responsible for acquiring knowledge and skills throughout your life through education, training, employment and life experiences. If you expect your tutors and mentors to expound all the knowledge you will need to become the practitioner of the future, you are in for a shock. Think beyond the elements of your course that are assessed and strive to become the best you can be by going that extra mile for yourself. You will make decisions about why, what, when, how and where you will study, so choose wisely – your future success will depend on the choices you make (Figure 1.1).

The reality for many students is that higher education is hugely bureaucratic and run by individuals who often manage administrative and research responsibilities along with their teaching roles. Try to learn something of the systems and people who shape your institution and influence your learning opportunities. You can do this by attending orientation days, speaking to staff, becoming a course representative, attending staff–student committees or by getting involved with your local Royal College of Nursing (RCN), Royal College of Midwives (RCM) or the National Students' Union.

Alongside the culture of your institution, you will also need to negotiate the culture and expectations of your chosen profession (Marshall and Rowland, 1996).

WHO ARE YOU?

- What are your values? How might these impact on others, say your clients? How will they perceive you?
- Are you a young undergraduate, away from home for the first time?
- Will you continue to have domestic commitments on top of your study?
- Will you be taking a part-time course while holding a full-time job (with or without domestic commitments)?
- Will you need to take a part-time job to make ends meet?
- If it is a taught course, are there likely to be any problems about attending all the lectures and seminars?
- Can you cope with studying in isolation, say if your course is a distance learning one?

Your circumstances may well be different from these. Take some time to think how your life is going to be affected by your new role as a student:

- What effect is it going to have on others close to you and how might they have to adapt?
- Will they feel threatened and become unsupportive?
- Will they become jealous or suspicious of the time you spend away from home?
- Will they feel burdened by any financial pressures resulting from your student income?
- Can your caring responsibilities be managed if one person says no, or is ill?

Succeeding as a student is a balancing act. Your friends and family are probably very excited and supportive of you starting your course. This enthusiasm can begin to flag a few weeks down the line when there is no milk in the fridge, nothing for dinner and all you think and talk

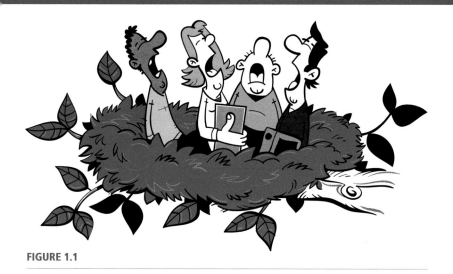

FIGURE 1.1

about is your course. For the first few months you might ride a roller-coaster of emotions and may feel exhausted most of the time. You will eventually find your equilibrium but, in the meantime, you will need to learn to say no to unreasonable demands with grace and confidence and know when you need to make time to have some fun (Common, 2007).

Before you start, be sure to find out about important things, such as what time your day starts and finishes; whether there is car parking nearby and how much it costs; and, if you are going to be late home, who will take care of your family (e.g. children and other dependants). Neglecting any aspect of your life will create an imbalance that might cause you additional stress and affect the quality of your work.

You are going to be developing existing skills as well as new ones, such as information technology skills or the power of language. This is demonstrated in the box below.

Imagine that at shift handover you are told that the client in bed 3 has been 'a hysterical nightmare all shift'. How does this make you feel about that client and how might it impact on the care you give him or her? What if your colleague had described the client as having been 'upset and tearful this afternoon' instead? Does this change how you feel towards that client?

Be aware of the powerful impact that value-laden and judgemental comments can have on you and those around you. Develop a communication style that avoids derisory language of any kind. Try to make your own assessments and decisions and look for something positive in everything you do and everyone you meet.

If you seek certainty in life and do not want to change your values or your ideas, then a career in nursing or midwifery might not be right for you. Higher education will confront you with questions that challenge your existing value systems. It will ask you to open your mind to both exciting and confusing possibilities. Explore your motivation for study and what you hope to achieve, then stay alert to all the ways that will lead to your success (Marshall and Rowland, 1996).

What is study?

Look at the following activities and think about what they might entail:

- problem-based learning
- attending lectures, reading, discussing, essay writing
- preparing presentations, group work, seminars and tutorials, literature searching
- critical thinking, reflection
- simulation and practice skills.

Some of these activities involve working with other students and some are solitary activities. To do them effectively, you will probably need to develop or enhance new skills, such as how to prepare for lectures or to read effectively; these are discussed in detail in other chapters. You need to think about what resources you need to become an effective student.

Your course should be designed to stimulate your curiosity and stretch your mind. There will be formal elements that require you master a body of knowledge in a particular way; but you should also be encouraged to ask your own questions. These may include:

- Why do I want to know about this particular subject?
- What is it that I want to find out?
- What are the interesting or most important aspects?
- What do I already know about it?
- What resources can I use to find more answers?
- How will I go about the task?
- When do I have to complete it by?

Asking 'why?' can help you to reveal fundamental questions. For example, asking 'why do we write information down about clients?' will produce more insightful answers than asking 'how can we improve handwritten records?' Asking 'why?' can lead us to understand, criticize and evaluate the status quo and inform our answers.

Nurses and midwives are researchers and innovators. Being able to ask experimental or cause-and-effect questions such as 'what happens if…?' or 'what might happen if…?' can help to influence how care is delivered. Equally, being able to free your imagination and ask speculative questions such as 'what if…' can lead to the development of practice in new and challenging directions. (Marshall and Rowland, 1996).

Preparation

How you learn, where you learn and when you learn will be determined by a number of factors. At university you will receive a timetable, which will tell you about the times and locations of lectures and seminars; do give yourself time to find where these rooms are, as arriving late is embarrassing for you and distracting for those who got there on time.

There may be minimum attendance requirements to pass modules – this will include time spent in practice – find out what these are and, if you are ill or away, be prepared to make this time up. There will be personal study time when you can choose 'how' and 'where' to study; use this wisely.

Making the most of study days

- With a whole day yawning in front of you, it is extremely easy for the time to slip through your fingers. Try to avoid the temptations of daytime television, online social networking or any unnatural urges to insulate the loft!
- Sit down with your diary and find your assignment deadline dates.
- Write in your diary that you will complete your final drafts by the week before the deadlines. This gives you time to put any finishing touches to them and earn those vital extra marks for presentation and referencing.
- Work out how many study days you have between now and the deadline.
- Plan how you will use each of your study days. Allocate a little time for you to get into the right frame of mind and set out your workspace with everything you need; then allocate reasonable amounts of time for tea and snack breaks; whatever is left you can use for a combination of creative and structured discussion, reading and writing.
- Devise a reward you will give yourself each time you follow your plan. This might be anything from a night out with your friends, to pampering yourself in front of your fireplace for an evening.

(Adapted from Siviter, 2008)

There is an assumption that you will spend time outside of 'university' hours engaged in activities related to the course such as reading, preparing assignments, collecting materials for projects.

Getting the balance right

Management of your time and the activities that fill it is a very important aspect of studying. When you are studying outside the time that has been allocated to you in university, you will have to make all the decisions; working at home means mixing your studies with all your other activities. Devoting time to your studies means that you will have less time for some of the other things that you already do. Northedge (2005) identifies three areas that generate activities that are likely to compete for your time: social commitments, work commitments and leisure activities.

- ■ Social commitments include going out to visit friends, time spent with a partner/family, attending parents' evenings or going to church.
- ■ Work commitments include housework and childcare as well as attending university and placements (they might also include any agency or part-time work you are engaged in).
- ■ Leisure activities include attending clubs or societies, concerts, sporting activities and going to the pub.

If you devote too much time to learning at home, or in university, then your social life and leisure activities will suffer. Embarking on a midwifery or nursing course can be life changing, and you need to be prepared for how it might affect people close to you.

- • Will they feel threatened and become unsupportive?
- • Will they feel jealous and suspicious of the time you spend away from home?
- • Will there be financial pressures due to a reduced income?
- • How will you manage the demands of the course and those of your partner and children?

You need to have balance between your social life, work and leisure. We are all different – some people like to leave things to the last minute whereas others plan ahead. Planning can help you organize your life and should lead to less stress. Planning/timetabling is very helpful; you can use a diary (online or paper based) or a year planner. Remember that:

- • You need to be realistic about what you intend to achieve
- • You need to strike a balance between studying and your other commitments

Being realistic will contribute to your sense of wellbeing. If you set yourself demanding goals and then fail to live up to your own expectations, it is possible that you will feel frustrated and disappointed; for example, not giving yourself sufficient time to write an assignment can result in you not answering the question, rushing it, making mistakes or having great ideas poorly structured (Siviter, 2008). If you set an achievable goal, you are less likely to fail and you can benefit from the positive feelings associated with a job well done. Don't be tempted to set goals that are easy to achieve; if they are too low, you may feel frustrated because you are not making the most of your abilities. You also run the risk of falling behind because you are not doing enough to keep up with the demands of the course.

What kind of learner are you?

Planning and setting realistic goals is a skill that is gained through experience, so don't be afraid to experiment and try out different things. First of all you need to identify what kind of learner you are.

- Are you a lark or an owl? Do you prefer to do your work early in the morning or in the evening?
- How many hours do you plan to work each day?
- Do you prefer to arrange set times for breaks (for meals, snacks, drinks, television programmes, etc.) or do you like to work straight through until you have finished?
- Are you going to do most of your work during the week so that your weekends are free, or are you going to work at weekends so that you can carry on with social and leisure activities throughout the week?

Break the task down to long-, medium- and short-term goals. For example, at the beginning of a semester you are given a 3000-word essay to be submitted in the last week of the semester; your long-term goal is to write it and submit it on time. Break the task up into smaller components, then ask yourself in what sequence they need to be done. So, for example, the first part of the essay involves undertaking a review of the literature – reading what various authors have written on the subject. By breaking the major work down like this you will be making it much more manageable, and also less daunting. Your medium-term goals include:

- the production of a draft for part one of the essay after 2 weeks
- an outline of the main points after 4 weeks
- a complete rough draft after 6 weeks.

For each of these there will be a number of tasks to complete (short-term goals). You will need to put time aside to search databases and visit the library (to borrow books or request library loans). Give dates when each task is to be achieved; this approach has the benefit of giving you positive reinforcement. You will see results for your efforts, be less daunted by the task and feel in control rather than being overwhelmed by the task.

Procrastination – delaying an action or task – is associated with university life, where you are required to meet deadlines for assignments and tests in an environment in which other activities are competing for your time and attention. Some students struggle with procrastination due to a lack of time-management or study skills, stress or feeling overwhelmed with their work. This can be overcome by having strategies for avoiding it.

- If you leave things until the last minute you might meet the deadline for your first assignment, but this could have a knock-on effect for other assignments.
- Extensions for assignments: these should be used only when necessary. Colleagues who use extensions are not the happiest or the most productive, and tend not to enjoy the course as much because they are always trying to catch up.
- Effective time management: it might seem nerdy but do you want to feel on top of things and in control, or under pressure?

Create a study place

The essentials are: your own desk, laptop or personal computer, box files and a filing cabinet or a bookcase. For most people, a place to study is a dining room table or some other shared space. You are more likely to get continued support if you can minimize the disruption that your need for space can create.

When you are studying you are likely to have a lot of material around you – writing paper, textbooks and journal articles, lecture notes, handouts and so on. Paperwork breeds, and needs to be organized so that you can find things again. Having a few organizational materials to hand can make life much easier: semi-adhesive tabs are useful for marking a page, so you can close a book and still return to the piece you were reading. Stray thoughts can pop into your mind and disrupt the creative flow – jot them down on a note pad or a Post-it note, so you know they won't be forgotten.

Try to develop good organizational habits, such as having only the material you need at hand. One fairly cheap but effective way of keeping everyone (including yourself) happy is to buy a box file and a few clear plastic wallets for your current project. Your own work to date can go in one wallet, lecture notes and handouts can go in another and any photocopied papers can be stored in another.

Using study periods

Having considered time and place arrangements you now need to think how you will use your study time effectively.

Think back to previous courses or times when you have had to study hard:

- How easy was it to just sit down and start?
- How long did you spend on each separate topic?
- How often did you take breaks – for how long – what did you do?
- How did you manage your tension?

There is a world of difference between studying effectively and just sitting in front of your books and papers paralysed with anxiety. Consider the following points.

Creating a suitable environment

When you have determined when and what you are going to study, you will need to decide where you are going to do it. Some activities require a specialized environment like a library or access to computers. On these occasions, you will need to plan ahead so that you are in the right place at the right time. On other occasions, you will be able to exercise more choice and select where you work. Some people prefer to work in the spaces provided by the university, such as workstations in a library or reading room. These places are set aside for studying so they are free from distractions. Other people like to work at home with familiar things around them.

- Make sure there is adequate light, heating and ventilation – you will not be able to work effectively if it is stuffy in the summer or freezing in the winter.
- Try and get a table or desk that is large enough to take all your books, papers, desk lamp, etc.
- Find a place close at hand to store dictionaries, files with notes and textbooks.
- Try and use a room where you can be on your own for a while so that you can avoid distractions.
- Choose a chair that will enable you to sit and read without causing you any discomfort.

The box on page 12 contains useful tips on getting started and planning your work.

Developing networks for support

Studying can become a big thing in your life; it can impinge on your social life, your family and your relationships with partners and friends. You might also be leaving home, your parents or your partner. You might be looking forward to the challenge or you may be anxious because you will have to make sense of all these changes on your own in an unfamiliar place. One way of reducing your anxiety is to talk to

Getting started

Students often say that this is one of the most difficult things to do. The range of avoidance strategies they give is fascinating: first, every pencil they own has to be sharpened, then a cup of tea or coffee is essential and then perhaps a look at the crossword to 'get the brain in gear'. This is procrastination. It is as if studying is a foreign process and these activities are the body's natural response to it.

The length of your sessions

Try to break up your study time into 30- to 40-minute periods and take short breaks in between. Now you can sharpen pencils or even iron a few clothes. You will be surprised how refreshed you feel after turning your mind to something trivial for a few minutes. It seems a shame that having conquered your fear of starting to study you should even consider stopping.

Long, unbroken study sessions are inefficient because they lead to fatigue; the longer you carry on, the less effective you are likely to be. Whether you are revising or learning new material, you will remember less of the later material. If you are writing an essay you will find ideas harder to develop and express the longer you go on.

Managing tension

Be aware of your body. Intense mental activity can generate tension, which can act as a barrier to learning. If you find your muscles tightening and your fists clenching then you need to relax because these are symptoms of adrenaline (epinephrine) release, which occurs when the body is under stress. Adrenaline prepares the body to deal with the causes of stress, and creates the 'fight or flight' syndrome, but you have nothing to fight and nothing to flee from – you are only reading and writing. You need to 'burn off' this adrenaline by doing something physical, like going for a brisk walk or a little light gardening. Ten minutes or so is not such a loss from your study time if it helps prepare you for another session.

people you know about the way you feel; they might not be able to make the unpleasant feelings go away but they can provide reassurance. Think creatively and stay open to all sorts of possibilities for help – words of wisdom and warm support can often come from unexpected sources (Marshall and Rowland, 1996).

Education can place enormous demands and challenges on relationships. Living apart from someone you are close to or changing other people's traditional role expectations of you, for example as a 'housewife' or 'mum', can be both emotionally and physically exhausting. Equally, while you are studying life will go on. People you love will have ups and downs and ask for your support; you might have to move house; you may start a new relationship or become a parent; or you might become ill or suffer a bereavement. At these times you may need to seek out the support of others to help you through.

Getting to know some of the other students you will be spending the next few months or years with is essential. If you feel shy about approaching others, try to imagine that they may be feeling the same way. Be open-minded and seek out friendships with people who are different to you: school leavers, mature students and everyone in-between can provide invaluable support and some unique insights. Courses in nursing and midwifery are very demanding and sometimes people drop out for a variety of reasons. If you have a good network of friends you will weather the storms more effectively than those who try to journey alone.

Your institution and students' union should provide a range of free, specialist advice and support services to you. They can offer guidance on everything from academic, housing and financial issues to counselling services that aim to help with issues such as mental and sexual health, alcohol awareness and eating disorders. There are often people appointed to look after disability issues, and study sessions to develop your skills in topics such as assertiveness, communication, using the libraries or computers. Do find out what is available locally by looking up 'advice' or 'support' on your institution's website and make use of these services when you feel the need.

 ## CASE STUDY

Joan has recently started a post-registration course. Her employers have agreed to give her study time so that she can attend the parts of the course that are taught at the university. She also knows that she will need more time to complete the project work and essays that are specified in the course requirements.

Joan has two children at school and she is worried about the commitments that she already has. These include managing her responsibilities at work, her work at home and childcare. Mike, her partner, has encouraged her to take the course and gain more qualifications but he has not said how he is going to support her while she is studying. Mike has done the housework and looked after the children when Joan has made a specific request for help but he has never used his initiative and done things without a request from her.

 Put yourself in Joan's shoes.

- Where should Joan go for help and advice?
- How should she sort things out with Mike?

Discussion

Joan seems like an intelligent woman with the capacity to undertake study at university. She is probably great at multi-tasking and is very resourceful. Mike probably imagines that she will take it all in her stride and that life will be pretty much the same. He knows that Joan is being given time off work to attend the course so may not have given any consideration to how she will find any extra time to research and write her assignments.

If Joan chooses not to speak up about her worries, it is likely that her mood, health and wellbeing will deteriorate and that will impact on Mike, her children and her job. If she feels she is neglecting her family duties when she studies, the quality of what she does will suffer; equally, if she cannot make time to study she risks failing her course. An alternative is for Joan to negotiate with Mike to take on more responsibility for the family duties in the short and longer term. Alternatively, she might look for help with childcare from friends and relatives or she might consider paying a cleaning service to come and help with some of the housework. By making small, incremental changes Joan can continue to balance her home, work and study commitments without sacrificing her sense of wellbeing.

If you are finding things difficult it might be helpful to talk to other people who are in a similar situation. Remember that some of the people you meet on the first day of the course are going to be in the same position as you. They may have ways of coping that you have not thought of. Even if they do not have solutions to your problems, they may be able to sympathize with you, which can be a source of comfort. If there are other people who share your problems and concerns it may be possible to form a self-help group, which will encourage group members to provide support and advice for each other.

Another strategy is to see what the university can offer. Some courses may allocate you a personal tutor who will be able to offer advice on personal problems as well as problems related to coursework. Some students' unions have health and welfare officers who can advise on problems related to accommodation or access to resources. You might also have access to a counsellor if you do not want to approach any of the people mentioned above.

- Look for references to any of these people in your university handbook.
- Look for references to them in any material that you receive from your local students' union.
- Look for information on notice boards.
- Make a note if they are mentioned in any presentations made by the staff during your introduction to the university.
- Listen to other students; they may recommend someone who has worked with them to overcome a problem.
- See if there are any clubs or societies that you want to join. They are a good way of making friends and meeting people who share common interests.

It is always worthwhile attending orientation sessions and picking up handbooks. You might not need to contact any of these people straight away but it is useful to know who and where they are in case you require their services in the future.

Making a timetable

You could spend time working out how much time is available for studying; however, this tends to get lost once you are working in practice and the typical week in university flies out of the window. Instead, use your diary and year planner to sketch out your work commitments.

Taught sessions (tutorials, lectures, clinical skills, etc.)
- Exams
- Hand in dates for assignments
- Practice placements

Social commitments
- Holidays
- Birthdays
- Parties, weddings, etc.

Leisure time
- 'Me' time
- Going to the gym
- Relaxing with friends and family

When you have entered all the information you will be able to see when the 'free periods' are; this will show you where there are chunks of time not occupied with leisure, work or social commitments. This will also show you if there are clashes between different activities. You will be able to see at a glance if your plan to start something new will involve stopping an existing activity or moving it to another time or day.

Daily, weekly and monthly calendars are useful when you start to make plans. Each calendar can perform a different function:

- monthly calendar: to plan long-range assignments
- weekly calendar: to learn consistency
- daily calendar: to help you set priorities.

Remember that no one week will be the same so when booking things in:

- Be generous when you estimate the amount of time allocated for each activity.
- When you recorded different activities, did you include time for travelling or changing clothes?
- Did you allocate time for any preparation that has to be done in advance or any tidying that follows an activity?
- Learn from your mistakes as well as your achievements.

It is better to make changes and modify your expectations than to abandon time management altogether. If the timetable that you have made is too tiring or too rigid, you could write in more leisure time and reduce your work commitments. If it is too loose and you do not feel that you are making any progress, then you might need to develop more structured activities.

Saying no

There will be times when you will need to refuse requests to do something at home, at university or in the workplace. This can be difficult if the person you are confronting is in a position of power or is more knowledgeable than you. Saying no assertively is an important skill to develop and even when you say it clearly, others may use tactics to make you comply with their demands. Your course might include a session on assertiveness but, if not, find out if your institution or students' union runs free workshops.

- Making your decision: get all the information you need to make an informed decision (who is involved, how long will it take, who will get the benefit, and what help and support will you get to do it).
- Take your time: do not be rushed into a decision and get back to the person when you have thought it through.
- Gut reaction: if you get a sinking feeling when you are asked you should probably say no.
- Saying no: practise a short statement that will make your message clear. This could be something like 'the answer is no' or 'my decision is no' or 'I'm not willing to…'
- Body language: use assertive body language (relaxed, upright, open, balanced) and give the person a chance to respond.

It is not always appropriate or necessary to explain your decision, particularly if you suspect that you will be pressed to change your answer. However, there are times when you will need to elaborate, such as when you are saying no to something that is in your job contract. It is polite to apologize and show concern, but beware of appearing submissive and creating an opening that will be manipulated. Often, you will have to be persistent in repeating your decision. You can do this by summarizing what the other person has said and ending with 'no'; this proves that you have listened. Alternatively, you can just repeat 'my answer is no', until the person gives up. (Adapted from Bond, 1988)

Prioritizing

Which learning skills do you need to help you prepare for each event? Think about the skills that you have already and then the additional skills you will need to learn. Does the programme show you where you will have opportunities to develop these skills? Does the programme show you where you will learn about research, information technology, statistics or drug calculations?

How frequently do you need to check your progress and preparation? This could become more than a checklist of things that you have or have not done. It is your chance to reflect on how things are going. Did you meet your learning outcomes? Were you told what they were or did you negotiate them? Did you enjoy learning? What did you enjoy? Why did you enjoy it? What didn't you like? Why?

Think about all the activities related to learning that you are likely to carry out in the next 2 weeks. Locate each activity on a chart (like the one below) so that you can see whether it is more or less urgent, important or not so important.

Important

Urgent   **Not urgent**

Not important

If you put activities near to the important and urgent poles it indicates that you need to think in terms of short-term, rather than long-term, goals. Long-term goals are not always less important. They may indicate something that is ongoing and does not need to be changed or reviewed immediately.

Another useful way of thinking about learning is to make a list of aims and objectives.

- An aim is a big, broad heading for something you want to achieve. It might involve a piece of work, such as the completion of an assignment, or it may be related to an aspiration such as 'I really want to work on my communication skills during my next placement'. A single aim may incorporate many objectives.
- An objective is one of the small steps you have to take to achieve your aim. A single aim might incorporate many objectives. Completing an essay will include objectives like carrying out a literature search, writing a plan, writing an introduction, and so on. Improving communication skills might involve objectives like using open questions instead of closed ones, paying close attention to body posture and non-verbal techniques, and improving listening skills.

One of the advantages of sitting down and working out a timetable is that you become more aware of the demands on your time. You will be able to see if there are periods when you will be under a lot of pressure. There may be specific times in the course when you are expected to do two or three things simultaneously. This could involve producing written work for assignment deadlines, changing practice placements or working with mentors and assessors on specific days.

One of the most anxiety-producing situations you can be confronted with is being given a list of submission deadlines and significant dates and not having a strategy for dealing with them. Without a plan you will find it hard to know whether you have done all the things you need to do, or what is the best thing to do next. When people do not have a very clear idea about what needs to be done they may be inclined to procrastinate, avoiding certain jobs or activities because they do not know how to go about them.

A task is more easily done if it is not urgent.

CASE STUDY

James is in the second month of the Common Foundation Programme (CFP). He has been told to do lots of reading and he has a formative essay of 1000 words to write for each of the three sciences represented in the CFP. The essays are not compulsory but he wants to do them because he would like to have some feedback on his essay-writing technique. James has not produced any academic work since the end of his course at college 3 years ago and he is worried because he is not sure what the tutors expect from him. He has 6 weeks to write the essays but he also needs to keep up with the reading that has been recommended for the psychology, biology and sociology components of the course.

- Put yourself in James' shoes. How would you arrange your study time over the next 6 weeks?
- How many hours does James need to study if he is going to get the work done?
- How will that time be divided between producing the essays and keeping up with his reading?
- James has stated that he aims to complete three essays within 6 weeks. What are the objectives that will help him to reach this aim?

Planning

A nursing course involves different themes or modules, which require separate assessments. It also involves practical work with other nurses and patients or clients. This range of activities means that it is not always possible to drop your other commitments so that you can complete a single task or assignment. If you do drop everything to meet the deadline it may have immediate repercussions on your other commitments. The pressure to meet all of these demands will accumulate and another crisis will develop. If this is the case, you are back where you started: under pressure and stressed.

If you think back to James (in the case study above), you will recognize that planning involves paying attention to many different aspects of learning. If you are going to reduce your stress levels and avoid rushing about at the last minute to get everything done, you will have to consider all of them at the planning stage. James needs to think about preparing himself for seminars by consolidating notes from lectures and reading, remembering to include the relevant module name, number and the date, as well as producing the essays. Organizing his notes – using files and folders (these can be hardcopy or electronic) – would be useful. If James is going to achieve this he needs to allocate time each week for his ongoing reading and consolidation, as well as time for the essays. Writing the essay will be the final stage of production. Before he can start this, James will need to research the subjects and produce an essay plan; both these activities could form separate learning objectives. James could also divide the time he spends on essays into preparation and writing time. Out of the 6 weeks available to him, 4 weeks could be spent on preparation and the remaining 2 weeks could be used for writing; not forgetting that resources might not always be available when he wants them.

Some people feel that they work well when they are put under pressure. They believe that they are most productive when they are up against a tight deadline. There is nothing wrong with this approach if you are sure that you have the skills to carry it off. However, there are some disadvantages that go along with it, which you may like to consider before you decide it is your preferred option.

Think about:

The availability of resources
If you leave everything until the last minute you can succeed only if everything you need is in the right place at the right time. If you need to borrow books from the library or require access to computers, you will be competing with everyone else who has put themselves (by accident or design) in the same position. There is more on this in Chapter 4, which looks at using information technology.

The research that you need to complete before you can start writing
The adrenaline that starts to flow if you leave things until the last minute may help you to write faster but you will not be able to produce good-quality work unless you develop a thorough knowledge of the material. Before you commit yourself to paper you will need to get to grips with the theories and concepts you are writing about. You will need to know what other people have written or said before you can establish your own point of view. Make sure that you allow yourself time for preparation, as well as for writing. There is more on this in Chapter 6, which looks at developing an argument.

Defining priorities

Effective management of your time will involve defining priorities. For example, when an assignment deadline is imminent it is noticeable how a number of students will not attend lectures because they are completing their work; however, they could be missing out on key sessions that will be important for their personal development. You need to be aware of the impact this has on your colleagues and lecturers.

Be aware that some of your peers will live their academic lives on the edge; turning up for lectures late or not at all, asking to borrow your notes from the sessions they have missed and then losing them, constantly asking for extensions, writing assignments at the eleventh hour and running around trying to find a working printer and a folder to present it in. By living in a constant state of chaos, they create headaches for everyone around them. When you are in control of your workload, you hear the announcements at the start of lectures, you read e-mails that warn you of timetable changes, you have time to seek out tutorial support, you access recommended texts from the library and you polish-up your assignment before handing it in. Effective time management means that you get the very best out of the opportunities your education has to offer and you get to enjoy life beyond your course.

Developing a special interest in a particular subject, or knowing that a subject is likely to be your Achilles heel, can be beneficial. Having this knowledge shows that you are aware of your strengths and weaknesses; however, it can become a disadvantage if preferences encourage you to avoid work related to other subjects. Remember that they have the potential to become problems as well. Being aware of how much time you dedicate to each area will help you to avoid getting hooked into a single theme. It may make you more conscious of the need to maintain a consistent approach to your studies. This does not mean that you have to spend equal amounts of time on each. It may involve making thoughtful decisions and keeping records so that you know how you are using your study time.

Thinking strategically

Creating a plan is useful, even if you do not stick to it. Departing from your schedule may be beneficial if an unforeseen event becomes a priority. Even if you find that you constantly have to change your plans or reorganize your priorities, it is still a productive way of working. Planning is evidence of thinking strategically, and developing a strategy for learning is an antidote to drifting aimlessly or bumping along from one crisis to the next. This can boost your self-confidence and allow you to take a more positive approach to coursework.

Students think about their work in different ways. Some people will visualize plans as a series of tasks arranged in a hierarchical order; the most important task will be at the top of an imaginary list. Strategies may involve devising ways of working down the list until all the tasks are completed. The following sort of questions may run through your mind:

- Where are there a couple of hours free so that I can visit the library?
- When can I find an hour to read about the composition of the blood?
- I need to make a plan before I can start writing this essay. Where will I find the time to make a start?

A successful plan will be built around a realistic appraisal of your own habits. You might decide to try and work using long periods for learning rather than more frequent shorter bouts. This can be useful if you want to tackle some big tasks in one go. This approach will not suit everyone. If you know that your concentration span is between 20 and 30 minutes then periods of between 2 and 3 hours will not be the best option.

Making an evaluation of your own progress is one aspect of reflection. Reflection is discussed in more detail in Chapter 12; you may like to glance at this chapter and make some notes on key points, or spend some time reading it when you have completed this section. Ask yourself the following questions so that you think about the effectiveness of your current study habits:

- Are other activities interfering with my study activities?
- Do my goals and priorities suit my current needs?
- Am I allowing myself enough time to study?
- Is my weekly timetable flexible enough to allow for the unexpected?
- Does my weekly schedule show that I am wasting time?
- Have I established a good balance between work and leisure in my schedule?

The answers to these questions might make you change your habits or amend your timetable. Adjustments and amendments are ways of adapting your original ideas so that they meet your current requirements.

This chapter has considered timetabling and organization. Remember the following key points when you begin to study:

- Acknowledge your other commitments
- Make realistic plans
- Think strategically
- Create a structure by setting aims and objectives, goals, or more urgent and less urgent priorities
- Evaluate and reflect on your learning
- Be prepared to seek and accept help and advice from other people

CHAPTER RESOURCES

REFERENCES

Bond, M., 1988. Saying no assertively. Nursing Times 84 (14), 63–66.

Common, L., 2007. Studying: ways to survive and thrive. Midwives 10 (10), 466–467.

Marshall, L. & Rowland, F., 1996. A guide to learning independently, 3rd edn. Open University Press, Buckingham.

Northedge, A., 2005. The good study guide, 2nd edn. The Open University, Milton Keynes.

Siviter, B., 2008. The student nurse handbook: a survival guide, 2nd edn. Elsevier, Edinburgh.

2

Learning skills and styles

Lisa Common and Sian Maslin-Prothero

KEY ISSUES

- What is learning?
- Understanding memory
- Responsibility for your own learning
- Learning styles
- Your existing learning skills
- Learning from life experiences
- Learning contracts
- Support networks
- Self-assessment

Introduction

Chapter 1 was about managing your resources so that you can study effectively. The overall aim of this chapter is to build on the previous one and develop your learning skills. This is achieved by identifying what learning is and how we do it. There is an explanation of different learning styles and how these can affect your studying, and an opportunity to identify your personal learning style. Knowing how you prefer to learn can help guide you through your course, although you need to be aware that your preference can change according to what you are studying.

Being an adult learner

It is important that you take responsibility for your own learning. Higher education is very different from school. As an adult learner, it is up to you to identify what you want to learn and how much effort you are going to give to learning – only you can successfully complete the course.

The aim of this book is to help you to become an independent and self-directed learner; this means you will be able to identify what you need to learn and to access the information you require without the assistance of a lecturer. Additional mechanisms in your place of learning will support and help you during the course, but you need to recognize how you take responsibility for your own learning.

When you enter a professional course in a university, you have earned the right to be there by a rigorous selection procedure. As an adult learner, you enter education with the status of an adult, a range of experiences and the motivation to gain a qualification; you are there because you choose to be – this is not compulsory education. Psychologists call this 'intrinsic motivation'; it is the strongest driving force there is.

A key proponent to any success is motivation – a sense of purpose is perhaps the most crucial aspect of learning, you must *want* to study. For example, if you are undertaking a pre-registration midwifery course purely because you couldn't think of anything else to do, you are not increasing your chances of success; your driving force – or motivation – may be weak.

Motivation is so important when you are embarking on something new and challenging. There are going to be times when you find the going difficult; regardless of what you have identified as motivating you at the start of a new course, your motivation will change during the course.

Briefly note down what has motivated you, either to start a new course or to learn a new skill.

Sometimes your motivation is going to be better, sometimes worse. This might be for a variety of reasons. You might have concerns about:

- financial insecurity
- meeting new people
- having reduced time available for family and friends
- making time for study
- not understanding the course and/or the academic language used by your teachers and peers.

A new course is exciting and will bring about a change in your life; this change might cause you stress. Stress is not always a negative thing, only when you are experiencing too much pressure – or stress – does it become a problem. A degree of pressure stimulates us and can be a very positive thing but, if not managed correctly, this pressure can become too much and we are unable to cope. It is important to be able to recognize these signs and symptoms in yourself and others; only through recognition and then doing something to create a change will you adequately address the problem. Chapter 1 identified some positive strategies that can be used to resolve some of these issues.

Remember what motivated you to start the course in the first place, and do something positive such as taking some exercise, finding a solution to your problem or talking to someone (either a professional – such as a counsellor – friends or colleagues).

What is learning?

Learning is something we do practically every day so it may seem a bit strange to be asking what we mean by it. However, knowing how learning occurs may help you to become a more effective learner.

- Learning is *any more or less permanent change in behaviour, knowledge or belief.*
- To experience this change we need to be exposed to new ideas or skills.
- Sometimes we are not conscious of the learning experience; examples such as reciting a television advert or singing a song prove that you can learn without deliberately trying. This is called 'passive learning'.

You can learn useful things by passive learning; for example, the signs and symptoms of illnesses frequently encountered in clinical practice. Such learning is superficial because you do not necessarily understand why it happens. So, although you might be able to copy the skills you have observed a more experienced practitioner perform, will you be able to modify the skill when a new and slightly different situation occurs?

Professional practice is more than just copying the behaviour of our predecessors and learning facts by rote. The Nursing and Midwifery Council's (NMC's) Code of Professional Conduct requires practitioners to '… take part in appropriate learning and practice activities that maintain and develop your competence and performance' (NMC, 2008, p. 4). This means actively engaging in the learning process, which occurs when you understand the principles behind the concepts and skills being studied. It can help to view learning as a progression from the acquisition of knowledge through to higher-level mental activities. Figure 2.1 represents this progression, starting from being able to remember straightforward facts, such as labelling a diagram of the heart (simple recall or knowing what the various parts are), through to being able to explain the function of the heart valves or the reason why the muscle layer of the left ventricle is thicker than the right, which represents a higher level of learning (the ability to comprehend the concepts you are studying).

Going beyond this level takes you to the stage of being able to apply your knowledge. For example, if you have a patient with damage to the left ventricle following a coronary thrombosis, you will be able to plan nursing care that takes the impaired circulation into account. By observing the effect of exercise on the patient, such as the degree of breathlessness after walking a prescribed distance, you will be able to evaluate the effect your plan has had on their heart.

Simply knowing and being able to perform are important but lower-order activities, and applies to someone who follows orders. However, midwifery and nursing students are studying to be able to act independently and to exercise professional judgement. You need to make

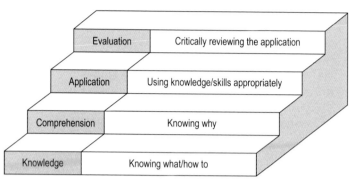

FIGURE 2.1 The progression from acquisition of knowledge to active learning.

links between theory and practice – what Mallik (2005, p. 320) refers to as the 'aha' moment; active participation in the learning process is essential.

Learning is more than the mere acquisition of facts, it involves a range of intellectual activities including the ability to make judgements on abstract matters such as topical issues or ethics.

Think about some of your political, religious or ethical beliefs.
- How did you acquire them?
- Do you understand the principles upon which they are based?
- How do they affect your practice?
- Have you at any time subjected them to serious critical scrutiny?

Often, we pick up our beliefs from influential people around us, such as parents, religious ministers or teachers, and we accept them because we respect the authority of the person teaching us; we expect that person to know what he or she is talking about. Such learning tends to be passive, resulting from being constantly exposed to the same ideas since childhood; and discussion and debate with friends or family with similar views will not encourage a critical perspective.

So how do we learn?

The concepts of learning and memory are closely related. When we need to perform a skill, recall an item of knowledge or explain something, we draw on our memory, but we can only draw on what is already there. Knowing how memory works can help you develop effective learning skills. Although memory is an incompletely understood concept, the Atkinson–Schiffrin model, described by Malim and Birch (1998, p. 291), explains memory as a series of steps (Figure 2.2).

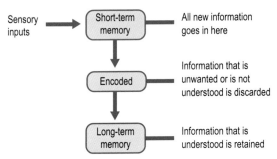

FIGURE 2.2 The Atkinson–Schiffrin model of memory (adapted from Malim and Birch, 1998).

The next activity demonstrates how we are constantly bombarded with sensory input.

Stop for a moment and focus on the information you are receiving via your five senses:

- What is happening outside your body?
- What is your body telling you about inside you – have you any aches and pains?

All of this information – most of which you don't need – is coming at you while you are trying to learn from a lecture or demonstration and is stored in your short-term memory. Sensory inputs are encoded, we try to give them meaning, and those that have no relevance are discarded. If you can understand lecture material, i.e. it makes sense to you, you can give it meaning in relation to your own experience, then you have successfully encoded it and it will enter and remain in your long-term memory. However, if you can't make sense of it, it will not be retained. Only information stored in the long-term memory can be recalled. Memory is dependent on making sense of information.

To make sense of new material (the encoding process), we have to work hard to establish links between what we already know and the new information. Consider the following example.

When studying orthopaedics you come across the term 'subperiosteal cellular proliferation'. At first glance, you may just see a complicated medical term but, when you look carefully, you will see that there are some familiar components:

- *sub* means 'below'
- *peri* means 'around'
- *cellular* refers to cells
- *proliferation* means 'production of a large number'.

So you can work out that a large number of cells are being produced, but where exactly? You have to try to understand the meaning of *subperiosteal*. At this point, you might need a dictionary to look up the meaning of *periosteal* (around the bone – *os* is Latin for bone). Looking at a diagram of a bone in an anatomy book will show you that the periosteum is the tissue that surrounds bone, so *subperiosteal* refers to the site below the periosteum where the cells are produced, hence *cellular proliferation*. Making sense of something like this is an encoding process – you are making sense of it.

If you are given pre-reading or worksheets before a lecture or seminar then be sure to complete them. If you do, then the session is more likely to make sense to you, and you can ask questions and clarify any points that you are not sure of.

Making new links does not always happen the first time you try to learn something, effort is required. If you can recall a time when you learned a skill, such as riding a bike, you will remember how you got some things right and some things wrong. Eventually, as you persevered you became relatively skilful and were able to perform in a fairly fluent way. It is believed that when we are learning we are making new circuits between our neurons (brain cells); these neural pathways are physical structures and are activated when we need to recall something. It may be helpful to use an analogy to explain this concept.

Think about a number of towns without any road or rail links; communication between them would be impossible. Laying down new roads and railway lines is a difficult and time-consuming job but, once they have been established, traffic can travel rapidly between the towns.

Once the hard work of understanding new concepts and developing new skills has been done, the neural pathways have been established and the information traffic can speed rapidly around the brain. This is why learning has been described as a more or less permanent change.

So why do we forget?

What are you good at remembering? Faces, names, what people say, football matches? I can remember people's faces and names – we are all able to recall certain things better than others. Spending time and effort does not necessarily guarantee success in learning, but it is how we use it that is important. Figure 2.3 shows the effect when students are stimulated to recall information, or practise skills, soon after being exposed to them. If this is done frequently, the chances of forgetting are reduced. Frequency of recall is the key factor in remembering.

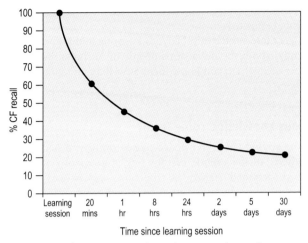

FIGURE 2.3 The Ebbinghaus forgetting curve – improving memory by recall.

The main principle is to give yourself as many opportunities as possible to rehearse: for example, practising a skill as often as you can and as soon as possible after being taught it (see Chapter 10). For knowledge and understanding, try to set yourself a series of short tests, based on the information you have read or been taught.

Get yourself a small address book that will slip in your pocket. Everything from passwords, door codes, how to document a palpation can be written here. Until this knowledge is second nature, you can flip to letter 'P', for example, and look up how to accurately document a palpation.

Sometimes, perhaps because we are anxious (e.g. during an examination), we fail to recall. You might have had the experience of not being able to answer a question in an exam and then, when you leave the room, the answer comes to you.

One way to overcome this is to visualize the brain as a channel that is constricted, preventing the flow of information; relaxation techniques can be helpful in situations like this. Imagining the walls of the channel relaxing helps you to imagine the flow of information returning. By relaxing and thinking loosely about the question, some ideas may begin to spark and these might lead to other relevant ideas – the information traffic starts to flow again.

Knowing things

How can we know anything? For example, how do you know that the South Pole exists? Or how do you know that oxygen moves into cells? The chances are that you 'know' because someone told you. This type of knowledge is second-hand knowledge – sometimes known as propositional knowledge.

Is there a difference between knowing and knowing about? You may know about the indigenous people of Australia, but how deep is your knowledge? Do you know them as well as someone who has lived with them?

Where does knowledge come from?

The second-hand knowledge passed on to you had to originate somewhere; all the science, history, bits of geography and information you have acquired started as someone's experience. Knowledge can be described as the articulation of human experience, and once someone has experienced something, such as the quickest route from one place to another, it can be described or made known to others. To gain knowledge that is more than second hand, you need to have a significant experience from which to learn.

Kolb, an influential thinker on experiential learning, stated that 'learning is the process whereby knowledge is created through the transformation of experience' (Kolb, 1984). He was referring to the development of personal rather than propositional knowledge; that is, that *you know* rather than merely *know about* something.

Learning styles

Learning underpins everything we do; for example, learning to drive, trying out a new recipe or learning to rock climb, yet we rarely stop and think how we have learned a new skill. During the course, your lecturers will support your learning through a variety of teaching and learning strategies including practice, lectures, seminars and tutorials.

Too often, both students and lecturers believe that the lecturer is the 'expert' and knower of all things. This is not true; we are all constantly learning new things and developing new skills. Becoming dependent on others will stifle your creativity and ability to make independent judgements and use new information. Your lecturers will expect you to take responsibility for your own learning, through making the most of every opportunity offered you.

We all learn in different ways, and this is based on your previous experiences and how you have learned to learn in the past. To be successful, you need to identify how you learn best and develop your learning style so that you can optimize any learning situation.

Honey and Mumford (1992) identified four basic learning styles: the activist, the reflector, the pragmatist and the theorist. These different styles are summarized in the box below.

LEARNING STYLES
The activist

- Enjoys new experiences and challenges
- Enjoys an environment of changing activities
- Likes being the centre of attention
- Appreciates the chance to develop ideas through interaction and discussion with others

The activist thrives and develops in an environment that utilizes some of the following teaching and learning strategies: group work, seminars, discussions, debates and workshops.

The reflector

- Appreciates the opportunity to reflect prior to making a decision or choice
- Prefers to listen and observe others debating and discussing issues
- Would choose to work independently of others

The reflector is someone who prefers to work on his or her own, through individual study and project work. Reflectors are likely to prefer lectures.

The pragmatist

- Likes linking theory with practice
- Enjoys problem solving
- Appreciates the opportunity to develop practical skills

The pragmatist will enjoy those learning experiences that involve problem-solving activities, practical sessions, clinical experiences and work-based projects.

The theorist

- Enjoys theories and models
- Thrives on problem solving, which involves understanding and making sense of complex issues
- Likes structure and making the link to theories

The theorist will benefit and enjoy those sessions that use problem solving, evaluating material and discussing theories with colleagues and teachers.

You have probably identified your preferred learning style from what has been listed. This will help to guide you and to recognize those situations from which you might learn more effectively. You will benefit from developing new skills, which may help you to learn effectively from every situation you encounter.

There are other learning styles. For further information, please see Fleming (2001). You will find that your preferred learning style might change depending on your needs or who is facilitating the session. The important thing is to learn to be flexible and to develop your skills.

Learning from practice

In many vocational courses, such as nursing or midwifery, there is criticism of the so-called 'theory–practice gap' (Rolfe, 1996). Practitioners often say that what is taught in the classroom is quite different from what is practised on the wards. In fact, what is taught within the university or college is a theoretical underpinning of practice. Practice itself, for the most part, is taught in the wards, departments and community by practitioners; that is why the courses are usually equally divided between university or college and clinical placements. However, this is not to say that clinical placements only provide opportunity for practice; it is my contention that a substantial amount of theoretical learning can be acquired through practice if certain conditions are met. This section will deal with:

- learning through experience
- student–mentor relationships
- using clinical assessments as learning experiences
- integration of theory with practice.

All of these relate to your forthcoming clinical learning opportunities.

Does having an experience necessarily result in learning?

In Kolb's view, experiential learning is a process that results in the generation of new knowledge, insights, ideas and even new skills. He described the process as an *experiential learning cycle* (Figure 2.4). How does this work in practical terms?

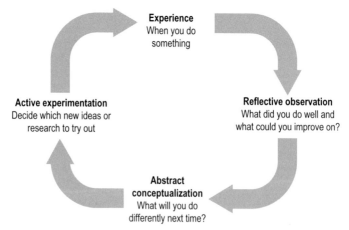

FIGURE 2.4 Kolb's experiential learning cycle.

- Experience: this could be something complex, like dealing with bereavement, or something straightforward, like learning to give an injection.
- Reflective observation: what did you do well and what could you improve on? You might be great at putting a patient at ease, but unfamiliar with the local medicines and infection control guidelines.
- Abstract conceptualization: this means thinking about what you will do differently next time. You might decide that you need to read-up on the appropriate injection sites for insulin or practise assembling syringes.
- Active experimentation: where you plan and apply your ideas to your practice.
- Experience: your new insights, ideas and skills will generate a different experience that you can follow through the learning cycle again.

A *concrete experience* is an event that happens to an individual, which, in the context of learning, provides the learning focus, for example, learning to play a musical instrument or learning to give an injection.

Reflection is the process of thinking about the experience in a structured way. Schon (1983) stated that reflection on action is 'a retrospective view of an experience to uncover the knowledge used in a particular situation'. Neither Schon nor Kolb describe in detail how individuals reflect. Other writers, such as Gibbs (1988), Johns (1994) and Boud et al. (1985) have offered ideas on how the reflective process can be structured (see Chapter 12). The model of reflection developed by Boud et al. (1985) is relatively simple but also academically rigorous. Boud et al. (1985) recommend that reflection should be on three aspects of the experience:

1. Actions: what you and any other participants did in the situation you are reflecting on.
2. Feelings: your negative and/or positive feelings, and the reasons why you felt the way you did.
3. Knowledge: the existing knowledge you had that was of use at the time, and the knowledge you realized you lack.

Reflection is not simply a matter of remembering an event and thinking 'that was interesting/unpleasant/embarrassing' or whatever. It is a structured process designed to enhance your own understanding and develop fresh insights.

Nursing is a practical job, so why is it important to spend time reflecting on it?

Abstract conceptualization follows on from reflection. A concept is an idea; abstract conceptualization is your understanding of a concept. For example, you may have some awareness of cultural differences and how they may be integrated within the healthcare context. When we reflect in a systematic way, we gain new insights and develop knowledge and understandings that we did not have previously. This may be in the form of theoretical knowledge, such as understanding the basic beliefs and customs of different religious traditions or it may be through gaining experience of caring for individuals and families from different faiths. We may gain insights into barriers to effective communication or our own feelings and preconceptions. Once we have some deeper self-awareness, we can act to make ourselves more sensitive and open to meeting the needs of those in our care.

Once you have spent time reflecting and reorganizing your personal knowledge and insights, you will be ready for active experimentation, ready to have another go at the experience but with fresh ideas. Reflection, therefore, is a way of improving your insights into practice and improving the practice itself (see Chapters 12 and 14).

By using a systematic process, such as the one described by Kolb, allied with a structured model of reflection, you will be demonstrating an analytical approach to the practical activity of nursing. This will enhance your understanding of the theoretical principles that underpin practice. Obviously you will not be able to do this for every single activity you engage in, but if you can develop the habit of reflecting on certain events that have some significance for you, you will amass a great amount of useful knowledge to help you nurse patients with understanding, rather than as a matter of performing routines.

Becoming a reflective practitioner

Reflection should become an active and ongoing part of your life as a nurse or midwife. It involves looking at yourself and your practice objectively and will help you to integrate changes that will enhance your competence throughout your career (Siviter, 2008). Like any other skill, reflective practice can be learned and, once learned, can become second nature. To reflect effectively a number of conditions need to be met. You will need:

- to set aside some time: reflection is more than allowing the day's events to run through your head on your way home
- the support of a mentor: to help direct your thoughts, to pass on their own insights and generally to provide a sympathetic ear
- to create a framework to structure reflections: such as the one described by Boud et al. (1985)
- a predisposition to reflect: that is to say, a tendency to take a reflective view of significant life events. Many people have this predisposition but, without the other three factors, they tend not to develop their reflective skills.

Students often have a reflective predisposition. However, it is really important to structure your reflections in ways that develop, rather than

Reflection IS about ...	Reflection IS NOT about ...
✓ Gaining confidence in what you do well ✓ Recognizing when you could have done better ✓ Learning from your mistakes ✓ Learning about yourself and your behaviour ✓ Trying to see yourself as others see you ✓ Being self-aware ✓ Changing the future by learning from the past	✗ Blaming anyone, yourself or anyone else ✗ Berating yourself ✗ Being overly critical ✗ Complaining ✗ Being superficial and holding back what you are really thinking or feeling

FIGURE 2.5 Reflective practice (from Siviter, 2008).

diminish, your confidence and practice. You might find it helpful to copy Figure 2.5 into the front of your notebook or journal and, whenever you reflect, check that what you are doing does not drift into the right-hand column.

Analysis of the scores from a group of nursing students who had completed a 'learning styles' questionnaire showed that the most predominant learning style was the reflective style. Clearly, most (but not all) have the predisposition that will help them derive knowledge from practice. That is to say, they will have the advantage of developing personal knowledge and not merely rely on propositional knowledge. This knowledge is more permanent, useful in practice and invaluable in examinations.

Reflective diaries

As identified earlier, we all learn in different ways. Learning through reflection helps us to focus on the material that interests us. We can learn more quickly if the material is relevant and interesting to us. By drawing on your own personal knowledge and life experience, you can try out and test new ideas and concepts. This is learning by doing – practising and occasionally making mistakes. Through feedback from others, such as our mentors (as well as ourselves), absorbing what has been said and making sense of what has been said, we then progress. It is important to see this as a continuous process. We might not think of it consciously but when we stop and think 'how did I get here?' we are able to follow this process.

One way of assisting this process is through a reflective diary. Keeping a reflective diary will enable you to:

- record details as they occur
- remember things that happened

- organize and clarify thoughts
- apply your experiences
- assess your development
- take a longer-term view.

This reflective diary will be your own personal record, to record your thoughts and feelings about colleagues, teachers and clients. You will find it very therapeutic to express your thoughts and feelings and, throughout this book, you will be encouraged to record your experiences in a reflective diary. However, you need to be sure that confidentiality is maintained and that individuals cannot be identified, should anyone else read it.

How to go about developing your reflective diary:

- Set aside 5–10 minutes a day.
- Use a framework for reflection, such as the Boud et al. (1985) model described above.
- Discuss your thoughts and feelings with your clinical mentor.

An example of a student reflection using Boud et al. (1985) is given below.

Lisa's reflection

Using the Boud et al. (1985) reflective framework, together with my own reflective diary, I am able to examine in depth my reactions to incidents that have occurred during my training. I can consider how, with a different approach or greater knowledge, I could improve a similar situation if it arose again.

I have recently worked on a ward where many patients had suffered a cerebrovascular accident (CVA), which had resulted in severe communication difficulties. On two occasions on the same shift, different patients attracted my attention and, although I dealt with both people immediately, they did not initially appear distressed, so I assumed that their need was not urgent. The first patient, an elderly man, seemed to be motioning towards his table; my first conclusions were that he wanted either his drink or the medication that was waiting to be taken. Neither turned out to be the case, he was actually nodding towards the urine bottles that were stored under the sink opposite his bed. Fortunately, in this instance I discovered the need before any embarrassment was caused; he actually seemed to find the scenario quite amusing.

Sadly, this was not the case with the second incident, when an elderly woman had a similar requirement. Both another nurse and myself desperately struggled to identify her needs and it was evident that her urgency and our lack of comprehension were increasingly agitating her. We thought we had identified a desire to stretch her legs but, whilst I turned my back to fetch her walking frame, she became doubly incontinent; this caused considerable embarrassment for everyone in the ward, but most particularly for the patient.

Action

- Me: recognized that patients had a care-related need, tried to guess their requirements.
- Patients: tried desperately to explain what they wanted; one suffered severe embarrassment.

Feelings

Positive: I empathized with the patients, fully appreciating their frustration and embarrassment at the sudden lack of such basic skills, not only the communication aspect but also the need for help with toileting. My first reaction was to escape and get someone else to deal with the situation, but I'm proud that I acted professionally and persevered; at least I discovered the needs of one patient.

Negative: embarrassed at the suffering caused to the other patient. Extremely frustrated at the difficulties I encountered in trying to understand the patients. Annoyed that I didn't consider the elimination need first. I made wrong assumptions based on appearances and did not consider that the patients' condition might have influenced how they were acting.

Knowledge

Existing knowledge: I knew the patients had suffered a CVA and that their communication skills were impaired. It was my responsibility to try to identify their needs by questioning.

Knowledge deficit: the extent to which a CVA affects communication skills – are both reception and expression skills impaired? When accepting responsibility for looking after such patients I should determine from their notes or the nurse looking after them previously the exact extent of their abilities and comprehension.

I need to find out how best to deal with patients with communication difficulties, particularly when they do understand me but have difficulty in even responding with a 'Yes' or 'No'. Talking to a speech therapist would give me a greater understanding of the problems and would give me the opportunity to seek guidance over the difficulties in communication. As I have chosen child branch, this problem could arise frequently under different circumstances, such as with younger or handicapped children. I need to develop a strategy to identify needs as quickly as possible, perhaps starting with structuring questions to deal with the potentially most embarrassing requirements first. This would probably include the need to become more in tune with patients' non-verbal communication skills.

Learning from this reflection

Improving my knowledge as identified above, and making fewer assumptions will enable me to deal with this situation with more competence in the future, which in turn will save my patients from considerable embarrassment and make their lives in hospital easier.

The student has spent time thinking about her experience, using a systematic framework to help structure her thoughts. Although it is not evident from the reflection, the student had guidance from a mentor; and had a strong predisposition to reflect on practice.

Learning contracts

A learning contract is an agreement between two or more people. We are making informal contracts with people all the time; for example, 'If I look after the children while you go for your tutorial today, can I go climbing later in the week?' A learning contract is used when there is an exchange of something, and this can be skills or knowledge. In this context a learning contract is a more formal, written agreement between a lecturer and a student, or a group of students.

Learning contracts (Figure 2.6) are being used more frequently in education institutions. The philosophy goes hand-in-hand with students taking more responsibility for their own learning. Once you embark on any course you enter into a variety of informal, unwritten agreements, such as attending the course and completing the required number of assignments. Learning contracts are particularly useful when you have specific learning outcomes or need to negotiate how you are assessed. It can also be used when you want accreditation for prior learning (APL) or accreditation for prior experiential learning (APEL).

Learning contracts enable students to identify, plan, manage and evaluate their own learning. The learners and their supervisor discuss, agree and record what the student wants to achieve and how it is going to be achieved. Both parties then sign the document.

Learning contracts have a number of benefits:

- Everyone is clear about what the goals are and how they will be achieved.
- Everyone knows what is expected of them.
- Negotiating your contract not only recognizes your needs but also enables you to take responsibility for your learning.
- Learning contracts can recognize prior learning; for example, APEL, APL.

Learning contracts are useful for both the learner and the supervisor, and enhance their commitment to the learning experience. This form of contract can be used in conjunction with a placement or workplace experience, where more than two people are contributing to the process.

You need to consider a number of points prior to agreeing your contract:

- What do you want to get out of this experience (your objectives)?
- What skills and knowledge will you gain?
- How will you reach/achieve your objectives?
- What are the deadlines?
- How will you demonstrate that you have achieved your objectives?

It is important to see the learning contract as something important to you, a way of you achieving your goals, with help and support from your supervisor.

Some of you might have experienced undertaking an individual performance review (IPR). This form of appraisal is used frequently in the NHS. It is a form of learning contract and you can use it to ensure that goals that are important to you, as well as to the organization, are met.

Location and duration of placement: Community Midwifery, 6.10.2008 – 26.10.2008
Student: Su Lin
Mentor: Lesley Bryant

Student and mentor review learning needs at start of placement

1) To observe and participate in abdominal palpation and describe my findings, both verbally and in writing
2) To develop my urinalysis and venepuncture technique; including the selection and completion of correct sample bottles and envelopes
3) To undertake an informed discussion about antenatal screening choices with clients and familiarize myself with the NICE antenatal care guidelines

Reflection by student of progress at mid-point of placement

1) I have had opportunities to observe different mentors performing abdominal palpation and to practice with consent from clients. My mentor recommended that I review Chapters 1–3 of Johnson and Taylor's 'Skills for Midwifery Practice' (2005).

2) I am becoming more confident and successful with my venepuncture technique and making accurate assessment of urine samples. I plan to review the local infection control and sharps safety guidelines.

3) I have observed mentors conducting antenatal screening discussions and have read the NICE guidelines and screening leaflets. I hope to have an opportunity to practice a discussion under direct supervision from my mentor before the end of this placement.

Review of placement experience to draw together key issues which will contribute to the preparation of subsequent placements/experience

It was helpful to read the Johnson and Taylor chapters and I am becoming more confident with this skill and have tried different approaches. For my next placement, I would like to develop my skills in listening to fetal hearts with a pinard stethoscope.

After reviewing local infection control and sharps safety guidelines I have now improved my technique and create a safer environment for myself and clients. I can now offer the correct test at the correct time and understand how to complete the paperwork to the required standard. For my next placement I would like to practice giving anti-D injections.

With the support of my mentor I was able to conduct an antenatal screening discussion. For my next placement I hope to repeat the experience and undertake a full antenatal booking which incorporates this skill.

Mentor comments

Su and I have discussed the progress she has made during this placement towards achieving her objectives. Su has demonstrated abilities to evaluate and reflect on her learning and practice. Su was proactive in following-up on recommendations for further reading and applying this to her practice. She has also taken time to look at local and national guidelines demonstrating an awareness of legal and professional issues.

Su has a good standard of knowledge about normal midwifery. For her next placement I plan to support her in developing her confidence in undertaking antenatal bookings. I would also like to see objectives that include infant feeding support and antenatal education.

Su has worked hard to develop a good standard of clarity and relevance in her record keeping. She is also self-aware and has shown excellent communication and interpersonal qualities with clients and colleagues. I will look forward to working with Su again.

Signature of student: *Su Lin*   Date: 24.4.2009

Signature of mentor: *L J Bryant*   Date: 25.4.2009

FIGURE 2.6 Example of a learning contract.

Support networks

Chapter 1 referred to your expectations and fears when embarking on a course of study, and emphasized the importance of managing your time; this leads to a more balanced life where you are able to include socializing and successfully studying.

I want to move on and recognize how to get the most out of your supervisors. Supervisors come in a variety of shapes and forms, they can be your teacher, personal tutor, mentor, friend, colleague or research supervisor. A supervisor is an experienced individual who facilitates the development of a colleague both educationally and professionally, and is there to help you learn. This can be in a variety of ways, including: getting the most out of your practice placement, acting as a role model, a resource, a counsellor or as a teacher (Figure 2.7).

The following are key characteristics of a supervisor:

- a good listener
- constructive
- a resource
- a role model
- competent.

However, supervision is not a one-way relationship; your supervisor will have certain expectations of you as a student. Please also remember:

- That supervisors are not only responsible for you, they are usually busy and will have other commitments.
- To make appointments to meet your supervisor, and to turn up prepared and on time.
- To phone if you are unable to make an appointment and let your supervisor know you won't be attending.

The emphasis is on you being prepared to listen to the constructive feedback and act on recommendations made. This will require both commitment and work from you. Be prepared to assess yourself and your progress; your learning diary will help you do this. As mentioned

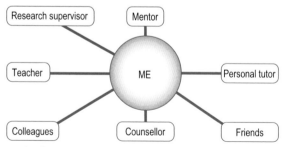

FIGURE 2.7 Example of a support network.

previously, supervisors are not gods; they are there to guide your learning, so be prepared and focused in tutorials.

360° feedback

Often, the best feedback on your clinical skills will come from your patients and clients. For midwives, vaginal examination (VE) is an essential skill when caring for a labouring woman, one that should be undertaken with sensitivity due to the intimate nature of the examination, but efficiently as the information gained will help assess progress and inform care (Johnson and Taylor, 2005).

 CASE STUDY

As a student midwife, I met a wonderful woman birthing her third child who had a very positive attitude towards students developing their skills. She consented to me repeating a VE after my mentor and gave me feedback throughout on what it felt like and how it was different to my mentor. This woman encouraged me to take my time and gather all the information I needed, while my mentor stood at my side and guided me. In such a supportive environment, my anxieties about causing discomfort or asking questions were minimized. My experience was enhanced by the client and my mentor enabling me to improve my confidence with VE and develop as a professional. I learned that by discussing my learning needs with clients, and seeking informed consent, they become valuable partners in my learning.

Managing the mentor relationship

Most practice placements will ensure that you have a mentorship scheme (see Chapter 11). The mentor is an experienced midwife or nurse who is there to help make the clinical experience a positive one. You need to establish your relationship, identifying your expectations for the practice placement. Your mentor is responsible for knowing what stage you are at in your course and for helping you to get the most out of your placement. It is important that you get to work with your mentor as much as possible: organize regular meetings and come to them on time and prepared. Additional points that you need to consider with your mentor include identifying your learning needs while on this placement, whether there is any assessment and when this might be occurring. You will be responsible for any assessment documentation, so look after it and don't leave it lying around.

What to do when it goes wrong

It is still the case that the majority of students are allocated to a mentor, rather than being able to choose one. Sometimes the relationship does not work and this can be for a variety of reasons, including: not liking each other, your mentor is unavailable, your requirements have changed. The most important thing is to do something about this. First, you should talk to your mentor and discuss how you are feeling; this might be embarrassing but it will be constructive and allow you to carry on learning. If you cannot resolve any difficulties between you and your mentor, then you need to identify a replacement.

Study networks

Another way of improving your learning is to form study networks with other students. Study groups are a form of self-help group, and can provide additional support to that which is provided by your teachers. With your fellow students you can:

- share resources
- pool ideas
- brainstorm
- meet and make more friends
- share tasks
- develop group working skills.

You might find you have to initiate the development of a study group. The following points might help you to develop a study network:

- organize a meeting
- explain the purpose of the group
- decide when, where and how often you will meet
- keep in touch, exchange addresses and phone numbers
- meet regularly.

Assessing yourself

Throughout your career in nursing there is an expectation that you can assess yourself, including your:

- personal skills and qualities
- strengths and weaknesses
- learning requirements.

You will also be expected to learn to evaluate your own work, as well as to evaluate that of others. The ability to assess yourself accurately will be useful in your professional career, as well as a valuable skill from a personal viewpoint. Self-assessment fits well with writing a learning diary; it will help you recognize your learning needs and how to achieve them. You will also be able to use it to support feedback received from supervisors, teachers and colleagues.

Conclusion

In this chapter you have looked at a variety of essential points necessary to help you with your learning. Having identified your preferred style of learning, you can use this information to enhance your studying.

In addition, there are costs to learning, and these are not only financial. Support networks are available to make your experience less painful. Finally, the use of learning contracts with supervisors can help you make the most of your learning, and ensure that you remain in control and that you pace yourself through the course.

Before moving on, take some time and record the following in your reflective diary.

- What is your preferred learning style?
- How will you use this preferred learning style to your advantage?
- List the requirements of your ideal supervisor. What do you think they might expect from you?
- Identify a supportive friend, with whom you could develop a study network.
- Talk to your teacher about learning contracts and developing a learning contract to meet your specific learning needs.

Acknowledgements

Thanks to Lisa Egerton, a former nursing student at the School of Health and Human Sciences, Liverpool John Moores University, for permission to use her reflective account.

 CHAPTER RESOURCES

REFERENCES

Boud, D., Keogh, R. & Walker, D., 1985. Reflection: turning experience into learning. Kogan Page, London.

Fleming, N.D., 2001. Teaching and learning styles: VARK Strategies, Honolulu Community College. Online. Available: http://www.how-to-study.com/LearningStyles.htm.

Gibbs, G., 1988. Learning by doing: a guide to teaching and learning methods. Further Education Unit, Oxford Polytechnic, Oxford.

Honey, P. & Mumford, A., 1992. The manual of learning styles, 3rd edn. Peter Honey, Maidenhead.

Johns, C., 1994. Guided reflection. In: Palmer, A., Burns, S. & Bulman, C. (Eds.) Reflective practice in nursing: the growth of the professional practitioner. Blackwell Science, Oxford.

Johnson, R. & Taylor, W., 2005. Skills for midwifery practice, 2nd edn. Elsevier/Churchill Livingstone, Philadelphia.

Kolb, D.A., 1984. Experiential learning: experience as the source of learning and development. Prentice Hall, London, p. 38.

Malim, T. & Birch, A. (Eds.), 1998. Introductory psychology. Macmillan, Basingstoke, p. 291.

Mallik, M., 2005. Getting the most from practice learning. In: Maslin-Prothero, S. (Ed.), Baillière's study skills for nurses and midwives, 3rd edn. Elsevier, Philadelphia, p. 298.

Nursing and Midwifery Council (NMC), 2008. The code. NMC, London. Online. Available: http://www.nmc-uk.org/aFrameDisplay.aspx?DocumentID=3954 [accessed 24/07/08].

Rolfe, G., 1996. Closing the theory practice gap: a new paradigm for nursing. Butterworth-Heinemann, Oxford, p. 127.

Schon, D., 1983. The reflective practitioner: how professionals think in action. Basic Books, New York.

Siviter, B., 2008. The student nurse handbook: a survival guide, 2nd edn. Baillière Tindall/Elsevier, Edinburgh.

3

Using the library
Sue Brain

KEY ISSUES

- Library resources and services
- Information resources
- Accessing library resources
- Electronic sources
- Literature searching
- Obtaining literature

Introduction

This chapter (and Chapters 4, 5 and 8) is about gathering information from a variety of sources. The emphasis is on your role in the process – how you can make the material and resources work for you. Gathering information can be broadly divided into two stages:

1. Locating the material.
2. Using the material.

This chapter deals with the first stage; Chapters 6 and 8 look in detail at the second.

One of the most valuable things you can do is to become familiar with your institution's library or learning resources centre as soon as possible. Libraries provide access to selected, high-quality information resources in various formats. They also provide equipment, technology and training for accessing information; for example, assistive technologies enabling people with disabilities to access information. Library staff are experienced knowledge navigators and provide training sessions and guidance in locating and making best use of the key information resources required for education, research or clinical practice.

The skills for finding the evidence and literature searching, together with skills to critically evaluate material, have received renewed emphasis in the light of the weight put on evidence-based health care (Sackett et al., 1996), clinical governance and clinical effectiveness (NHS Executive, 1999). Literature searching and information-literacy skills are a vital component of the evidence-based approach in health care. Access to information has been transformed with the advent of the internet, electronic publishing and the arrival of gateways such as NHS Evidence. Therefore, familiarity with information and communication technologies (ICT), a grasp of basic computer skills (see Chapter 4) and information-searching skills are vital.

Learning is nowadays seen as a life-long process and is no longer viewed as something that finishes with leaving school or college. Library and information-gathering skills will be important throughout your working career and beyond.

Critical process

Finding and using information is a process that involves critical thinking, understanding and constant interpretation. It is a questioning process and provides a good foundation for the reasoning skills you need to present a written argument (see Chapter 6).

Guiding principle: be clear about your purpose

Gathering information is done more effectively if you have defined your purpose. Whether you are deciding which database to search or which article to read, keep your purpose clearly in mind. For example, while preparing for an essay, keep the essay question clearly visible to prevent you from straying down interesting but irrelevant avenues (a useful tip for when you come to write it). Information overload means that there is a huge amount of material available and it is easy to be overwhelmed. Knowing your purpose keeps you focused and enables others – for example, library staff – to help you.

Information sources

As a student (and professional) you can expect to use the following:

- Libraries for:
  - books: general and specialized texts
  - journals: also known as periodicals or serials; professional, academic or specialized
  - audiovisual material: DVDs, videos, multimedia packages
  - reference material: dictionaries, directories, encyclopaedias, etc.
- The internet (access via the library or from home) for:
  - databases: MEDLINE, CINAHL, etc.
  - publications: electronic or e-journals, e-books, government publications, etc.
  - patient information: patient organization websites, newsgroups, etc.
- Professional associations/specialist information centres for:
  - contacts
  - specialist information
  - patient information.

This chapter concentrates on how to access the information sources generally found in libraries. The aim is not to turn you into an expert but to give you the confidence to use the resources and staff available.

Library resources and services

Why use a library? Many people assume that nearly all the information they require is now available via the internet. However, it is still important to become familiar with the resources and services offered by libraries. It is true that many traditionally library-held resources (books, reports, journals, databases, etc.) are increasingly becoming available, and are easily accessible, online via the internet. Most libraries would describe themselves as being in a hybrid situation at present, i.e. they hold both print and electronic resources.

It is important to remember that not all sources of information have been digitized yet and that access to traditional print resources is still necessary. Newer publications are increasingly being published both electronically and in print form but there are still huge gaps in the literature and, in particular, sources published some time ago will only be available in print.

It is true that libraries are gradually moving away from the concept of being repositories and housing large physical collections of printed documents and journals. In the electronic age, the librarian or information specialist's role is increasingly concerned with facilitating access and guiding users and researchers to the appropriate resources. We are facing an information explosion in all subject areas, and it can be difficult to know where to begin with your information gathering. Librarians, subject specialists and knowledge managers all have a role in offering guidance through the bewildering amount of information that exists, in whatever format – electronic, print, audiovisual, etc. Many libraries are developing their own portals or websites, which offer guidance to their users on the most useful and appropriate sources of information. These websites typically contain links to the library catalogue (also known as an open-access public catalogue, OPAC), user guides, other useful websites, listings of new resources and contact details. Try to find out whether your library has a website and add it to your Favorites or Bookmarks (depending on which internet browser you use; this allows your web addresses to be saved so that they can easily be visited at a later time).

Library services

The following is a list of services typically offered by libraries. Your library will offer some or all of these:

- Loans service, reservations, short-term loans for items in heavy demand.
- OPAC.
- Document delivery and interlibrary loans (access to resources held in other libraries).
- Enquiry facilities and subject-specialist librarians.
- Registration and guidance on how to access specialist electronic resources.

- Library website or portal.
- Photocopying facilities.
- Computers and printing facilities.
- Quiet study space.
- Laminators and binding facilities.
- DVD/video/CD-ROM viewing facilities.
- Assistive/adaptive/accessible/enabling technologies for students with disabilities and special needs.
- Current awareness and alerting services.
- Training; for example, copyright and plagiarism guidance, literature searching/information literacy, evaluating and critically appraising information, reference management software.
- Induction sessions for new students.
- Library guides and searching guides for specific databases or subject areas.
- Specialist collections.
- Outreach services; for example, in a hospital there may be a clinical librarian who gets involved in the ward rounds and who aims to provide quick and easy access to clinical information.

It is important to get to know early on in your studies what services the library offers. These should be listed in the general library guide (available online or in print).

Adaptive technologies

Libraries will do their best to ensure that all their users are able to access the information they need. Various adaptive technologies (also known as assistive, accessible or enabling technologies) are provided to ensure that disabled and users with special needs are able to access information. These technologies include:

- magnification software
- screen-reading software
- text-to-speech software: for people with dyslexia
- voice-recognition systems
- text highlighting
- spell checkers
- word prediction
- thesauri.

Training and help with using these technologies will be provided on a one-to-one basis.

Resources

Most libraries will have the resources listed in Table 3.1, which offer material appropriate to different search needs. How do you know which to use when, and how do you access them?

TABLE 3.1 Resources typically available in a library

SOURCE	ACCESS	PURPOSE
Books		
Textbooks Handbooks Research reports Government publications Theses Guidelines	Online public access catalogue (OPAC) listing details of collections, shelf location and access information, e.g. shelf marks OPAC accessed via library workstation or library website (remote access, e.g. at home) Print, e-books and online	Core reading Background Context Factual Original research details and conclusions Policy documents Skills and guides Historical
Reference books		
Dictionaries Encyclopaedias Directories Yearbooks and almanacs Atlases Statistical publications (official and unofficial sources) Bibliographies	OPAC as above Print and online, e.g. NLH, Credo Reference	Definitions Factual information Concise overviews Further reading or bibliographies Contacts Geography Population, socio-economic and numerical data
Journals		
Research and popular Print and e-journals (also known as articles, periodicals or serials)	OPAC, as above, or separately printed or online journal list gives titles, length of holding, location, access details Indexed – print or online indexes, internet databases with links to full text Internet	Current and specific material Current awareness Primary research papers Literature review News Information exchange Reviews Contacts Events Jobs
Newspapers		
Broadsheets Tabloids	OPAC as above or listed with journals as above Titles, length of holdings, location and access details Indexed Microfilm indexes CD-ROM indexes online Print, CD-ROM or online	Current and contemporary Lay/popular material News and reports of latest research Reviews Factual Statistics Online indexes and full-text
Audiovisual		
Videos or DVDs CD-ROMS Audio tape or digital Computerized assisted learning (CAL) packages Online e-learning packages	OPAC as above for titles, holdings, location and access	Instructive and learning packages Factual Visual documentaries TV programmes Current and contemporary

Table 3.1 gives a general picture of sources, means of access and purpose, but it is not meant to be exhaustive. Your own library may hold other resources. You can probably begin to see how the type of information you need, that is, your purpose, determines which source you use.

Take the two following questions and, referring to Table 3.1, think (for about 5- to 10-minutes) where you would look for the material for the answer to each. There could be more than one source:

1. Describe the structure and function of the skin.
2. What causes the skin condition psoriasis and how is it now treated?

Both questions deal broadly with the skin. The first concerns basic anatomy and physiology, factual information that is unlikely to change greatly. Textbooks and audiovisual material (i.e. DVDs, CD-ROMS, videos) would probably provide excellent information for this question.

The second question deals with a specific skin condition and requires current information. Textbooks would provide some material and a medical dictionary would give an introductory definition but you would need to use journal literature to discover the up-to-date treatment and care, and any research, findings or discussion/controversy concerning them. There might also be recent TV documentaries (recorded and held in the library) or relevant, current newspaper reports that might aid your understanding of the more clinical material in the health journals. Look for guidelines, for example, the National Institute for Health and Clinical Excellence (NICE), the British Association of Dermatologists and Clinical Knowledge Summaries (CKS), and evidence-based summaries; for example, Clinical Evidence (*BMJ* subscription service), Bandolier, the Cochrane Library (systematic reviews).

What resources does your library offer?

If you don't already know what your university and/or professional library holds, where books and journals are kept and how you access electronic resources – find out! It's best to familiarize yourself with such things early in your course before you need them. All libraries should offer induction and tuition in the first few weeks of a course. Make the most of such opportunities – seek them out.

The library catalogue

This resource must be mastered as soon as possible. The catalogue tells you what stock the library has and where it is shelved. The type of material listed will depend on the library but will certainly include books and government publications. Audiovisual materials may well be in the catalogue but there may be a separate listing of journals and newspapers.

Nowadays, libraries have computerized catalogue access, often known as OPAC, WebCat WebOPAC, etc. OPACs can tell you what material the library holds by author, subject or title, where any item is shelved or whether it's out on loan. Other facilities are dependent on the system used by the library. Quite often it is possible to put a hold or reservation on items via the catalogue. Most university, college (and public) library catalogues are now accessible via the internet, usually via the library's website.

Journal literature

What is a journal?

Essentially, journals are the way you communicate with your fellow professionals nationally and internationally. All professions and trades have journals. The medical and health professions have thousands. From this you will deduce that your library will not have all of them; more on that later.

You may come across journals referred to as 'serials' and/or 'periodicals', because they are published periodically and because each issue is part of the whole. A journal may be published weekly, monthly, bimonthly, quarterly (four times a year) or occasionally less frequently. Generally, the issues appearing in one year are described as one volume, each year having one volume number. The *Journal of Advanced Nursing* is an example of a research journal that is published twice a month and consists (unusually) of four volumes per year (24 issues) with each volume consisting of six parts or issues; for example, there were four volumes in 2003, volumes 41–44. The October 2003 volume started with volume 44 part 1. The standard way of writing this is 44(1). The volume number precedes the issue number, which is in brackets.

How is the material in journals different from that in books?

Journals differ from books in five important ways:

1. Currency: books can take 2–4 years to reach publication; journal literature is usually published within months, depending on the frequency of the journal itself. Increasingly, journals are being published electronically via the internet, making them even more immediately available. Open access journals make the research articles freely available via the internet; for example, BiomedCentral, BMC Nursing, Public Library of Science (PLoS).
2. Specificity: articles are condensed material and are therefore focused on specific areas. When you search the literature, your subject headings can be correspondingly precise.
3. Ongoing: reports of ongoing, long-term research projects are to be found in the relevant journals, information otherwise unavailable for perhaps years.
4. Peer-reviewed: research reports published in academic and scholarly journals are subject to the peer-review process and subject to scrutiny by a panel of experts.
5. Contemporary: literature from journals published in the 1960s, for example, directly reflects the tone, attitudes and knowledge of the time, unmuddied by hindsight.

What sort of material do the different journals contain?

You can expect the more frequent (weekly, monthly) journals to contain current affairs, jobs and listings, and articles that are informative, wide ranging but not necessarily research based. The name of the journal is a fair indication of its broad aim, standards and content. So, the *Nursing Times* and *Nursing Standard* aim to inform the nursing profession and will cover anything they consider relevant. The *European Journal of Oncology Nursing* clearly has a narrower remit; articles are longer, specific and often research based. Published bi-monthly, its material is less immediate and more analytical.

Accessing the journal literature

When you need to find out whether a book contains information on a topic, you use the index at the back. This tells you if the topic is covered, on which pages and in how much detail. The principle is the same with journals, i.e. you use an index. It tells you what articles are available on a subject and in which journal you will find them. The chief difference is that journal indexes are generally published as electronic bibliographic databases accessible via the internet; they also index many different journals simultaneously. Quite often, databases provide links to the full text of selected electronic journals (e.g. services such as Thomson Dialog, Ovid, ProQuest, EBSCO), depending on the services or journals subscribed to by your library or resources purchased on behalf of NHS staff by NHS Evidence.

There are advantages to this. Remember that there are thousands of health and health-related journals, hundreds in nursing and midwifery alone. If these were indexed individually instead of collectively, searching the literature would be an enormous task and you would be restricted to the journals your library held. (The flip side is that using journal bibliographic databases means you will probably require some articles not held by your library or subscribed to electronically; most libraries recognize this and will request articles from other sources via the interlibrary loans system.)

How much information does a database give about articles?

Index information consists of the basic bibliographic details about any one item. For a journal article these details should be:

- title of article
- author(s)
- journal name
- volume and part numbers
- date
- page numbers
- abstract (not always included)
- descriptors, indexing terms or subject headings.

This information makes up the citation or reference. Depending on the indexing service used, you may be told more about the article; for example, how much further reading it includes or how many references it has cited, whether the content is research based or statistical, and so on.

Abstracts

Many databases provide a summary of content. This summary is called an abstract. Abstracts help you to make a more informed decision about the value to you of an article, paper or report. They are not a substitute for the original text and must not be treated as such. You must not quote them in your own writing as if you had read the original full-length work. In addition, the indexing terms (descriptors or subject headings) may also be listed. These are the terms used by the person who indexes items and may be useful in helping you to find similar articles.

Electronic databases

Finding journal article citations used to involve searching through a printed index or abstracting publication. This was very labour intensive and time consuming. With the advent of CD-ROMs and – more recently – the internet, this task is made much easier, more flexible and much faster. Electronic bibliographic databases have replaced the traditional print indexing and abstracting services. The publishers of CD-ROMs and printed indexes now make their services available via the internet, either by subscription services to institutions, or freely available, as in the case of PubMed (the free version of MEDLINE produced by the US National Library of Medicine). It is now possible to perform a literature search and gather source material from an integrated service such as Thomson Dialog, ProQuest or Ovid. Your library will provide its students with access to one or a number of similar services. These enable a search for citations to be run on various databases and from there to link directly to the full-text of journal articles.

Electronic databases allow you to search terms in combination (e.g. 'breast cancer' and 'case studies' and 'post-operative care'). Searching electronic databases gives you the advantage of more means of access to the information, and therefore greater control over your search. There are other benefits, including being able to print out your search results, e-mail or download them to disk or to reference management software (e.g. EndNote, Reference Manager), together with the added advantage of being able to access full-text articles in some cases. Your library will most likely provide training sessions, in groups or on a one-to-one basis, on how to use specialist databases, downloading information, copyright, reference software and other aspects of using online resources. Again, find out now what your library offers and start using it!

As mentioned above, there are so many health journals and other types of health literature that no single bibliographic database can cover

TABLE 3.2 Some of the best known databases (most are available via the internet or CD-ROM)

NAME AND PRODUCER	ACCESS	YEARS COVERED	DESCRIPTION
MEDLINE US National Library of Medicine	PubMed (Internet with free access) NLH – NHS National Core Content Clinical Databases Information aggregators, e.g. Thomson Dialog, Ovid	OLDMEDLINE 1953–1965 MEDLINE 1966– 'In process citations' are very new citations and provide basic citation International coverage information prior to receiving full indexing and MeSH headings	Indexes 5200 biomedical journals Medicine, nursing, midwifery, dentistry, veterinary medicine, healthcare systems 18 million citations Bibliographic records, abstracts. Uses MeSH subject indexing
CINAHL (Cumulative Index to Nursing and Allied Health Literature)	CINAHL Direct Online Service NLH–NHS National Core Content Clinical Databases	1982–	Indexes 1200 publications, nursing, midwifery and allied health Bibliographic records, with abstracts Uses CINAHL subject headings
EBSCO Information Services	Information aggregators, e.g. Thomson Dialog, Ovid		International coverage
EMBASE	Elsevier bibliographic database	1974–	A biomedical and pharmacological database with strong UK and European coverage
Elsevier	NLH–NHS National Core Content Clinical Databases Information aggregators, e.g. Thomson Dialog, Ovid		Indexes 5000 journals 12 million citations Subject indexing using EMTREE (similar to MeSH) Some overlap with MEDLINE
BNI (British Nursing Index) Bournemouth University, Poole Hospital NHS Trust, Salisbury Health Care Trust, RCN	NLH–NHS National Core Content Clinical Databases Information aggregators, e.g. Thomson Dialog, Ovid	1985–	Nursing, midwifery and community healthcare database Bibliographic but does not include abstracts Indexes 250 journals UK coverage and updated monthly UK coverage
AMED (Allied and Complementary Medicine Database) British Library	NLH–NHS National Core Content Clinical Databases Information aggregators, e.g. Thomson Dialog, Ovid	1985–	Complementary medicine, palliative care, occupational therapy, physiotherapy, podiatry and rehabilitation, speech and language therapy Uses the AMED thesaurus of indexing terms Indexes 400 journals

(continued)

TABLE 3.2 (continued)

PscyINFO American Psychological Association	NLH–NHS National Core Content Clinical Databases Information aggregators, e.g. Thomson Dialog, Ovid	1987– Psychology and the psychological aspects of related disciplines, e.g. medicine, psychiatry, nursing, sociology, education, pharmacology, physiology, linguistics, anthropology, business and law Indexes 200 journals
DH Data Department of Health Library (UK)	NLH–NHS National Core Content Clinical Databases	1983– Health service and hospital administration, NHS, nursing, primary care
ProQuest ProQuest Information and Learning	NLH–NHS National Core Content Clinical Databases	Various dates Three databases offering access to 1000 full-text journals: ProQuest Medical Library, Proquest Nursing Journals, ProQuest Psychology Journals
National Research Register Department of Health	Free access via the internet	2000– Some records from 1990s A database of ongoing and recently completed research projects funded by, or of interest to, the UK National Health Service Over 110000 records
ASSIA (Applied Social Sciences Index and Abstracts) Cambridge Scientific Abstracts	Cambridge Scientific Abstracts	1987– 426575 500+ journals US and UK Health, social services, psychology, sociology, economics, politics, race relations and education
NLH is now known as NHS Evidence		

all the material published. Most are fairly comprehensive and cover a number of subject areas but are designed for specific disciplines. For example, nursing and midwifery databases include the British Nursing Index (BNI) and the Cumulative Index to Nursing and Allied Health Literature (CINAHL); MEDLINE and EMBASE cover biomedical subject areas, including nursing and midwifery, but have a stronger emphasis on clinical medicine.

It is your information needs that determine which indexes are best and when. Table 3.2 lists some of the databases available in the health-information field, but there are many others. It is always advisable to run a literature search on several databases and not to rely solely on a single source. Despite some overlap between databases, different results will be produced. CINAHL and MEDLINE have some overlap but will also produce unique citations.

Starting the literature search

The first step in any literature search is to be clear about the meaning of the overall question and the meaning of the words or concepts contained within it. In other words, right from the very beginning it is essential that you are clear about what it is you are looking for. You will need to return at intervals and remind yourself of the question. Successful searching depends on a careful analysis of the title, the choice of search terms and the way these are combined.

Often, a good place to start is using dictionaries, encyclopaedias, subject handbooks, companions or textbooks to get a general grasp or overview of the topic. Doing a brief search on the internet using a search engine or directory site can also help you to get an overview of the subject and might lead to some useful ideas to get you started. When answering a question, consider carefully which aspect or facet of a subject is being asked about. If you are responsible for setting an area to study yourself, narrow it down to a particular aspect if you find that your initial subject area is too large.

Are you working to a deadline? Leave enough time to plan, search for information, order materials if necessary, and read material. Don't forget, you still have to write your essay.

Consider your search/information needs

What sort of information do you need?

- Research: primary original research studies or secondary studies, i.e. material derived from the primary research. Also consider whether qualitative or quantitative research is required
- News reportage
- Factual
- Reviews/overviews of the literature

- Opinion
- Theory, ideas, philosophical perspective
- Government policy or reports
- Historical
- Personal experience
- Surveys or statistics
- Practice guidelines (NICE, Royal Colleges, SIGN, CKS, RCN, Royal College of Midwives, etc.).

Search terms

The first step is to break the question down into its main concepts. Have you thought about your search terms/subject headings? Think carefully about what headings you might use and how the thesaurusi and indexing terms might express your subject. It is useful to brainstorm this, creating a spider map of your subject area. This helps to identify specific and broad terms, and provides a rough, visual hierarchy of the subject.

Limits

You also need to decide on the limitations to apply to the search. Think about how you might want to limit your search by:

- Age group: neonate, infant, child, adolescent, adult, elderly
- Study group (human or animal)
- Gender
- Language
- Publication date: within the past year, 2 years, 5 years, 10 years or further back?
- Country: international or specific country?
- Publication type: clinical trial, systematic review, etc.

Most databases have the facility to limit searches in some way, such as by year (e.g. publications published within the last 5 years) or they enable you to search on specific journal titles. They may also enable you to search by study type, e.g. clinical trial, review.

Evidenced-based health care and clinical questions

When asking questions that relate to clinical questions it is worth considering a number of aspects. Think about the way you ask the question. PICO is the recommended method of framing your question:

P: Patient/population
I: Intervention or exposure
C: Comparison: intervention/no intervention
O: Outcomes.

The next step is to consider whether you are looking at therapy, diagnosis, prognosis or aetiology questions. Various search strategies can be employed for searching the literature; these include search filters. PubMed Clinical Queries is an example of a service with predefined filters that enable you to type in search terms, indicate the category and specify the emphasis on either a sensitive search (broad) or specific search (specific).

Research study types or the hierarchy of evidence/levels of evidence are important when considering clinical questions. The highest level, 1, is normally a systematic review (the Cochrane Library being a prime source) while level 2 includes well-conducted randomized controlled trials, right down to level 5, which is expert opinion. See the websites mentioned above for further information (addresses at the end of this chapter).

Further information on using search filters and the different types of study can be found at the ADEPT website (ScHARR). The websites of the Centre for Evidence-based Medicine, based at Oxford, and the Center for Evidence-based Medicine, University of Toronto, contain useful information on conducting evidence-based searching and the skills of critical appraisal. The Critical Appraisal Skills Programme (CASP) website contains a selection of tools or checklists that will assist you in critically appraising the different types of research study (e.g. systematic reviews, randomized controlled studies).

Being aware of these considerations is helpful before attempting a search for clinical information. The type of research study, its methodology and design, and its applicability to your practice are all important considerations in evidence-based health care. *How to read a paper* (Greenhalgh, 2006), originally based on a series published in the *British Medical Journal* in 1997, with chapters from the 1997 edition available via the BMJ website, is worth reading. *The evidence-based practice manual for nurses* (Craig and Smyth, 2007) is a really useful resource covering the evidence-based process from asking the right, clearly focused question, effective literature searching, evaluating evidence retrieved and deciding on its applicability.

A good starting place for finding evidence-based resources and information is NHS Evidence, described later on. This contains links to some invaluable resources and is regularly updated. The Turning Research Into Practice (TRIP) database is a free resource that cross searches a range of evidence-based clinical resources.

Which database?

You will have realized by now that your search needs dictate your choice of database or resource used! The exercise below (maximum 10 minutes needed) gives you some practice at this.

This exercise involves matching search needs to the right database. Using Table 3.2, decide which database might be most appropriate for finding the necessary material for the search questions below. There is no right or wrong choice exactly but, clearly, some databases are better than others.

As you match search and databases, note the reasons for the choices you have made. This may help to clarify the thinking behind your decision.

1. What effect does a hip replacement have on patients' self-image, and how might that influence their recovery?

2. Does nurse education equip students to cope with the emotional stress of nursing terminally-ill patients?

3. What, if any, relation is there between inequality in health and social class?

1. This question encompasses two issues: the psychological and social effects – psychosocial factors – of a condition and the role of the carer in recognizing and dealing with these effects. There is a clear nursing angle, so the databases CINAHL or BNI would all be useful sources. A combined search of CINAHL under hip surgery and self-image (or whatever the correct search terms might be) would swiftly reveal what, if any, material is available.

   The nursing indexes are the obvious source for the caring angle. However, you might want to read current material on the subject of self-concept, and explore its psychology. PsycINFO would then be a useful source.

   It is probably immaterial whether the articles you find are American, British or Australian, as there is no particular cultural slant to the search. Your main concern is the subject, which is universal.

2. Again, this is clearly a nursing issue. CINAHL or BNI would be appropriate routes to the relevant material. However, the question is also about stress, death and education. The educational element needs you to be aware of the country of origin of the material you might find; it could well still be relevant for the sake of contrast or proposed change, but if you require only UK material use the UK indexes first.

   You could search MEDLINE for information on how effective medical education is in this regard. General material on occupational stress can be found in any of the sources mentioned, but add DH Data for a management angle.

3. This question is primarily sociological. A database with sociological content, e.g. Applied Social Sciences Index and Abstracts (ASSIA), would be an appropriate source. DH Data or the King's Fund database (formerly the Health Management Information Consortium or HMIC) might provide information on monitoring the quality of the delivery of health across society. Again, the country of origin might be important, although American, etc., material could be useful for comparison.

Which search terms?

Having identified the appropriate database, you need to clarify your search terms or subject headings. These are the words you use to look up your subject in the databases. They may also be referred to as key-words. Identifying your search terms happens in two stages:

1. Highlighting the key terms (or main concepts) in your essay question.
2. Ensuring that they are the terms used by the databases you intend to search.

For the first stage, look again at the questions in the exercise above.

Take 10 minutes to identify what you consider to be the keywords for the search (then check them against those below):

1. Hip replacement; self-image; recovery
2. Nurse education; students; stress; terminally ill
3. Inequality; health: social class

It is possible that your keywords are not exactly the same as those used by any of the databases you intend searching.

It is helpful at this stage to spend a few minutes brainstorming for alternatives. Alternative terms/keywords might be: hip replacement: hip surgery/hip prosthesis/artificial hip; self-image: body-image/self-concept/self-esteem; recovery: rehabilitation/postoperative care.

It is likely that, in some cases, the terms you use will be different depending on the database, despite the fact that you're looking up the same subject.

These differences are due to cultural differences, terminology, spelling and diversity of language. For example, look at the two lists in the box below, both full of terms related to their subject.

Cancer	Ageing
Cancer	Ageing/aging
Oncology	Aged
Neoplasm	Elderly
Tumour/tumor	Old age
Growth	Geriatric
Carcinosis	Gerontology
Melanoma	Older person/people

A database could use a quite different term to the one you have chosen to search. If your search terms do not match the database you are using then you are wasting your time. If you search for 'geriatric nursing' and find no material, there are two possible explanations:

1. There might not be anything published/available.
2. The database has used the indexing term 'care of the elderly'.

But, how do you know which explanation is the true one?

It is essential when you are searching a database that you speak its language, even allowing for electronic databases' increased flexibility over the printed index. Some databases automatically convert your 'free-text' or natural language terms into the subject terms or keywords of that database. This is known as 'mapping'.

Most databases try to help by providing a list of their terms for you to check before you begin to search. Called a thesaurus, or subject headings list, this has two functions:

1. To provide you with the correct search terms for that database (see the first entry in the box below).
2. To introduce you to narrower (more specific), related or broader search terms, i.e. to alert you to other headings, which may be equally or more relevant (see the second entry in the box below).

Thesaurus entries

- Nurse education:

  see Education, nursing

- Education, nursing:

  see also:

  Education, nursing, Baccalaureate

  Education, nursing, continuing

  Education, nursing, post-registration

Such a list is essential not only to you, the searcher, but also to those compiling the database. They need to standardize their headings so that related material is clustered under the same term, ensuring that you will find all the material available on a subject. New subject terms are added every year; this reflects the growth of information, the need for more specific terms and the changing language. Consulting a database's thesaurus or list of keywords informs you of the best search terms for that database. If your terms are wrong you will not find the material. Subject headings/search terms are really keywords.

Medical Subject Headings (MeSH) is the MEDLINE thesaurus and is available on the US NLM National Library of Medicine Medical Subject Headings website. MeSH is an example of a controlled language with a very well-defined structure, e.g. the MeSH tree structure.

When you find useful references as a result of a database search it is worth looking at the descriptors or indexing terms that have been used. You can then refine your search terms to incorporate these into your search as appropriate.

A thesaurus or subject headings list is not infallible. It won't always list your original search term and therefore alternatives. In this instance, you need to be your own thesaurus. This is where brainstorming possible subject headings is helpful. Another source of help is, of course, the librarian.

Use the following steps:

- Identify your search terms from your essay question, or write down your search need in a way that helps you to highlight the keywords. Brainstorm for alternative keywords/search terms.

- Browse the database's list of indexing terms or use the thesaurus; it ensures you are using the correct search terms and those most appropriate to your search.

- Be aware of variations in American and UK spellings and allow for these.

- Identifying your search terms properly will retrieve relevant material, or confirm its absence.

Searching electronic databases

Mastering a few basic search techniques, such as how to use Boolean operators, will prove invaluable when searching electronic databases. These techniques can also be applied when using internet search engines. Some search engines allow quite sophisticated search techniques to be used, similar to the methods used when searching databases. Wherever possible, it is advisable to spend some time looking at the search help pages. Most databases or internet search engines include a help facility. The library may have prepared a user guide to searching specific databases, which is either printed or available online. These will contain useful tips and enable you to get the most out of the source being used.

Boolean operators

Using Boolean operators offers more control and the ability to refine searches. The main operators are AND, OR and NOT. Plan how the concepts are going to be linked in your search statement. Use Boolean logic to narrow, widen or exclude when combining terms. Link your terms by using AND to narrow, OR to widen or NOT to exclude terms.

- AND is used to narrow a search statement. This ensures that all the search terms appear on the web page or document; for example, 'cancer AND lung AND patient AND nursing' results in all of these terms appearing in the citations retrieved.

- OR is often used to widen a search. Using OR between words (e.g. 'nursing OR nurse') results in either one or both words appearing in the reference. It enables you to specify more than one word, term, phrase or synonym in a search statement (e.g. 'cancer OR neoplasm

OR tumour OR tumor'). It is useful, for instance, where a database includes both American and UK spellings.

■ NOT enables the exclusion of a word or phrase from a search statement. Combining terms with NOT (e.g. 'child NOT adult') means that the first word must be present but not the second.

■ Proximity searching with NEAR or WITH or ADJACENT (sometimes abbreviated to 'adj') is often used to specify how close terms should appear to each other (e.g. 'palliative NEAR care'). It is possible to specify that words should appear within the same sentence or paragraph.

Truncation and wild cards

Using a truncation symbol such as *, ? or $ after or within a word enables you to pick up words with a variety of spellings. Many words have a common stem or root, which can be used as a search term. Using a truncation symbol allows you to broaden the search to include all records that contain any variation of the stem. This is particularly useful where you are unsure of the exact spelling, when including plurals or where there may be alternative spellings.

■ Using hospital* will find references with the words hospitals, hospitalization, hospitalization, hospitalized, etc.

■ Using nurs* will find nurse, nurses, nursing, etc.

Some databases allow truncation or wild card symbols to be used in the middle of words or at the beginning of a word.

■ Using wom*n will find the words woman or women.

■ Using *ye* will find stye, styes, eye, eyes, etc.

Use these symbols with caution, particularly if a word might appear quite frequently in a database. It will slow the computer down when searching and may result in a large number of irrelevant items being found!

Nesting

Nesting, or the use of parentheses – brackets ( ) – around search terms or set numbers (search terms are allocated numbers as the search progresses) allows complex queries to be constructed. The brackets indicate the order in which the logical operators or commands are to be carried out by a computer. These are used with multiple Boolean commands and need careful planning; for example, '(child OR infant) AND (cancer OR tumour* or neoplasm*) AND pain control'. The terms in brackets will be searched as queries in their own right, one at a time, before being linked to the phrase pain. Without the use of the parentheses confusion would ensue and irrelevant results would be found.

How useful is that reference?

It is difficult to deduce the potential value of an article from the basic information given in a database; that is, from the citation. However, there are indicators:

- Is there an abstract?
- Check the authors' credentials: they may be well known in their field and have written other material.
- Is the journal cited academic, scholarly, research based or more news based?
- How long is the article? If long, consider the time necessary to read and understand it; if short, how informative will it be?
- How many references does it cite? These may lead to other material on your subject and may indicate the authenticity of the author/s' work.
- What type of paper is being cited? Is it original research or a review of the literature? Is it a systematic review, meta-analysis or randomized controlled trial? Where does it sit in the hierarchy of evidence?
- Is the article itself cited by others? Check a citation index if possible (ask your library staff); this will tell you if, and how often, this particular article has been referred to by other published authors.
- Ask tutors and fellow students or colleagues if they have read, seen or know of a certain work or author.
- Practise critically appraising the article and considering the applicability and appropriateness of research results (see the section on evidence-based health care).

Judging the relevance of an article is a skill, which will come with practice. You will make mistakes because you cannot be 100% certain of any material until you have read it. There won't always be an abstract, authors and journals are numerous and many will be unknown to you. However, if your search terms are accurate and well thought out, you are more likely to retrieve relevant material.

The internet

The internet is an increasingly important resource for anyone undertaking research. It makes information available to a wide audience at a relatively low cost. It has had a tremendous impact on the provision of health information both for professionals and the public alike, and it is developing at a phenomenal pace. Access to the internet is via the library or from home. Your library will probably provide help with searching the internet. It will also provide you with the means – registration (providing you with a username and password) – to access specialist and scholarly online resources, e.g. databases and online full-text journals, subscribed to by your college or institution.

Internet resources

Many resources traditionally available through a library are now accessible via the internet. These include newspapers, journals, databases (as already mentioned), encyclopaedias, dictionaries, books, atlases, government publications (such as policy documents and reports), statistical data, drug information and patient leaflets. Using the internet is not a substitute for using a good library. With regard to research material it lacks the coverage, depth and span of holdings that a good library can provide, but may be a useful adjunct to research.

The internet contains information from a wide range of bodies, including educational establishments, government departments, institutions, societies, companies, voluntary organizations, professional organizations, the media, health consumer groups and individuals. The main problem with the internet centres on its democratic, but unregulated, nature. As already mentioned, quality and reliability of information is a major concern and you must always bear this in mind when using web sources (see Chapter 8). Internet Detective on the Intute website's internet training page is an excellent general online tutorial on how to use the internet for education and research purposes. This online learning resource covers advanced internet skills, looks at quality issues around information on the internet, describes how to critically evaluate information found and covers copyright, plagiarism and citation issues. Your college or university library will also provide similar tutorials or printed guides.

The principles established by tools such as Health on the Net Foundation (HoN) and Discern (developed to assess the quality of consumer health publications) are worth bearing in mind when using web-based resources. A degree of caution is required when using the internet and it is important to consider the reputation of the originator of the content and whether commercial or other interests are involved. Individual pages should always be dated and the author's name should be clearly displayed.

Finding information on the internet

Health information gateway sites

It is always advisable to start your internet search using a reputable gateway website. These sites contain links to resources that have been either evaluated or quality checked. NHS Evidence is being developed, with librarian involvement, as an NHS gateway for UK health professionals and aims to provide easy access to best current knowledge and know-how, with the aim of improving health and health care, clinical practice and patient choice. NHS Evidence links to key resources such as:

- the Cochrane Library
- National Library of Guidelines Specialist Library

- CKS Clinical Knowledge Summaries (incorporating Prodigy)
- the National Institute for Health and Clinical Excellence (NICE)
- the *British National Formulary* (BNF) and the *British National Formulary for Children* (cBNF)
- clinical databases (UK users via Athens)
- full-text journals (UK users via Athens)
- electronic books (UK users via Athens)
- medical dictionaries
- specialist libraries (by subject: women's health, child health, cancer, health management, etc.)
- 'Behind the headlines' (critically appraised news stories from NHS Choices website).

Some of the resources available through NHS Evidence are not password protected but for NHS staff, if you login using your Athens username and password then the full range of resources becomes available (listed under My Library). A revised search 2.0 facility was launched in 2008, which allows advanced searching of the NHS Healthcare Databases from within this same interface.

From NHS Evidence there are other useful links, including the NHS Choices website (For Patients), which is rapidly becoming the preferred gateway to information for the public, and is replacing the NHS Direct website at the time of writing. There is a health A–Z, a facility to compare hospitals, Behind the Headlines, a facility to receive personalized information (registration required), a Live Well section and videos, etc.

There are American equivalents to NHS Evidence and NHS Choices: the US National Library of Medicine has a Health Information page containing links to MEDLINEPlus, MEDLINE/PubMed and the US National Library of Medicine (NLM) gateway (which provides cross-searching of NLM resources). MEDLINEPlus, produced by the NLM, aims to link the public to the most reliable and authoritative information. It has a comprehensive medical encyclopaedia, a medical dictionary and a health topics section covering over 750 topics with links to resources produced by authoritative bodies, institutes and organizations; news; directories and other resources. Healthfinder is another gateway developed by the US Department of Health and Human Services. It has links to evaluated health information for the general public.

HealthInsite is the Australian equivalent, providing quality-assessed information originating from a variety of sources. Sections cover lifestyle; conditions and diseases; life stages and events; population groups; expert groups.

Intute (formerly OMNI/BIOME) is a free online service providing you with access to the very best web resources for education and research. The service is created by a network of UK universities and partners. Subject specialists select and evaluate the websites in our database and write high quality descriptions of the resources. Intute organizes web resources by broad subject categories: Nursing, midwifery and allied health, Medicine including dentistry, Biological Sciences, Social Sciences, Psychology. Conduct searches by keyword or browse using MeSH or RCN headings to obtain details of evaluated websites. Intute provides various internet training resources including the Virtual Training Suite, a set of internet tutorials in specific subject areas designed to help with the development of internet research skills. Tutorials are provided in nursing, midwifery, allied health, medicine and other disciplines.

Evaluating health information on the internet

A number of accreditation or evaluation tools, codes, or kitemarking schemes are available for assessing the quality and validity of general internet health information, particularly aimed at assessing health information provided for the general public (please see the section 'Evidence-based health care and clinical questions' on p. 57 for suggested resources for evaluating and appraising research studies). One of the original codes is HoN, a not-for-profit Geneva-based organization that has developed a code of conduct for health websites. These eight guidelines cover aspects such as authority, confidentiality and transparency of sponsorship. Its website includes a medical search engine, MedHunt, a medical documents finder and HoNselect, a medical search engine that uses MeSH headings. Other criteria, codes and kitemarking schemes for evaluating internet resources are: Discern and Judge, which are websites for health. See also the Intute collection development framework and policy, which describes the criteria for selecting suitable websites for the Intute gateway.

Internet search engines

Search engines allow you to type in keywords to search the worldwide web. They act as indexes to the vast amount of information available on the web. A word of caution, though: they can lead you to totally misleading and inaccurate information! You need to develop skills to evaluate the results produced by search engines. Remember that the internet, or more precisely the worldwide web, is largely unregulated and unmediated. Search engines employ robots or 'spiders' to trawl the net for new content and then index words from the pages they find into vast databases. Typing in keywords enables you to search an index of websites. Even the best of these is only able to index a limited percentage of the rapidly growing web content. Search engines do not search everything (e.g. the deep web or invisible web). One of the best-known search engines – Google – searches only the visible web and not, for instance, records held in specialist databases (as subscribed to by libraries). Google Scholar does contain details of scholarly articles and references but even this does not index the full range of academic literature.

For general internet searching advice and tutorials, see the tutorial 'Finding information on the internet: a tutorial', produced by the Teaching Library at the University of California at Berkeley.

When using a search engine, remember to look at the search help pages. These contain useful tips to give you more control over your searching. For instance, when searching for phrases, or where you are searching for words that must occur together, enclose the search terms in double quotation marks (e.g. "Tourette's syndrome").

Databases

The US National Library of Medicine launched its free PubMed database service (MEDLINE) on the worldwide web in 1997. This is directed at both health professionals and consumers and gives access to one of the premier biomedical databases, with records dating back to the 1950s. Currently there are over 18 million citations or references in this database. Its covers the biomedical sciences, including medicine and nursing. Access to the majority of databases is still mediated by your library, online via a subscription services (Ovid, Dialog, etc.). These require you to register and acquire a username and password. The library will be able to advise on registration and access requirements.

Journals

As previously mentioned, many research journals are available through services such as ProQuest, EBSCO, and so on. Find out which services your library subscribes to. NHS staff have access to electronic journals via NHS Evidence, as part of packages bought on behalf of the NHS, together with additional titles purchased by local Trust libraries. Many journals are also available, individually and separately online, via their publishers' websites. Many make contents pages, together with abstracts, or selected articles from the current issue freely available (e.g. the *Nursing Times* and research articles from the *BMJ*). Quite often, they require registration in order to access limited content. Many operate free alerting services that help you stay in touch with the latest contents of that particular title.

Newspapers and news services

Most newspapers, both national and local, have websites. Many provide access to their daily content and some have a limited search or archive facility. These sites do not provide total access to their contents, nor do they have a comprehensive search facility (as with an online subscription services available via library services). Nevertheless, they are still useful for finding news stories or for providing an overview of the daily news. Newspapers such as *The Guardian*, *The Independent* and *The Times* categorize news stories into sections including health, society or science news. Newspapers from around the world are available via services such as The Paperboy. General news services abound, including specialist health news services: the BBC, Reuters, CNN Health News, ABC. TNMSI Health News gives a quick overview selection of daily news stories relating to health, together with links to newspapers home pages.

Library catalogues

Most universities and colleges, and some professional societies and associations, make their library catalogues available via the web. The HERO (Higher and Research Opportunities in the United Kingdom) website has links to the UK library OPACs in higher education. There is free access through the Consortium of University Research Libraries (COPAC) to the merged catalogues of some of the major university research libraries in the UK and Ireland. The records include books and periodicals (but not periodical contents). The British Library, a national deposit library, provides a facility to search its catalogue (both reference and lending collections) on the web. The Royal College of Nursing (RCN) library database is available online and includes references to books, journal articles (from 1985), theses and videos. The Royal College of Midwives catalogue is not currently available online.

Access to these catalogues is useful for checking references and you should be able to request books from other libraries through your local library interlibrary loan system (check with your library).

Government and official publications

The UK Directgov website offers a useful gateway to government departments and publications. The UK Department of Health (DoH) website is a good starting point for anyone needing health and social-care policy documents, including statistical reports, white papers, green papers, health circulars, legislation publications, government responses, leaflets and booklets, news, and so on. Many health-related publications can be found at the Stationery Office UK Official Documents website and can be viewed by date, title or department. Acts of Parliament and other government department publications are now published on the internet. Parliamentary publications, including Hansard (the daily debates), public and private bills and select committee publications, can be accessed in full at the UK Parliament website.

Statistics

The most obvious starting point for finding statistics is the Office for National Statistics (ONS) website, which is part of the UK Statistics Authority. The ONS is the government agency responsible for gathering and publishing statistical data. The DoH website contains details of statistical and survey publications. This includes data on public health, health care, social care, the workforce and expenditure. There are links from the DoH website to the NHS Information Centre, the main agency involved in providing facts and figures to health and social care. A good all-round guide to health statistics can be found at *Health statistics: a guide to printed and online resources* (London South Bank University). This contains numerous links to useful documents and websites.

Using other libraries

It may become necessary to extend your search for material to other libraries that house specialist collections or resources your library does not hold. The Royal College of Nursing (telephone: 0207 409 3333 or see the RCN website) has its own library, including specialist historical and nursing research collections. Only RCN members and students attending courses at the RCN Institute are eligible to borrow items. Non-members can use the library for a charge and should contact the staff before visiting. The Royal College of Midwives (telephone: 0207 312 3535) also has a library but this was mothballed for 18 months from 17 February 2008.

The King's Fund Library (telephone: 0207 307 2568 or see the website) welcomes visits from the public as well as enquiries in writing or by telephone or e-mail. It specializes in health management and policy The library is reference only and this means that you will be unable to borrow material. As with most specialist libraries it is advisable to phone in advance to check opening hours and to make an appointment to visit.

The British Library is the national library and receives publications by legal deposit. It is split into a number of different collections. The St Pancras site includes the humanities reference collection together with the science, technology and business collections. These are available to those whose research needs cannot be adequately met by other libraries. Access is restricted and certain criteria have to be met. Contact the Reader Admissions Office (telephone: 0207 412 7676) or see the website for details.

You will need to telephone in advance if you want to access libraries at other universities and colleges. You will only be allowed to use these at the discretion of the library staff if you are not a registered student at that institution.

Public libraries make access to their reference collections freely available, although to borrow items you have to study, work or be resident in the local authority's area. Reference collections are usually located in large central libraries and offer access to special collections such as local studies material. They usually house a wide range of encyclopaedias, dictionaries, directories, yearbooks, journals, reports and government and statistical publications. They also provide internet access and electronic resources. You may have to book in advance to use special facilities such as internet. It is always a good idea to phone in advance if you want to use these facilities.

What if you find little or nothing?

Information retrieval is a frustrating business. There will be times when there appears to be nothing published on your subject – nothing that answers your need. And it is also true that failure to locate any material can never be attributed with certainty to the fact that there is nothing. There will always be a niggling doubt that you didn't seek hard enough, or for long enough, in the right places; that the very item you require exists somewhere. This is when you have fallen prey to the myth 'I've thought of it, therefore it exists'.

Certainly, there will be times when you have to accept the awful truth and readjust your search (or do some research and get it published to fill the gap!). But don't give up straight away: first, be resourceful and adaptable in the following ways:

- Check your search terms: use the thesaurus, library staff or fellow students.
- Make sure you are using the most appropriate source: appropriate database, textbook versus journals, general versus specialist libraries/ information centres.
- Is there comparable information available? For example, in the activity on p. 58, question 1 could use research material from studies on breast cancer or AIDS – the key element is the patient's self-perception and response to his or her condition.
- Talk to colleagues, fellow students, tutors and library staff: they have expertise, contacts and knowledge not available via established channels.

The box below contains a checklist that condenses the main points of this chapter and the steps of a literature search.

Preparation

1. Define your purpose: why do you need this information and what precisely do you need? Write this out.
2. Plan your time: allow for search setbacks, for obtaining items from elsewhere and for reading the material.
3. Familiarize yourself with your library's facilities and services as soon as possible: opening hours, catalogue, CD-ROM and internet access, photocopiers, journals in stock, procedures for requesting items.

Defining your search

1. Identify your keywords from your search statement/essay question.
2. Brainstorm your keywords for alternative headings.
3. Identify appropriate sources.

Ask for help at any point.

Starting the search

1. Check your search terms in the subject headings list/thesaurus for each database or index you use.

2. Record the search terms you used and the sources searched; for example, BNI 1999 under nurse education or CINAHL 1998–2000 under education-nursing and death-education. This saves you repeating parts of your search and can inform library staff if you need further help. Electronic databases generally allow you to print or save your search, giving you an excellent record of what terms were used and how; that is, your search strategy. You might have access and be able to download references directly into bibliographic management software, such as EndNote, Procite or Reference Manager. This enables you to capture references from a wide range of sources, to insert them into documents and produce bibliographies with ease.

3. Record the full citation details of items, articles, etc. that you wish to locate and read. This information is necessary for swift location and for your own final reference list. Noting each citation separately on index cards enables easy filing with space for annotation, i.e. brief notes on its usefulness and content.

4. Locate/order and read your material, noting further search needs and ideas.

5. Adapt your search as necessary – modify search terms, explore related subject areas, use comparable material. This is developing your strategy. Record such developments.

6. Stick to your time plan and your purpose. Literature searching is time-consuming and full of distractions. Your time for searching and reading is limited. Be realistic and have a clear cut-off point (although you can note items of interest for another time).

7. There are twists and turns in the literature search, but you are not alone. You're not expected to struggle on without help. Professional help and expertise is to hand – use it! But help the professionals to help you by being clear about your purpose, your information need.

- Get to know your library and its resources
- Ask for help whenever you need it
- Make full use of any library tuition
- Allow time for library and literature searches
- Identify your information needs
- Define and stick to your purpose
- Your best sources of information will change according to your needs
- Spelling and terminology differ according to origin and source
- Journals contain much more current material than textbooks
- Your library is unlikely to hold everything you will need
- Your library can obtain material from other libraries
- Allow time to order material
- Keep references and records
- Practise these skills

Conclusion

In this chapter we have discussed and tested the process of information finding. At all stages, you have had to make decisions based on your needs, acting critically and reflectively. To do so, you have had to keep your purpose to the fore. The growth of electronic information sources, particularly the rapid development of the internet and the worldwide web, is markedly improving access to information. There is an enormous range of information available to you via libraries and the internet. In Chapter 5 we will see how knowing your purpose also applies to using the information you acquire during your studies.

 CHAPTER RESOURCES

REFERENCES

Craig, J.V. & Smyth, R.L., 2007. The evidence-based practice manual for nurses, 2nd edn. Churchill Livingstone/Elsevier, Edinburgh.

Greenhalgh, T., 2006. How to read a paper: the basics of evidence based medicine, 3rd edn (rev). BMJ Books, London.

NHS Executive, 1999. HSC 99/065 Clinical governance: quality in the new NHS. Department of Health, London. Online. Available: www.dh.gov. uk/en/Publichealth/Patientsafety/Clinicalgovernance

Sackett, D.L., Rosenberg, W.M.C., Gray, I.A.M. & Richardson, W.S., 1996. Evidence-based medicine: what it is and what it isn't. British Medical Journal 312, 71–72.

WEBSITES

ABC news: www.abc.net.au/

ADEPT: www.shef.ac.uk/,scharr/ir/adept

BBC news: www.news.bbc.co.uk

BioMed Central: www.biomedcentral.com

British Library: www.bl.uk

British Medical Journal: www.bmj.com

Canadian Health Network: www.Canadian-health-network.ca

CASP (Critical Appraisal Skills Programme): www.phru.nhs.uk/Pages/PHD/resources.htm

Centre for Evidence-Based Medicine (University of Oxford): www.cebm.net

Centre for Evidence-based Medicine (University of Toronto): www.cebm.utoronto.ca

Centre for Evidence-Based Medicine: Hierarchy of Evidence: www.cebm.net/index.aspx?o=1025

CNN: www.cnn.com

Consortium of University Research Libraries (COPAC): www.copac.ac.uk/

Daily Telegraph (newspaper): www.telegraph.co.uk

Department of Health: www.dh.gov.uk

Directgov: www.direct.gov.uk

Discern: www.discern.org.uk

Finding information on the internet: a tutorial (University College Berkeley Library): www.lib.berkeley.edu/TeachingLib/Guides/Internet/FindInfo.html

Free Medical Journals: www.freemedicaljournals.com

Google Scholar: scholar.google.co.uk/

Google: www.google.com

Guardian (newspaper): www.guardian.co.uk

Health on the Net Foundation: www.hon.ch

Health statistics: a guide to printed and online resources (London South Bank University): www.lisa.lsbu.ac.uk/004_health/healthstats/hs.htm

Healthfinder: www.healthfinder.gov

HealthInsite: www.healthinsite.gov.au

HERO: www.hero.ac.uk/niss/niss_library4008.cfm

How to read a paper (by Trisha Greenhalgh and Rod Taylor): www.bmj.com/channels/education.dtl (search for 'how to read a paper')

Independent (newspaper): www.independent.co.uk

Ingenta: www.ingentaconnect.com

Intute: www.intute.ac.uk

Judge: Websites for health: www.judgehealth.org.uk

King's Fund: www.kingsfund.org.uk

National Research Register Archive (see UKCRNP for recent data): www.nrr.nhs.uk

NHS Choices: www.nhs.uk

NHS Direct: www.nhsdirect.nhs.uk

NHS Evidence: www.evidence.nhs.uk/

NLM Gateway: www.gateway.nlm.nih.gov/gw/Cmd

NLM Medical Subject Headings: www.nlm.nih.gov/mesh/

Nursing Standard: www.nursing-standard.co.uk

Nursing Times: www.nursingtimes.net

Office for National Statistics: www.statistics.gov.uk

Paperboy: www.thepaperboy.com

Pinakes: www.hw.ac.uk/libWWW/irn/pinakes/pinakes.html

Public Library of Science: www.plos.org

PubMed Clinical Queries: www.ncbi.nlm.nih.gov/entrez/query/static/clinical.shtml

PubMed: www.ncbi.nlm.nih.gov/pubmed/

Reuters: uk.reuters.com/news/science

Royal College of Midwives: www.rcm.org.uk

Royal College of Nursing: www.rcn.org.uk

The Stationery Office (UK official documents): www.official-documents.co.uk

Times (newspaper): www.timesonline.co.uk

TNSMI Health News: www.presswatch.com/health/index.php

TRIP: www.tripdatabase.com

UK Clinical Research Network Portfolio: www.public.ukcrn.org.uk/search/
UK Parliament: www.parliament.uk

GLOSSARY

Abstract: summary of the contents of a journal article, research paper, conference report or book.

Audiovisual: non-print items that need to be viewed or heard, such as videos or audiotapes. Sometimes known as media.

Bibliographic: relating to the details of the book or article. Bibliographical information, e.g. title, author, publication date, volume number, page numbers, etc. is necessary for the location of the item.

Boolean operators: logical operators (AND, OR, NOT) used to link keywords or search terms when searching a database.

CD-ROM: compact-disk read only memory. A computer-read disk with the capacity to store an enormous amount of digital data. DVDs have an even greater capacity to store data.

Citation: the giving of bibliographical information.

Current awareness: bulletins that provide information on recently published journal articles, books, reports, etc.

Database: a collection of, for example, bibliographic electronic records accessible via CD-ROM, online or internet.

DVD: digital versatile disk.

Index (journals): list of articles by subject.

Internet: a network linking millions of computers across the world and making vast amounts of information available from these computers.

Journals: regular publications (e.g. monthly, weekly, bi-monthly) that act as a forum for newly published research, news, articles and the professional exchange of information.

Literature search: search of mainly journal and research literature for material relating to a topic.

Online: live database, journal, etc. which is constantly being updated.

OPAC (online public access catalogue): system that makes library catalogues accessible via a computer and replaces card catalogues.

Periodical: *see* Journals.

Reference: unit of bibliographical information.

Search engine: a computer program that enables the user to search the worldwide web using keywords. Search engines index documents on the web and compile vast databases of web content, which are searchable.

Serial: *see* Journals.

Thesaurus: list of subject headings or indexing terms used by an index or database. It will often show the hierarchical relationship between terms, e.g. broader, narrower and related terms.

Website: a location on the worldwide web, usually containing a home page and other pages, documents or files. It is compiled or managed by an individual organization or company.

Worldwide web: Consists of documents or pages written in a special language known as hypertext mark-up language (html). This enables links to be made to other documents and it supports graphics, audio and video files.

4

Using information technology
Denis Anthony

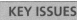

KEY ISSUES

- Applications: spreadsheets, statistics packages, qualitative analysis packages, bibliographic packages
- Data Protection Act
- Searching the internet
- Reference management
- Systematic reviews and clinical guidelines
- Online courses
- Electronic portfolios

Introduction

This chapter gives an overview of the common information technology (IT) applications that you may find useful as a research-aware clinical nurse keen to keep your clinical practice evidence based. IT is also useful for managers, educators and researchers; all areas relevant to nursing.

Information technology can help you in your studies and enable you to use your study time more effectively. Although more and more nursing students at pre- and post-registration level have access to and understanding of computers and information technology, this chapter is aimed at the student who has little experience with computers. Those of you with some experience of using computers to help your studies will probably be able to skim quickly through some parts of this chapter.

The European Computer Driving Licence Foundation (www.ecdl. com) has ten products, one of which is the European Computer Driving Licence (ECDL). This 'is the global standard in end-user computer skills, offering candidates an internationally recognized certification that is supported by governments, computer societies, international organizations and commercial corporations globally'. The syllabus covers basic IT, word processing, spreadsheets, databases, presentation software and web browsing and communication. This is a large part of the content of this chapter. If you are a complete beginner then the ECDL Foundation offers 'EqualSkills', which covers even the most basic skills such as turning a computer on and using the mouse, and so on, up to using word processors and e-mail.

Hardware

Hardware is the physical machinery, e.g. the computer itself and anything attached to it. I am not going to discuss hardware in detail. You will need a computer that has:

- A fast-enough *processor:* the main computing element of the computer, the engine of the computer.
- Enough *memory:* space on the computer for storing data that can be accessed quickly but is lost when the computer is switched off.
- Enough *disk space:* where data are stored for later use; for example, data that were in memory and now need to be kept.
- *Peripherals*: items attached to the computer such as printers, scanners, CD-ROMs, etc.
- *Internet access:* to access the worldwide web and e-mail, typically using a modem and a dial-up link or broadband. Broadband is becoming standard due to it being much faster than dial-up, and increasingly wireless connections are being used.

Your supplier will be able to advise on an appropriate set-up for your needs.

I am assuming that you can use a keyboard and mouse, can copy to a disk drive, print to a printer and access the internet to use e-mail and the worldwide web (a massive resource, where huge amounts of information are available from the internet). This is all you really need to be able to do to get started.

Operating systems

All computers need an operating system, which performs the basic functions of the computer and allows programs to be run on it. In practice, you may not care about the operating system and many users do not even know which one they are using. The look and feel of the computer will to some extent be affected by the operating system chosen, so a Macintosh computer looks and behaves slightly differently from a Windows PC. However, you will probably be more interested in the applications (programs) that run under these operating systems.

You will probably be using a PC or a Macintosh computer. If you are using the latter, you will be using one of the Macintosh operating systems. If you have a PC, you may be using one of the Windows operating systems. Alternatively, you may choose to use Linux, a version of the operating system UNIX that runs on PCs.

Which operating system you employ will be in part personal preference and in part dependent on the sort of work you do. Many graphic designers prefer the Macintosh, as it has particularly good facilities for this sort of work. Most business and general-purpose work is conducted on a PC under Windows. Many academics, especially in computing, engineering and pure science, like Linux. As Linux has a huge amount of *open source* software, it is increasing in popularity even among non-technical users (open source software is freely available and may be copied and even adapted; it is not necessarily free, although much is available at no cost).

Software

'Software' is the term for all the programs (also called applications) that run under a given operating system on the computer. I am assuming you can use a:

- word processor, to create and edit text documents
- web browser, to access the worldwide web
- e-mail application to read and send electronic mail.

Antivirus software

Computer viruses are malicious programs. They are typically spread by e-mail (opening attachments in e-mail is a particular hazard, and you should not open an attachment unless you are happy that it is free from viruses) or by using an infected disk (i.e. a disk that has a virus on it). Most of the time they are simply irritating, accessing your e-mail directory and e-mailing everyone in it with some message (although even this can be very damaging to your reputation, or embarrassing – some viruses take bits of text from your computer and send them out by e-mail) and possibly infecting their computers. Some of them are physically damaging, and you could have all your data deleted by a virus.

It is very important that you have antivirus software installed on your computer. Examples include Symantec (www.symantec.com), McAfee (www.mcafee.com) and F-Secure (www.Europe.F-Secure.com). Some antivirus software is free to download and install; for example, in addition to commercial programs, Avast has the free home edition (www.avast.com). These will protect your computer against known viruses and, if you keep them updated, emerging viruses are unlikely to infect your computer either.

Databases

Creating and using databases can be necessary to you as a student if the work you are doing for your course involves listing and sorting information. If you are undertaking a research project, for example, you might wish, as part of your study, to ask questions and record the answers in a way that allows you to retrieve these answers at a later date. Additionally, you may wish to keep a list of names and addresses of useful contacts. You could undertake both of these tasks manually with pen and paper. However, if you are handling large amounts of information, the process of checking your information and retrieving it at a later date is tedious and time consuming if you do it by hand. For example, if your list of contacts contains over 100 names, think of the time it will take you to write each name (last name and first name), and additional data for each, such as address, phone number, job title, place of work, area of expertise – and to do this in alphabetical order! Obviously, you could write all this information, person by person, on individual cards and place them in a box file in alphabetical order. However, in 4 months time you might remember that one of the 100 people on your list has a particular area of expertise that you need. If you do all of this manually, you will have to read through the entire card file, name by name, to find the person who has the expertise you are seeking. Equally, you may need to categorize each of your 100 people by job title or by place of work. If you do it manually, you will need to write a whole new list or set of cards for these 100 people under the heading you want.

Database software provides a very simple solution to the above situation. A database is like an electronic filing system where any one piece of information stored acts as a basis for sorting and retrieving any information that has been stored in the database (or electronic filing system).

For example, Let us go back to the list of 100 contact names that you want to keep in your filing system. For each of the 100 people you can create a database that records the following (Figure 4.1):

- last name
- first name
- address

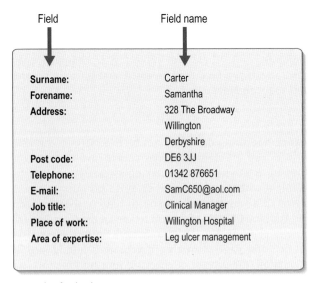

FIGURE 4.1 Example of a database entry.

- post code
- telephone number
- e-mail address
- job title
- place of work
- area of expertise.

Each of these bullet points is called a 'field name'. Next to each field name is a space (which is called the field) into which the appropriate information is entered. All the fields together make up a record, which is unique to each of the 100 people. A group of records is a file and one or more files collectively make up the database.

To summarize, think of a database as a filing cabinet. Each drawer in the filing cabinet is the same as a file. Each document in each of the suspended 'slots' in each drawer is the same as a record and each 'name tab' clipped on to the top of the suspended 'slots' in the filing cabinet drawer is the same as a field name.

Once you have created the database with all your 100 names, addresses and so forth, you can then sort and retrieve the information in any form you want using any one of the fields:

- You can call up a list of all people whose job title is 'clinical manager'.
- You can call up a list of all people with expertise in leg ulcer management.
- You can call up a list of all people who work in Willington Hospital.

Calling up a list based on a particular field is known as undertaking a search or query.

Setting up a database needs some careful thought. For example, if you think that in the future you might want to retrieve a list of all the people in your database who live in a particular county, then you need to make sure that you create a separate field called 'county'. If in the future you will want to contact everyone on your list over the age of 40, then you need to create a separate field called 'age'.

Most database software packages can print out a report for you so that you have a hard copy of the results of your search or query. Most can also perform basic statistical calculations, which is useful if you are undertaking research. However, if you are dealing with a large amount of data, especially figures, you are probably better off using a purpose-designed statistical software package, or a spreadsheet.

Spreadsheets

A spreadsheet is a particular piece of computer software that enables you to both record and process numerical information and to undertake arithmetical and statistical operations on these numerical data. The basic appearance of a spreadsheet is shown in Figure 4.2.

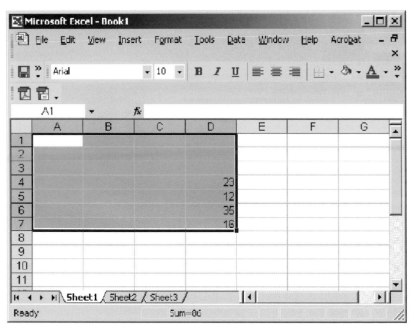

FIGURE 4.2 A basic spreadsheet (reprinted with permission from Microsoft Corporation).

Each column of the spreadsheet is identified by a letter and each row by a number. The box where a column and a row meet is called a cell. Each cell has its own 'address', which is derived from the letter column and row number (e.g. A6 or B4).

If you look at Figure 4.2, what is the address of the cell that has the number 16 in it?
If you answered D7, then you are right.

Cells may contain text (titles, headings), values (numbers) or formulae (for mathematical or statistical calculations). Spreadsheets are particularly useful for formulae and it is in this area that they are far more useful than electronic calculators.

As an example, look at the four numbers in column D of Figure 4.2. You could easily add these up manually and record the sum of the four numbers in cell D8. You do not necessarily even need a calculator to do this as there are so few numbers that it is an easy task to complete manually. However, look at Figure 4.3.

Here you will see a spreadsheet with a list of numbers. You could add the 16 numbers up manually but it would take a while to do it. You could use an electronic calculator for greater speed. Or you could use the spreadsheet to add up all the numbers and record the sum of all 16 figures in cell D18.

	A	B	C	D	E	F	G	H
1				54.89				
2				95.37				
3				2.6				
4				23.67				
5				66.12				
6				34.67				
7				21.09				
8				39.88				
9				40.05				
10				79.99				
11				23.11				
12				13.9				
13				54.33				
14				98.37				
15				51.22				
16				78.39				
17								
18				777.65				
19								

FIGURE 4.3 Spreadsheet with calculation (reprinted with permission from Microsoft Corporation).

You may ask 'Why should I use a spreadsheet to do this addition when a calculator is almost as quick?' The answer is because a spreadsheet is particularly useful when any numbers in the cells change for any reason. Unlike a calculator, where you must type in the figures individually to get the sum total (54.89 + 95.37 + 2.60 + 23.67, and so forth), with a spreadsheet you instruct the computer to add the cells together (D1 + D2 + D3 +D4, and so forth). In this way, if you later change any figures in the columns, the spreadsheet notices this and recalculates the total automatically.

Is there any way that a spreadsheet might be of use to you at work or in your studies?

Spreadsheets are typically used for things like keeping accounts, planning budgets and dealing with wages. They can also be used for planning off-duty rota sheets and are often used effectively by managers to make projections. For example, if there is a 4% rise in nursing salaries, a spreadsheet can quickly show the manager how this will affect the total salary bill.

At home, you can use a spreadsheet to keep track of your bank accounts, or to record the income and expenditure of a local club or organization.

Graphics and drawing

You will probably have noticed the clever use of title sequences before a television programme begins, or the cartoons and moving logos that are so eye-catching in television advertisements. These are made possible through sophisticated graphics and software drawing packages. Smaller and less expensive graphics and drawing packages are available for individuals to use on their own desktop or laptop computers. These can be used to add diagrams or pictures to your project work, reports and essays, or to produce greeting cards, posters and brochures for home or work.

The word 'graphics' refers to everything from a simple black and white drawing using shapes (Figure 4.4) to complex colour images that can move. Most of the illustrations in this book have been produced using some sort of graphics software package.

Graphics packages come in different forms and can be used in different ways. The simple drawing in Figure 4.4 can be produced by the drawing tools that come as part of standard word processing packages. If you have time, patience and skill, you can use graphics packages to produce your own pictures and diagrams from scratch, and these may be quite detailed, complex and sophisticated.

A graphics package called 'clip art' often comes as a standard part of the software provided when you buy a computer. You can also buy various clip art graphics packages. These contain hundreds of images and pictures – some in cartoon form, others not – which you can retrieve and use as they are or customize to suit your needs. They are usually free of copyright so you can use them without seeking anyone's permission.

An alternative is to use an electronic scanner, which can be attached to your computer and allows you to reproduce a picture electronically

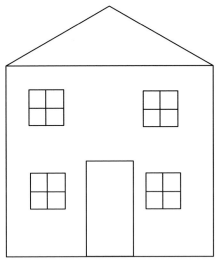

FIGURE 4.4 Picture of a house using tools in a word processing package.

and use it in your own report, essay or document. Care must be taken, however, not to infringe copyright law.

A useful resource is the ability to download photographs and graphics images from the internet so that you can then include them in presentations, posters and assignments. However, there are copyright implications in doing this. Sometimes a website will say that anyone is free to use any of the material (including pictures and graphics) without seeking any further copyright clearance. Where there is no mention of this on a particular website, you are obliged under copyright law to seek clearance from the webmaster of that website to download the material on to your own computer for your use. The webmaster is the person who controls, builds and updates the website.

Digital cameras and digital video cameras are now relatively cheap and can be connected to a computer, allowing pictures and video to be loaded onto the computer. They usually come with software to edit the images or film clips.

In summary, graphics and drawing packages, as well as the internet, can be used to enhance your presentation, whether this is for an assignment, poster, seminar or group presentation as part of your studies or your work.

The Data Protection Act

Anyone who uses a computer to store, retrieve and use personal information about other people needs to be aware of the Data Protection Act (1998). This Act of Parliament replaced the earlier Data Protection Act (1984) and was passed to create tighter standards of practice for people and institutions that hold, in an electronic format, potentially sensitive data about people. The Data Protection Act lays down the responsibilities of those who hold the data (users) and the rights of the people on whom data are electronically held (subjects). All those who store, use and retrieve potentially sensitive data about other individuals should have a copy of the Data Protection Act. The information section at the end of this chapter tells you how to get a copy of the Data Protection Act (1998).

The Act indicates that all data users must register with the Data Protection Register and must comply with the principles of data protection as laid down in the Act. A summary of these principles is given in the box below.

SUMMARY OF THE PRINCIPLES OF THE DATA PROTECTION ACT

Personal data should be:

- Collected and processed fairly and lawfully
- Held and used only for specified and lawful purposes
- Adequate, relevant and accurate
- Held for no longer than is necessary for the registered purpose
- Protected by proper security

Failure to comply with the provisions of the Act can lead to prosecution. Information about the Act can be found on the Information Commissioner's Office (www.ico.gov.uk).

Searching the internet

How can you access information on the internet for your studies?

The first thing you need to do is to gain access to the internet. If you are studying at a university, this will be possible through the computers in your university. Hospitals and health practices generally have computers with internet access.

If you have your own computer at home, you will be able to get internet access from a huge number of companies (including Orange, Sky, Microsoft, Virgin, AOL, BT and even WH Smith and Tesco). Most of us are constantly reminded of this, with free offers of internet access coming through the post, on television and on advertising hoardings. Telephone/broadband deals are available that are cheap enough to make considering dial-up an obsolete choice. Access via cable may be available to you, depending on where you live, and you might also be able to access the internet via a wireless connection. If you are an occasional user of the internet, dial-up on an ordinary phone line with a modem is acceptable. If you use the internet a lot (daily for more than half an hour) or if you need to download large files a lot, broadband is the only viable alternative. Broadband costs about £20 per month, but there are typically no extra charges however long you are on the internet, and you don't need to have a separate telephone line for the internet.

If you are a personal subscriber to an internet provider, the instructions for how to access the internet will be given to you when you subscribe to that internet provider. In a university, internet access is through the university's internet server, and all networked computers should have access to the internet at all times.

All websites on the computer have a dedicated 'address' called a URL (uniform resource locator). If you know the URL of a particular site, all you need to do to access the site is to access your internet server's website and then, where you see the box labelled 'Address' at the top of your internet server's home page, type in the URL and press the 'return' key on your keyboard. Depending on the speed of your server's link, you will quickly see the home page of your selected website come up on the screen. You then follow the instructions on the home page to access other pages on that website. This usually is through 'clicking' (using the left-hand button on your mouse) on to a word or picture with your mouse or through typing in some words in a particular box and then pressing the 'return' key.

If you have access to a computer with internet access, try the following:

1. Access the home page of the internet server: this may happen automatically when you turn the computer on. Alternatively, there may be an icon (symbol) on your screen that you can 'click' on to get into the internet.

2. In the 'Address' box, type in the following URL: www.ask.co.uk

3. This takes you to a website called 'Ask'. The website asks you to type in a question.

4. In the 'Question' box, either type your own question to ask or else type in 'Where can I find a map of London?'

5. When you have typed your question, click on the word 'Search' next to the question box.

6. What have you found?

You have just used one of the many search engines for the internet. Others include Cuil (www.cuil.com), Google (www.google.co.uk) and Yahoo (www.yahoo.co.uk).

What does a search engine allow you to do?

Search engines allow you to find things on the internet. You type in key words related to the information you would like to find and a search engine will give you a list of the websites where you can find the information you are seeking. The activity you did (above) is an example of one search engine called 'Ask'.

There are many search engines available; each is located at a different website. Some search engines are US based while others are UK based. Some of the most common search engines are listed in Table 4.1.

Although these websites look quite different from each other, they all work in almost the same way. Towards the top of each of these search engine web pages will be a box that says 'Search'. You will be able to type a key word or phrase in that box. If you type a phrase (rather than an individual word) in the search box, it is helpful to type it in double quotation marks (" ") to avoid the search engine finding information about

TABLE 4.1   Examples of search engines

NAME OF SEARCH ENGINE	WEB ADDRESS (URL)
Cuil	www.cuil.com
Google	www.google.co.uk
Yahoo	www.yahoo.com
Lycos	www.lycos.co.uk
Excite	www.excite.com
MSN	www.msn.co.uk
Alta Vista	jump.altavista.com
Ask	www.ask.co.uk

the separate words rather than the phrase (i.e. if you want to search for information on health education, type it as "health education").

Next to the search box where you have typed in your key words is a button that says 'Go' or 'Search' or 'Go get it'. Click on this button using the left-hand button on your mouse. This tells the search engine to find the information you are seeking.

What will come up on your screen is a list of websites related to the key words you typed in the search box. Using the mouse, you can click on any of these websites and immediately go to that site to get the information you need. Not all websites will automatically have what you are looking for but this will depend on the nature of the search and how specific you were when typing in your keywords. General, broad key words will give you hundreds or thousands of websites that will prove to be of little or no use to you. Very specific search instructions will probably provide you with information you really can use.

Alternatively, instead of using a search engine you could access a directory, where information is stored in a structured format on a given subject. For nursing, midwifery and allied health for example, there is Intute (formerly known as NMAP). Intute 'is a free online service providing you with a database of hand selected web resources for education and research,' which offers useful links. An example of links found for pressure ulcer is shown in Figure 4.5, compared with a search conducted on Cuil.

How do I know if the information I find on a website is accurate and valid?

The internet is a free place and, provided you know how to set up your own web page, you can publish anything on the internet with little or no academic scrutiny or critical review. There is an extremely wide variety of information available on the internet, of varying degrees of accuracy, reliability and value. No one has to approve the content before it goes on the internet. Therefore, it is up to individual users to critically evaluate internet sources of information and research. Harris (2007) has posted a guide for evaluating the quality of internet sources on to the internet and it is essential for all students to become familiar with this skill. Harris identifies several things that need to be looked at to evaluate sources from the internet:

- *Screening information:* matching a site with what you are looking for. Looking for papers that are factual and well argued with supported claims, considering whether you have enough information about the source of the website to feel that the material might be reliable and accurate.
- *Tests of information quality:* the CARS checklist for information quality: credibility, accuracy, reasonableness and support. These are explained comprehensively on www.mhhe.com/socscience/english/ allwrite3/seyler/ssite/seyler/se03/cars.mhtmland www.lib.uct.ac.za/ Training/Infolit/infolit/cars.htm.

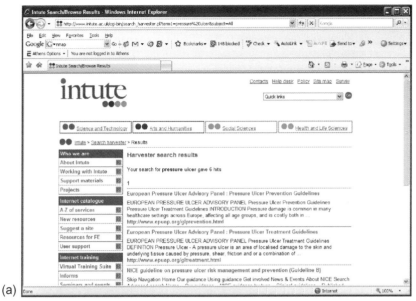

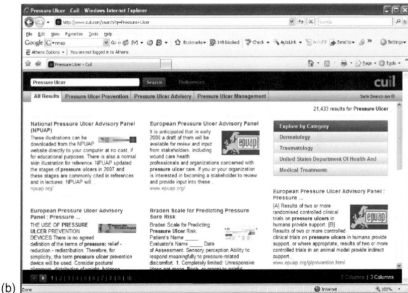

FIGURE 4.5 Links found for pressure ulcer on (a) Intute and (b) Cuil. ((a) Reprinted with permission from The Intute Consortium; (b) reprinted with permission from www.Cuil.com.)

One problem that has worsened with the internet is plagiarism. It is possible to download material from the internet and pass it off as your own. This is considered to be an academic offence in all universities, and proven plagiarism will normally lead to disciplinary action. If you always reference any material that is not your own, and make it clear when you are quoting from another work, you should have no problems.

Clinical problem

For the remainder of this chapter I will consider a clinical problem, and see how IT can help to solve it. Applications shown in these sections are important if you want to conduct research and may be useful if you have to write a dissertation for your study.

The problem to be investigated is the importance of different risk factors for the development of pressure ulcers in immobilized patients. The Waterlow score (Waterlow, 1985) is widely used in the UK and consists of eleven subscores, including gender, age, mobility, continence, recent surgery and other special risks, and other factors thought to be relevant in pressure ulcer incidence. Only certain components of the Waterlow score are relevant in any specific clinical area, different components being relevant in different areas. It has also been shown, beyond reasonable doubt, that serum albumin (a measure of nutrition) is relevant over and above the Waterlow score in predicting those patents who are at risk of pressure ulcers (Anthony et al., 2008).

But what does this mean in practice; that is, how does this impact on the care of a patient? In principle, if we know who is at most risk, we should be able to allocate resources to those patients to reduce that risk (e.g. pressure-relieving devices) but there is little evidence that this in fact is the case.

If you were to deal with the issue, you would want to assess the impact of reduction of pressure ulcers, and it would be helpful to first assess what happens to a patient who has one, compared with one who does not.

Consider what different outcomes two patients may have. One has a pressure ulcer, one does not.

Many different outcomes may be seen in the two patients. The patient with a pressure ulcer might develop infection at the wound site, suffer pain or feel depressed about the ulcer or embarrassed by the smell of the wound. One major impact may be that it is difficult to discharge the patient, and he or she might stay in hospital longer.

Using the internet to conduct a literature review

Let us explore the problem of increased length of stay (LOS) in hospital, as this is important to the patient, who probably wants to go home, and to the hospital, which wants the bed to treat more patients. First, we need to find out what is known about pressure ulcers and LOS. We need to conduct a review of the literature. Increasingly, we are asked to conduct reviews systematically. A systematic review is one in which we are precise about how we conduct the review and state how we have performed it so that another person using the information we record would come up with an identical set of papers and a similar view of the literature.

How would you plan such a review? Where would you search for this information, from what date would you want to explore the literature, in which languages, in which type of journal, what type of study, using what types of database? You might look at www.library.nhs.uk or www.york.ac.uk/inst/crd for ideas.

As the subject is clinical, you would probably look in medical, nursing and allied health bibliographic databases, such as MEDLINE and CINAHL. As pressure-ulcer research is not as time sensitive as (say) policy issues or technological innovations, you would probably search from the start of the databases, which is from the 1960s for MEDLINE and the 1980s for CINAHL. You would be most interested in empirical studies with data on LOS, using an appropriate methodology. You might also explore the Cochrane Library (accessible via www.library.nhs.uk) for systematic reviews. You might look through every issue of relevant specialist journals such as the *Journal of Wound Care*. You would probably restrict yourself to one or a few languages (although most articles indexed in MEDLINE and CINAHL are in English).

You could use a CD-ROM in the library but it is probably easier to use the internet to access the bibliographic databases. For example, you could go to www.library.dmu.ac.uk and click on 'databases' and then select the databases you wish to access – ones to do with health, possibly MEDLINE or CINAHL. I recently searched MEDLINE for the medical subheadings (MeSH) key words 'length of stay' AND 'pressure ulcer' and obtained 91 articles.

In addition to the bibliographic database search, you should consider using the web as a resource. Employing a search engine (see above) you may find further information that is not published (possibly in researchers' own web home pages), or not found in my previous search.

What problems might there be with information found on the web? What quality assurance criteria might you employ to check the validity of these pages?

In many, although not all, cases, material on the internet has not been subject to peer review scrutiny, and there may be bias. The author's authority might be questionable; the information may be purely marketing material. However, if you employ a good checklist you should still be able to use web-based material. There are many such checklists available in textbooks or on the web, or you could use the CARS checklist discussed earlier in this chapter. Essentially, you want to consider the authority of the authors (are they competent, qualified, attached to a respected institution, etc.?), the timeliness, relevance and level of the material (is it up to date and to the point: do you understand it, or alternatively, is it too basic?).

In many cases, the papers are available in full text, typically in portable document format (PDF), which you will probably not be able to view on your word processor. You need a separate, but free, package called Adobe Acrobat Reader, which you can download from www.acrobat.com. There is a more complete version of Adobe Acrobat, with added features, for which payment is required, but you probably only need the simple free program. PDF files show you the paper exactly as in the printed page of the journal, which is why they are used often in preference to (say) web files (HTML), which differ depending on your screen size, resolution and how your computer is set up. PDF files have a major advantage in that, if you refer to a page or set of pages, any reader will be able to access the correct pages.

Some articles I located were worth getting in full. These are the articles that appear to be relevant, based on the titles, keywords and, where available, the abstract. I could in many cases get these from my library, which is about 50 yards from my office in the university. This is not going to be convenient to most clinicians, and is only of use to me if the article is in the library. An alternative is to use the internet to download the text, which may be free, if my institution subscribes to the text, or I may need to pay for it. Rather than access the site of the journal, it is better to use the Athens system. The advantage is that, instead of having to register and use a different password for each journal, Athens give you one user code and password, and all journals signing up to Athens (a very big proportion of the ones I care about) are available in full text. I access electronic journals through my university library pages at www.library.dmu.ac.uk, which offers me a list of electronic journals. If my library subscribes to the journal I will be linked through to it, normally using the Athens system.

I can now go through the references, which include the abstracts. What I discover is that there is a lot of material suggesting that pressure ulcers and LOS are related and that patients with pressure ulcers have greater LOS.

Can you describe the typical patient with pressure ulcers? How might he or she differ from a patient without pressure ulcers? Does this have any bearing on LOS?

The typical patient is more likely to be older, incontinent, diabetic, confused, immobile, a smoker, have had recent surgery or trauma or have higher scores on any of the Waterlow subscores. As typical patients are more ill, they may stay in hospital longer because of their greater morbidity rather than because they have pressure ulcers.

Reference management

Having done my review, I needed to store my references so that when I later write a paper or report I can refer to them.

How would you store these references?

You could take hard copies of any full papers you photocopied, or downloaded over the internet, and put them in a folder, in a box or on a shelf for later use. You could take the details of each paper and put them in a card index box, or listed on paper, stored in a word processor document, or on a database such as Access. However, there is a better way – use a reference management system, which is a database specifically designed to store bibliographic references.

Reference management systems have been available for decades (I used one for my studies in the 1980s). A reference management system allows you to store references in a database and insert them as needed as citations into an essay, paper, thesis or other document. The program typically operates from within your selected word processor, and can automatically produce the correct format of citation and the appropriate reference list. You can change the output reference list and the citations referring to it by directing the program via a simple 'switch' to, say, use the Vancouver or the Harvard system.

This is useful for a variety of reasons. It is simple, it is efficient, you can use the same references in more than one document with no extra typing, the reference list is always complete, and all citations refer to a reference and all references have a citation. This is particularly useful in long documents.

Early reference management systems included Refer and BibTeX, originally designed for the UNIX operating system. An early reference management system operating on DOS (a basic operating system used on PCs before Windows) was Papyrus. However, these systems are not as easy to use as the more recent Windows-based systems. Many reference management systems run on PCs and on Macintosh computers;

examples include Procite, Reference Manager and EndNote. These systems are all functionally similar, and probably all the modern systems do much the same thing. The use of EndNote within Microsoft Word is shown in Figure 4.6. EndNote and some other reference management software, when it is installed, creates a new item in the Tools menu in Microsoft Word (for example) and from within Word I can ask for a reference that is already created in EndNote. Some reference management software (EndNote and Reference Manager, for example) allow you to directly import references from bibliographic databases, so you do not even need to type them in once.

Hospital information support systems

From my literature review, I am not sure whether LOS is caused by pressure ulcers or merely associated with it, as patients with pressure ulcers are in any event much more ill and frail. My colleagues in Burton have a Hospital Information Support System (HISS) on which is recorded patient data. This is a computerized system.

HISSs are databases, although very large and complicated ones. Clinical data are stored on an HISS, and may include medical notes, nursing notes, laboratory data and other patient data. The great advantage of

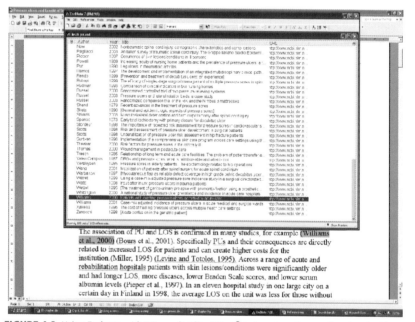

FIGURE 4.6 Using Endnote with Microsoft Office Word® to insert a reference (reprinted with permission from Microsoft Corporation).

HISSs is that authorized users can access data as soon as they are entered on the system. Furthermore, multiple copies can be read, so more than one health professional can see the data at the same time. For example, both the ward manager and the doctor can access the laboratory results on the same patient simultaneously. HISSs or similar systems can be the basis for an electronic patient record (EPR). The aim of an EPR is to allow all health professionals to be able to access relevant data at any time and from any location. The EPR can automatically follow the patient, as it will still be available if the patient is transferred and should be immediately available when the patient is admitted. The doctor cannot take the patient notes off the ward, and there should never be missing notes.

While the HISS is typically used to treat patients, here I want to use it for audit or research.

Statistical packages

I use the Statistical Package for Social Sciences (SPSS) and want to analyse these data. SPSS is like a specialized spreadsheet with additional statistical, graphical and reporting facilities. SPSS is a complex package but there are many texts discussing its use; for example, one I like is by Bryman and Cramer (2005), and one favoured by many of my students is by Pallant (2007).

SPSS is useful for small datasets. For example, if you have data on even a few dozen patients it is easier to use SPSS than to conduct the analysis manually. Burton had data on hundreds of thousands of patients, and using a statistics package is the only practical way to conduct the analysis. Also, once data are entered, I can produce tables, plot graphs and conduct statistical tests very easily. Some differences between manual statistical analysis and the use of a package are shown in Table 4.2.

It would be great to download the data straight into SPSS. This is probably possible, but I know it is possible to download the data from the proprietary software to an Access database, which is an industry standard. SPSS did not at the time support Access, but Access can export data into the Microsoft Excel spreadsheet, and SPSS can read Excel files. The upshot is that, with a bit of fiddling, I can download patients' data into my chosen statistics package. I have of course, prior to this, applied to the relevant ethics committees and obtained permission to use their data, and I have had the data anonymized (see the earlier section on data protection) prior to receiving it, so no patient is identifiable.

In this section I am using a graph called a boxplot. It is not necessary here to fully understand the boxplot, what is important is that it gives useful information on groups of patients. First I perform a boxplot of those patients with pressure ulcers against those with none. A boxplot show you a lot of information on some variable, such as LOS in days

TABLE 4.2 Statistics conducted manually versus using statistical software

	MANUAL (PEN AND PAPER) STATISTICS	STATISTICAL SOFTWARE
Inputting data	You will want to have data in an optimal form for conducting analysis This might mean having several forms of the data on paper	Input data once
Statistical formulae	You will need to know these and be able to manipulate them	You only need to know the test you want to conduct, not how to compute it
Errors in calculation	You may not know you have made an error, and if you do you will need to recalculate	The software should not make errors of this type
New data, or input data corrected	You will need to recalculate	The computer will recalculate when you ask for the analysis again. You can save analyses into a special file and simply call it up
Inappropriate test used	You can use the wrong test but if you know statistics well enough to compute manually, it is likely you will know when to use a given test	You can ask the computer to conduct almost any test on almost any data. The software is in general not able to detect that you are doing the wrong thing
Many different statistical approaches needed on data	You will need to recalculate for each test, or plot each graph or produce each table individually	You can ask the software to conduct many tests, plot graphs and produce tables once the data are input

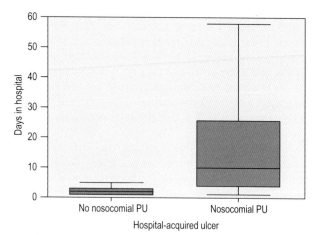

FIGURE 4.7 Boxplot showing the effect of pressure ulcers (PU) on length of stay in hospital.

(Figure 4.7). The range of values – from lowest to highest – is shown as two short horizontal lines. In practice, extreme values (outliers) are removed, so we see the range of the overwhelming majority of the data, missing possibly a few really odd values. Between these high and low points is a vertical line with a box in it. This box contains half the data. Within the box is a straight line, which marks the median value.

So a lot of information is seen in a boxplot. Here we can see that the patients with pressure ulcers have in general a much greater LOS. The range for pressure-ulcer patients shows that the bottom and top values for LOS are higher, as the nosocomial (i.e. occurred in hospital) pressure ulcer has a range of 1–58 days, compared with 1–5 days for those with no ulcer. Also, the box showing where 50% of the patients lie is much higher, and the median is higher. So all three measures show that pressure ulcer patients have greater LOS.

However, we know that there may be confounding factors. For example, the various risk factors of the Waterlow score could mostly be associated with greater LOS. What if I were to try to allow for these by taking only patients in a given risk group, say only those with a high risk? Then if it were the risk factors rather than the pressure ulcers that were causing greater LOS the plots should be similar. In fact, when I selected only those patients with the same Waterlow score, there was still a greater LOS associated with the pressure ulcer group. It looks as if pressure ulcers may cause greater LOS rather than just being associated with it.

Presentation software

Suppose that, having explored pressure ulcers and LOS, you decide that we need to get the hospital Trust to support further work. It would be useful to get the chief executive of the Trust on board. You might need to do a presentation, and here presentation software will help. You might later want to give a lecture at a conference, or a teaching session. All of these could be helped using such presentation software. You could use Microsoft PowerPoint, but other packages, including those running on Linux (an alternative operating system to Windows), are functionally similar.

I have taken some graphical output from SPSS and copied it directly to PowerPoint. There are several ways to do this, but one very simple way is to use the 'Edit' then 'Copy' pull-down menu in SPSS (and most other Windows packages, such as Word and PowerPoint) from within SPSS. This copies the graph into the Windows clipboard (an area copied to and from Windows programs). In PowerPoint I can do 'Edit' then 'Paste' and the graphic will appear in my PowerPoint presentation (Figure 4.8). I could also have done this to include the boxplot in a Word document; for example, an academic paper I intended to send to a journal.

Qualitative analysis packages

Thus far, we have assumed that our data are quantitative and have employed SPSS for the analysis. However, suppose that, instead of taking numerical data about patients, I interviewed them. Let us assume that I want to know what it is like to have a pressure ulcer. I have a set of questions I want to ask, possibly asking patients to rank their pain on a

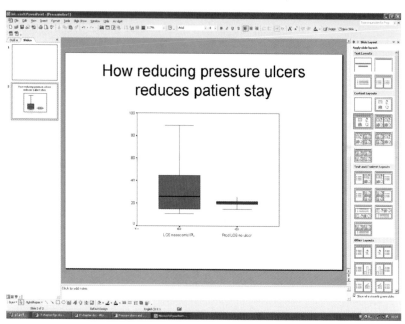

FIGURE 4.8 Using Microsoft PowerPoint® (reprinted with permission from Microsoft Corporation).

1–10 scale, for example. This is clearly quantitative data (although based on subjective assessment). However, I may also ask them to put in their own words how they feel. What I get back will not be analysable with a statistics package like SPSS. There are a whole range of qualitative packages. If you access one of the web pages for qualitative analysis, such as www.qualitativeresearch.uga.edu/QualPage/, you will see a list of them.

Just because the technology exists, it is not necessary to use it. You can perform qualitative analysis manually. However, if you are going to do a lot of qualitative analysis, or will be working in a team, it may be advantageous to learn to use a qualitative analysis package. For a discussion of the advantages and disadvantages of qualitative data analysis software, specifically in a nursing context, see McLafferty and Farley (2006) or St John and Johnson (2004).

You can download a demonstration package of one of the market leaders, NVivo, from www.qsrinternational.com. There are also free packages from the Centers for Disease Control and Prevention in the USA. AnSWR is on www.cdc.gov/hiv/topics/surveillance/resources/software/answr/index.htm and CDC EZ-Text is on www.cdc.gov/hiv/topics/surveillance/resources/software/ez-text/index.htm.

Clinical guidelines

By now, I think I know that pressure ulcers are a big problem, and I would like to institute some intervention that reduces the incidence of pressure ulcers. What I need is a clinical guideline. A clinical guideline is the result of a systematic review that is used to inform clinical practice by creating an evidence-based document.

Consider a nurse on a medical ward, who may need to have the most up-to-date practice for diabetes, heart disease, rheumatoid arthritis and many other diseases. All nurses should base their practice on research but no clinical nurse has the time to personally review the academic press on any given subject, let alone all the areas they may need to address.

Clinical guidelines are produced by teams of experts to deal with specific conditions. Increasingly, these are available on the internet; for example, the National Library for Health (UK) on www.library.nhs.uk, the National Guideline Clearing House (USA) on www.guideline.gov and, my personal favourite, the Scottish Intercollegiate Guidelines Network on www.sign.ac.uk, are all sites that offer clinical guidelines.

Suppose you want to reduce the incidence of pressure ulcers. If a clinical guideline exists that would help to reduce pressure ulcers then I could use this in an audit programme. Indeed, on searching via NHS Evidence (www.evidence.nhs.uk), which has a clinical guideline finder (www.library.nhs.uk/guidelinesFinder/), I can find a clinical guideline for pressure-ulcer prevention (Figure 4.9).

Web page design

Suppose you have now written a paper based on the work on pressure ulcers and LOS. At this point, you want to add the paper to your curriculum vitae (CV). It is common practice for academics to do this, as others may want to know, for example, the type of work a given academic or team is involved in. If I come across a paper that is of interest, I may access the personal web page of the author to see what else he or she has published, or even not yet published. My (short) CV is on the web – you can see it at: www.dmu.ac.uk/research/hls/staff/professor_denis_anthony.jsp (Figure 4.10). How do I do this?

There are several ways. You might use a specialist web authoring program, such as Microsoft FrontPage, although there are many other such packages. Some of these are free and freely available on the web, and many are available on the Linux system. Using such a package, you can create hyperlinked documents fairly easily and, if you have your own webspace via your organization or your internet provider, you can upload the document. Most providers will give you some webspace, many of them at no extra cost, which you can access with a user code and password. This is called publishing the document in FrontPage, and is a simple process, involving putting in the user code and password for

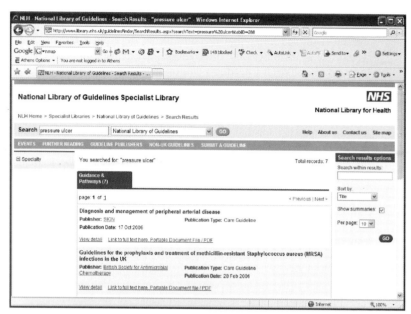

FIGURE 4.9 Locating a clinical guideline (reprinted with permission from NHS Evidence).

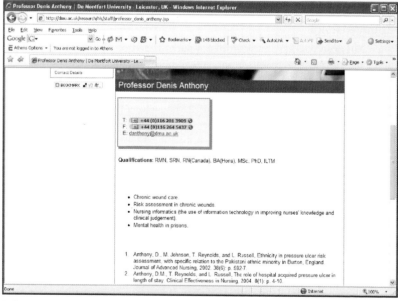

FIGURE 4.10 My web page (reprinted with permission from De Montfort University; www.dmu.ac.uk/hls).

your webspace. Once uploaded, the file can potentially be viewed by anyone with a web browser, i.e. virtually anyone at all. They will need to know what the file is called, or much more probably you will have linked the document into a special page called the home page, which is the one all users access automatically when they access your site.

Web authoring packages can be complicated, not very easy to use, not robust and with many features in which you are not interested. I often want to update a page when I do not have the software with me (I travel and use internet cafes a lot). You may not wish to purchase further software (although increasingly FrontPage comes as a standard on new PCs). You can edit many web pages perfectly adequately in Word or other word processing packages, although some complex pages are difficult because Word is not designed specifically for web page editing and can produce some strange results. Nonetheless, Word does support basic web page editing. Word, and other packages, even create a link for you if you enter what appears to be a web page or e-mail address. Thus when readers browse your page and see the address, they may click on it and automatically (if connected to the internet) access that page. So I could have made my changes to the file in Word. Also, if I had a pre-existing Word file (if, say, my CV was in a Word document) I could save it as a web file, using 'file' and 'save as' options in Word and choose to save as a web file. Thus I have avoided the necessity to learn any HTML (the language used to create web pages).

But how do I transfer the file?

As described above, you could have a specialized web authoring system that will do this for you. Alternatively, most computers have a file transfer protocol (ftp) program. Some of these are Windows based, but at the very least you should be able to use a DOS based one, which should be installed on most or all PCs, called simply ftp. You can also find ftp packages via the web, freely available, and some at no cost (Figure 4.11). In this figure I am using FileZilla, which is freely available at www.filezilla-project.org.

The ftp allows you to copy files from one computer to another. Here, I have used it to copy some course notes to my website. In the first screen you can see that I am connecting to one of several ftp sites, in this case my own personal site on www.danthony.talktalk.net, which requires me to give a user code and a password. Once connected, the second screen is shown, which now allows me to upload files on to the site. The files already on the site are shown in the right-hand side of the screen. I am copying from a part of my hard disk, and this is shown in the pop-up dialogue box in the middle of the screen.

Online courses

An outcome of the web is increased interest in online courses. These use the power of the internet to allow distance learners to access material. However the added benefit of using web-based material is that the look and feel are familiar to anyone who is familiar with web pages.

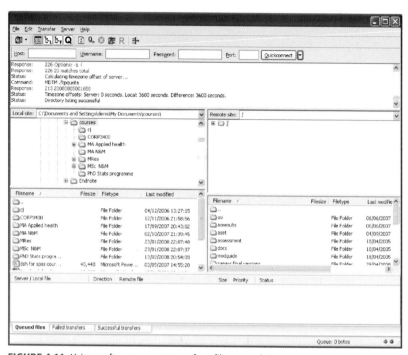

FIGURE 4.11 Using an ftp program to transfer a file to a website.

Several virtual learning environments (VLEs) now invariably use web-based technology. The market leaders include Blackboard (incorporating WebCT), which is a commercial product, and Moodle, which is open source. They are functionally similar. A course I teach on is illustrated in Figure 4.12. This shows a menu and icons that represent various parts of the course on qualitative and quantitative analysis, here from the former part of the module. For example, there is a discussion board and e-mail facilities where students can talk to each other or engage in seminars. Figure 4.13 shows one of the content pages, which happens to be from the quantitative part of the module.

The use of such a course could help provide ward staff with the critical skills necessary to evaluate papers on pressure ulcer treatment and prevention or any other clinical research topic.

Electronic portfolios

Portfolios are commonly used in education. Disciplines as diverse as engineering, education, nursing and medicine employ portfolios. Part of the purpose is to record and assess achievement, but reflective practice is also an important element. Portfolios are normally part of personal development planning (PDP). While many portfolios are paper based

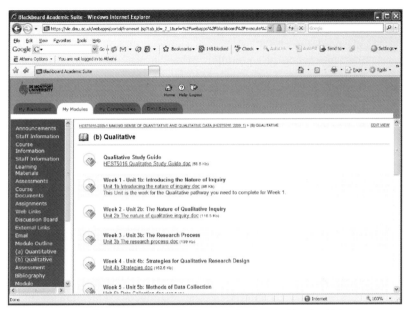

FIGURE 4.12 An online course (reprinted with permission from De Montfort University; www.dmu.ac.uk/hls).

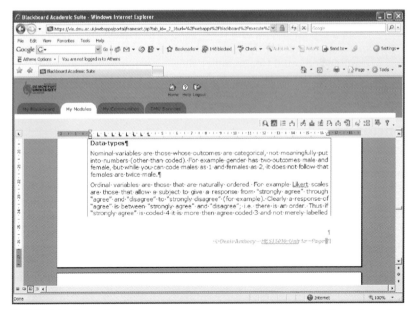

FIGURE 4.13 A page from the research methods online course (reprinted with permission from De Montfort University; www.dmu.ac.uk/hls).

(p-portfolios), electronic portfolios (e-portfolios) are widely used in universities, schools, employers and by individuals. For a good overview of e-portfolios and a comparison with p-portfolios see Butler (2006). For a discussion of e-portfolios in use in placements in nursing and business courses, see the latest ASET report (Duffy et al., 2008).

There is a blurring of the boundaries between p-portfolios and e-portfolios for the following reasons:

- People's p-portfolios are normally written using word processors, are often sent to tutors or mentors via e-mail and can be stored as webpages, so they are rarely based solely on paper.
- People's e-portfolios typically allow paper output because students value the paper product and mentors (often employers) will often only look at paper, so they are rarely purely electronic.

Many universities are implementing, or planning to implement, e-portfolios using VLEs. Others are using specialized e-portfolio products such as PebblePAD or specialized PDP systems that include e-portfolio development such as PDSystem (University of Ulster: www.pds.ulster.ac.uk).

In Figure 4.14, I show the PebblePAD interface. One of many things I can do is create a webfolio, which is a portfolio available on the web. See Figure 4.15 for a page I created that has recent references and a CV linked to it. Clicking on recent references gives the screen seen in Figure 4.16 and clicking on CV gives the screen in Figure 4.17. This webfolio was created for me by going through a simple webfolio builder in PebblePAD and needed no knowledge of web authoring or programming. I can share this with other people, in which case they are automatically e-mailed with a link to the webfolio. This allows collaborative learning and could (for example) allow a mentor to view my portfolio. In PebblePAD any 'asset' (which could be a thought, a CV, a blog and many other items) can be shared with other people.

Conclusion

This chapter has outlined some basic IT facilities – hardware, software, antivirus software, databases, spreadsheets, graphics, the Data Protection Act and searching on the internet. Some applications were then demonstrated with the aid of a clinical problem: pressure ulcers. After a literature review, conducted over the internet, and some papers downloaded over the internet, the relevant references were downloaded into a specialized database, a reference management system. A clinical guideline that would be useful was also downloaded from a specialist site. Online courses were introduced that could improve patient care by educating healthcare staff. Finally, I discussed how e-portfolio packages can be employed to create a webfolio.

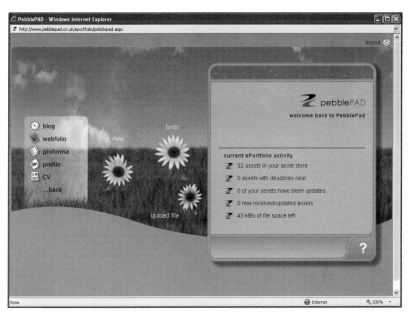

FIGURE 4.14 PebblePAD interface (PebblePAD product screen shots reprinted with permission from Pebble Learning Ltd).

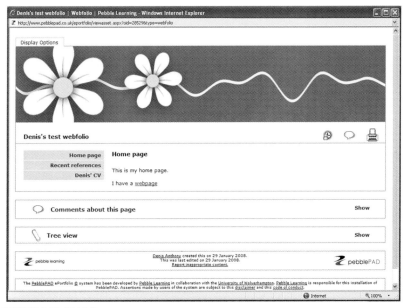

FIGURE 4.15 Webfolio.

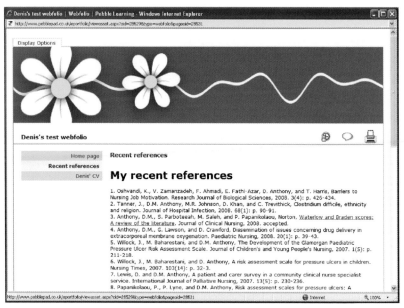

FIGURE 4.16 Current references.

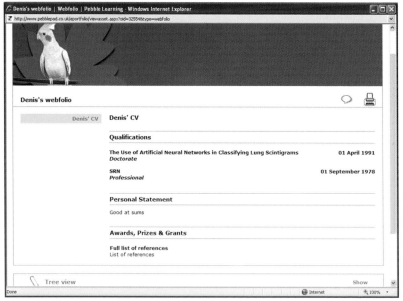

FIGURE 4.17 Current CV.

CHAPTER RESOURCES

REFERENCES

Anthony, D.M., Parboteeah, S., Saleh, M. & Papanikolaou, P., 2008. Norton, Waterlow and Braden scores: a review of the literature. Journal of Clinical Nursing 17 (5), 646–653.

Bryman, A. & Cramer, D., 2005. Quantitative data analysis with SPSS 12 and 13: a guide for social scientists. Routledge, London, UK.

Butler, P., 2006. A review of the literature on portfolios and electronic portfolios. Massey University College of Education, Palmerston, New Zealand.

Duffy, K., Anthony, D.M., Vickers, F., 2008. Are portfolios an asset to learning and placement? A report of a project funded by ASET. Online. Available: http://www.asetonline.org/documents/AreE-PortfoliosAnAssetToLearningandPlacement-ASETandDMUReport-March2008_001.pdf. ASET. Sheffield.

Harris, R., 2007. Evaluating internet research sources. VirtualSalt [version date: 15 June 2007]. Online. Available: www.virtualsalt.com/evalu8it.htm.

McLafferty, E. & Farley, A.H., 2006. Analysing qualitative research data using computer software. Nursing Times 102 (24), 34–36.

Pallant, J., 2007. Title SPSS survival manual: a step-by-step guide to data analysis using SPSS for Windows. Open University Press, Maidenhead, UK.

St John, W. & Johnson, P., 2004. The pros and cons of data analysis software for qualitative research. Journal of Nursing Scholarship 32 (4), 393–397.

Waterlow, J., 1985. Pressure sores: a risk assessment card. Nursing Times 81, 49–55.

5 Getting the most from reading and lectures

Kym Martindale

KEY ISSUES

- A critical approach
- Reading skills
- Reviewing and recording
- The role of the lecture
- Note taking
- Engaging with the material

Introduction

Understanding information requires effort at any level of study, and within any discipline. Your role is not passive; for example, good note-taking skills make all the difference in the ultimate value of any material to you. Nor is your role confined to the time spent in the lecture or reading an article, although both these activities are essential. However, the process of learning is greatly helped by you knowing what you want. As in Chapter 3, the rule is 'define and stick to your purpose'.

A critical approach: subjectivity and interpretation

A critical approach initially recognizes that all information is presented in an edited form. No matter what the medium – text, broadcast or web based – contents and presentation are chosen by authors, editors, producers, website designers and others. Such selectivity is partly in response to the constraints of the medium, and the understanding that any material must be 'written' for its recipient.

Two obvious examples of frame of reference influencing information are politics and newspapers. You are aware of the values and beliefs through which that speaker or journalist operates so you listen/read in a questioning light. But politicians and newspapers hold stated positions (officially or not). Most authors and contributors of internet material are first and foremost professionals in their field. They operate, like you, through a complex system of values, beliefs, ethical concerns and cultural influences, which are not easy to detect or define. Combined with the air of authority that the media (especially print) seem to bestow, they can lull you into a false sense of acceptance.

How do you know who to believe?

Approaching material critically understands that to say, 'A is right, B is wrong' is often naïve. A critical approach asks, 'What made A reach that conclusion when B decided this?' B may have differently researched, differently experienced and differently interpreted the subject from A.

You must weigh these factors, considering how they might affect the information given. You must question the author/editor/producer and bring their possible frame of reference to the fore – if you can. In Chapters 6 and 8, deciding which material might be of use involves examining the author's credentials. This is similar, but in greater depth.

Your questions won't all have answers

This is important. You might not be able to find out everything you'd like to know about a piece of research or an editor's influences. You won't even know if you have uncovered everything. In some cases you will have to argue that there is no hard 'yes' or 'no' answer. But the questioning is the critical and important act and shows that you can think beyond texts and lectures.

Nor will you always know who to believe. You must appraise the evidence, both stated and implicit, and either decide for yourself or present a well-researched and clear argument as to why you cannot decide.

- Being a critical and active learner involves questioning:
  - Who is giving you your information?
  - What is their purpose and agenda?
  - What are their sources and methods of research?

- Our individual frame of reference influences our work. Objectivity is only an attempt to be disinterested; it is never possible to be utterly neutral. Remember, you too work within a frame of reference.

- You won't always be able to provide answers to questions you raise, but raising them demonstrates that you have thought around the subject.

Question … Concentrate … Understand

We have spent several pages addressing this issue, but it is important preparation. A questioning reader/listener is thinking and concentrating on the material. It follows that such a student stands a better chance of understanding and, in the long run, remembering.

Reading: being practical, realistic and prepared

This section looks at how reading skills vary depending on the material and your need, at how to be selective and at how to ensure you focus on your information need while reading.

Different skills for different material

You already have sophisticated reading skills and apply them every day to the various types of material you encounter. Table 5.1 lists some examples, their possible purpose and the level of reading skill you would require for each.

Consider Table 5.1 for 5–10 minutes. Note in your reflective diary:
- What types of reading you have done this week?
- How you went about this, i.e. how did your approach differ in each case?

From Table 5.1 and the notes, you can see how, perhaps unconsciously, you employ a range of reading skills. However, you might not be using them as well as you could. For instance, how selective are you in your reading? Do you try and read as much as possible or give close attention to carefully chosen material? Do you understand the content? If not, what do you do about it? Reflect on this for 5 minutes.

The active reader

Look again at Table 5.1. Most of the tasks require active reading involvement. However, the two whose purpose is understanding – that is, the article and the textbook – require several readings, notes/diagrams and

TABLE 5.1 Material types and skills involved in reading different material

TYPE OF MATERIAL	PURPOSE	READING SKILL
Article on inequalities in health	Understanding and knowledge of issues, relevant theories and views	Slow reading and re-reading, noting own ideas, linking to other reading, questioning the material
Library opening hours	Factual information	Note/memorize for future reference
Technical instructions	Accurate completion of task	Step-by-step reference
Anatomy textbook and diagrams	Informed, factual understanding	Slow and concentrated, re-reading, making notes
Encyclopaedia	Specific definition/information	Specific search under heading
Travel guide	General information	Use of index/contents to locate relevant information

an intelligent personal response. Within that, you would consciously have to apply different levels of reading skills:

- Skimming/scanning the material for the gist. You can quickly decide what parts you need to concentrate on; that is, which sections contain the information you need. Use the layout of the material – contents page, headings, index, tables/charts – to help you.

- In-depth reading/re-reading of the denser material. Be prepared to spend time on this and use reference books; for example, a dictionary for unfamiliar words. Have pen and paper to hand for your notes.

- Inferring as you read, i.e. reading between the lines with awareness of the context. You already do this when you read anything: no written material is without context and the same statement in different contexts can have different intent (see box below). Inference and context are related to subjectivity and interpretation.

- Paraphrasing important or difficult points and ideas in your notes. This means you record *your* understanding of, and response to, the material. It forces you to engage with the material, which is far more effective than simply highlighting passages of text: not only do you achieve better understanding of, and concentration on, the material, you are also honing your writing skills. The notes you make now may provide ideas for your essay.

How context can change intent

- Statement: 'I blame the parents'
- Context 1: Letter to local paper complaining about vandalism
- Context 2: Slogan on T-shirt sold at a Gay Pride event

In Context 1, we have a straightforward reference to a perceived decline in family values and its effect on society.

In Context 2, the statement becomes ironic.

Preparation and purpose

Remember: *define and stick to your purpose.* Active readers do this by identifying what they need from their material. Writing these needs down as a series of questions clarifies and keeps them visible so you don't digress. If you are clear about the answers you need, you are less likely to waste time on irrelevant material. If you do have less relevant but interesting ideas, note them down for exploration later, but stick to the task in hand.

The activity below (which should take 10–12 minutes) asks you to read an extract, first without and then with identified information needs; that is, questions. You may then reflect on the effectiveness of your reading in each case.

The passage below is from *Teratologies: a cultural study of cancer* by Jackie Stacey and, as the book's title suggests, begins to place a medical condition in a cultural context. Read it through as you would any text for study.

Heroes

Books about cancer always tell stories. Those who write them offer recognizable narratives of diagnosis, of treatment and of prognosis. Those who read them often do so in search of the comforting hope of survival. Faced with a sudden change in the story of their lives following a cancer diagnosis, many rehearse the possible trajectories which now present themselves through the accounts of those who have been there before them.

There are books written by doctors about 'the facts' you need to know; they tell of the different types of cancer, the typical prognoses and the likely treatments and their side effects. There are books written by alternative practitioners encouraging a holistic approach to the disease, advising on diet, therapy and a change of lifestyle. There are books written by spiritual evangelists who write of cancer as an opportunity for salvation.

There are also, of course, books written by patients, or their friends and relatives, which offer personal accounts of the experience of living with cancer. If the person with cancer has lived to tell the tale, the story is often of a heroic struggle against diversity. Pitting life against death and drawing on all possible resources, the patient moves from victim to survivor and 'triumphs over the tragedy' that has unexpectedly threatened their life. These are often the stories of transformation in which the negative physical affliction becomes a positive source of self-knowledge. The person who has faced death and yet still lives, who has recognized the inevitability of human mortality, now benefits from a new-found wisdom. Accepting the fragility of life itself, the cancer survivor sees things others are not brave enough to face (or so the story goes). Cancer offers the chance to reassess. It allows the person to pause and to re-evaluate their life: having cancer teaches us that life may be shorter than we thought and that it may be time to decide to live it differently. These are the kinds of wisdoms which are told and retold in books about cancer.

If, on the other hand, the person with cancer dies, the story told is one of loss and of pain, but also tends to be a celebration of their courage and dignity. It may be written by friends, lovers or relatives. Stories of pointlessly shortened lives, lost opportunities, or of medical or industrial malpractice and ineptitude, warn others to try to avoid a similar fate. The late diagnosis, the misread X-ray or the high levels of radiation near nuclear power stations are some of the motivations for authors to tell their stories. But few write (or publish) accounts which tell only of disaster and depression, suffering and unbearable loss. For there is always room for heroism in tragedy and many such stories offer accounts of stoicism and of a fighting spirit. They document the triumphs along the way, even in the event of death.

The market for books about cancer is enormous. Amongst the expanding health and fitness/self-development/New Age and spirituality sections of highstreet [sic] bookstores and the increasing number of publications for sale in health food shops, books about cancer are not hard to find; in fact, they are hard to avoid. Once the news has been broken, books about cancer surface from all directions: they are on every friend's bookshelf, in every shop window. A veritable 'cancer subculture' proves to have been thriving, but, like so many others, it remains invisible until it becomes relevant and then, as if by magic, it seems suddenly all-pervasive. For many people with cancer these books are the starting point of coming to terms with the diagnosis. They are read in the hope of finding a story that fits, of finding a story that offers hope, of even finding a story that ends happily. They are also read for information about the disease or about the treatment: some offer the chance to learn the language of oncology, to understand the principles of chemotherapy or radiotherapy; others educate their readers on the workings of the immune system, the anti-cancer diet or the negative effects of stress on the body. Read all of them and you can become expert in your field, an expert on your particular disease and an expert on yourself.

Given the changes in health cultures in 1990s Britain, the proliferation of this market of 'self-health' cancer books is hardly surprising. As the government cuts in public health provision become the source of endless stories in everyday life (patients returned home prematurely after surgery, beds not available for emergencies, newly equipped wards standing empty because there's no money to staff them, nurses' threats of unprecedented industrial action signalling intense desperation and frustration), people are increasingly encouraged to look elsewhere for reassurance. The introduction of internal markets into the National Health Service in Britain through the National Health Service and Community Care Act (implemented on 1 April 1991) fundamentally changed its principles of organization and management, placing health firmly within a world of competition and consumerism. In these emergent health cultures, where the language of the market has come to dominate ideas about health provision, the scope for appealing to individuals to take charge of their health is ever-widening.

(*Teratologies: a cultural study of cancer*, Stacey J, pp. 1–3, ©1997; reproduced by permission of Taylor and Francis Books, UK.)

Now re-read the passage with the following questions in mind:

1. The author lectures in Women's Studies and Cultural Studies; how is this evident in this passage?

2. Can you think of cancer accounts you have read that fit these descriptions?

3. What links does the passage make in order to suggest that cancer is a cultural and political concern?

The above activity should have helped you to concentrate on the passage in the following ways. The first sentence and the chapter's heading should alert you to the author's approach: it is not conventionally medical; the words 'heroes' and 'stories' imply a cultural rather than scientific discourse. You are confronted immediately with a different way of thinking about how society copes with cancer. In addition, it is difficult to tell whether Stacey is using the word 'stories' here to suggest fabrication. You will need to ascertain this, and why she uses this term.

1. Thinking beyond the text, questioning and making connections are what the active reader does: here you might list and reflect on other accounts of terminal illnesses. Do they match Stacey's descriptions? (You might also reflect on how illness and disability are reported in the media.)

2. First, Stacey classifies cancer accounts under types of narrative: the 'hero' battles, overcomes/dies/achieves redemption/wisdom, not unlike heroes and heroines in myths, movies and novels. Storytelling, a cultural exercise, helps us to structure the messy, frightening business of cancer, and simultaneously blurs the line

between fact and fiction, or if you like, provides us with frames of reference. Second, Stacey links the growing interest in self-health to the increasingly consumerist and market-led policies in the NHS during the 1990s. You might need to refer to other documents – for example, reports, articles and contemporary journalistic commentary – for a richer context here. The book was written and published in the late 1990s, and this places its concerns in a particular cultural and political moment.

Identifying information needs enables concentration on the relevant sections of the passage, and precision concerning your wider information needs. Being selective, i.e. focusing on several well-chosen readings, is essential. However, be prepared: sometimes your information needs won't be apparent until you have read the text several times, and perhaps other texts.

Your time is limited – you can't read everything.

In-depth reading is time-consuming, but you will understand material better by giving it close attention.

Quality not quantity!

Reviewing and recording your reading

Reviewing your reading helps in summarizing what you have learned and ensures that you have answered your questions as fully as possible. Your review should be recorded with bibliographic details.

Recording the bibliographic details (i.e. the citation) is necessary for your references and enables future location of that material. This also applies to non-textual and internet material. Brief notes on content and value are helpful towards future essays. All this creates an annotated bibliography of material that you have used throughout your course, which can be arranged and stored. The box below shows the possible content of such a record (see also Chapter 4).

Stacey J (1997) Teratologies: a cultural study of cancer. Routledge/Taylor and Francis Group, London.

pp. 1–3, outlines cancer 'genres' and characteristics and relates growth of such books to NHS in enterprise culture/Thatcherism – extensive notes – used for essay on perceptions of terminal illness and treatments; rest of book combines personal experience and sociocultural critique of cancer, treatments and (sexist) attitudes in orthodox and alternative medicine.

Related reading – see Cancer Help Centre/Laura K. Potts/Sontag?
Uni. library book, class. no?

The active reader recognizes that:

- Reading is work – to be done at a desk, not in an armchair
- You read to learn – keep a dictionary to hand
- You read at different levels – select material, scan for relevance, read the relevant material in depth. Purpose and preparation help concentration and understanding
- Understanding means time spent re-reading and referring to other works
- Understanding means engaging with the material, paraphrasing and re-interpreting in your notes
- You must read critically, constantly aware of context and the author's frame of reference
- You keep records of your reading, recording the bibliographic details, reviewing the contents and value
- Your responses and ideas from your reading are the beginning of your essay

Plagiarism

Keeping records of your reading is essential for references. If you quote or refer to the work or ideas of another person, whether published, broadcast or spoken informally, you must acknowledge your source. To claim, even accidentally, the ideas of others as your own, is intellectual theft. If discovered you could fail your course.

Several referencing systems exist. Your university should give you guidelines on which to use in your written work (see also Chapter 9).

Lectures

This section looks at learning effectively from lectures. Many of the principles from reading apply, but some of the techniques are different.

The role of lectures

You could be forgiven for seeing lectures as the most important part of your course. They are given by the 'experts' and have an air of authority. You might also see lectures as being the responsibility of the lecturers. Their job is to package and impart knowledge to you, after all. Both perceptions are unhelpful, however. Lectures are important; their aims are to:

- introduce material (terminology, ideas, theories, a line of argument)
- explain the above
- complement your reading.

Time spent in lectures should be far less than that used for private or group study.

Lectures are of little use unless you are an active participant. Before the lecture, treat its contents as new terrain. You wouldn't go to a strange city without a map: preparatory reading is like mapping what you are going to hear. During the lecture:

■ ask questions
■ take notes – effectively.

You might see the similarity between being an active reader and an active listener. The key is taking responsibility for your own learning.

Preparation can help understanding and concentration. Think back to a TV documentary you have watched recently. In your reflective diary, reflect on:

• What, if any knowledge did you have prior to the programme?
• Either way, how did this affect your understanding and concentration?

Note taking in lectures

You cannot control the pace of a lecture, as you do when reading or viewing. This can be stressful as you try to do several things simultaneously:

■ listen
■ understand
■ take notes.

To get the most out of lectures you should:

• Prepare: get some idea of the content of the lecture, read background material
• Identify the purpose in your preparation: note areas on which you want to concentrate and ask questions about
• Summarize the content of the lecture briefly in your notes: this will help your review
• Review from your notes and handouts whether you achieved your purpose and plan further reading/discussion

Unfortunately, this is impossible. You cannot listen *and* take notes. You cannot understand without giving thought to something, and if you're thinking you're not listening. Don't try! But if you have identified areas of interest, you can focus on what is being said and summarize it your notes when the lecturer moves on. Summarizing demands your interpretation, which aids your understanding, like paraphrasing when reading.

Don't try and write down everything: it impossible, and not the purpose of the lecture

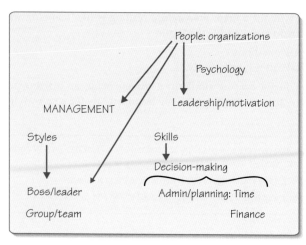

FIGURE 5.1 A visual approach to note taking.

Styles of note taking

There are as many different ways to take notes as there are students, but they fall broadly into two categories:

1. visual
2. linear.

Note taking is a matter of personal choice. A visual approach might look like that shown in Figure 5.1. A linear approach might use headings, indentations and personal shorthand. It might look like that shown in Figure 5.2. Both approaches allow you to map your subject (see Chapter 3),

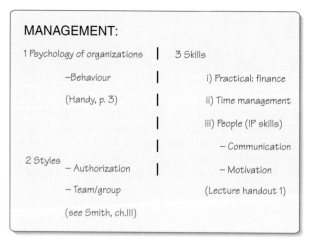

FIGURE 5.2 A linear approach to note taking.

organizing it in your mind, enabling you to note areas for further reading. You can code or highlight areas or topics with different coloured pens according to their importance. Experiment with styles; adopt one that suits you.

As an active listener you recognize that:
- You need to prepare for lectures
- Identifying your purpose helps you to focus on the relevant areas during the lecture
- You will need to ask questions during the lecture
- You take notes to understand
- Lectures must be supported by reading and discussion
- Reviewing your notes and handouts will help to identify areas for further reading
- Summarizing a lecture is part of the review

Conclusion

Both this chapter and Chapter 3 stress the importance of your role in seeking and using information effectively. Learning takes place not only in the lecture or from reading masses of titles from your reading list, nor is it solely the responsibility of your tutors. Your involvement is the key.

Lecture preparation
Look at your timetable for a lecture that will cover a subject new to you. Note in your reflective journal:
- the lecture title
- the subject to be covered

The day before/of the lecture read briefly round the subject – a chapter or an article. You may not understand it – don't worry. Note in your reflective diary:
- the reference for the material read
- the time spent on it
- your understanding of it, e.g. poor, good

After the lecture consider in your reflective diary:
- Did your pre-lecture reading familiarize you with terminology, concepts, etc.?
- Was your understanding of the lecture enhanced?
- Were you able to make clearer notes?
- Were you able to ask questions of the lecturer from a more informed position?
- Did you have a better idea of which points you needed to have explained further?

You should have answered positively to some of the above points. It is surprising how a little reading can lay the groundwork of understanding for a lecture on a new subject.

Finally, re-read your pre-lecture material. It should now begin to make sense. It may even round out your lecture notes.

Main points to remember:
- be critical
- be selective
- different reading needs require different levels of study and skill
- prepare for lectures
- engage with the material

CHAPTER RESOURCES

REFERENCES

Stacey, J., 1997. Teratologies: a cultural study of cancer. Routledge/Taylor and Francis Books, London.

WEBSITES

Florence Nightingale School of Nursing and Midwifery, Kings College London: http://www.kcl.ac.uk/schools/nursing/vc/studyskills

Student Help: a resource for students of nursing and health care: http://www.attu70.dsl.pipex.com/student/ or http://www.richard-ingram.co.uk

University of Central Lancashire, Faculty of Health: http://www.uclan.ac.uk/facs/health/nursing/documents/handbook/sectionb/index.htm

FURTHER READING

Cottrell, S., 2008. The study skills handbook. Palgrave Macmillan, Basingstoke, UK.

Cryer, P., 2006. The research student's guide to success. McGraw Hill/Open University Press, Maidenhead, UK.

Fairbairn, G.J., Fairbairn, S.A., 2001. Reading at university: a guide for students. Open University Press, Buckingham, UK.

Redway, K., 2004. Beat the bumf!: cut clutter, read rapidly and succeed in the information jungle. Management Books, Cirencester, UK.

Rose, J., 2001. The mature student's guide to writing. Palgrave, Basingstoke, UK.

6

Writing skills and developing an argument

Netta Lloyd-Jones and Abigail Masterson

KEY ISSUES

- Developing an effective writing style
- How to develop an argument
- Distinguishing between fact and opinion
- How arguments work
- Reviewing the evidence
- Structuring arguments
- How arguments can go wrong
- Learning from feedback

Introduction

As students and practitioners, we need to be able to communicate effectively in writing. This is necessary to meet the requirements of professional practice not only in assessing, planning, implementing and evaluating care, but also in completing nursing and midwifery notes and in supporting and justifying changes in practice to managers and other multidisciplinary colleagues. In addition, you might want to write for publication in order to share good practice and innovative developments with a wider audience. Remember that there is probably no such thing as a born writer. The successful writer is the one who regards writing as a skill to be learned, refined and constantly improved.

Successful writing is about using ideas and information to say something in a clear, unambiguous way that others will understand. Many different types of writing are required in professional practice; for example, 'academic' style, report writing and protocol development. The focus of this chapter is on developing an academic style.

Academic style is important in the development of learning skills in two ways: (1) you will come across it in your reading; and (2) you will be learning to develop it yourself through your assessed pieces of coursework. Therefore, it is necessary to understand its 'rules'. Academic writing in its purest form is cautious and tentative in approach and depends on argument supported by strong evidence. The aim is to be as exact as possible and to say only what can be justified. Academic writing is designed for a very critical reader who is interested only in whether the arguments make sense and not in appeals to the emotions.

Take something you have written recently, e.g. an assignment, a formal letter or minutes from a meeting. Read it through carefully and 'mark' it against the following criteria:

- Has all the relevant information been included?
- Does it make sense?
- Is it simple and to the point?
- Is it legible and easy to read?

Having marked it in this way, you should be able to begin to see where some of your strengths and weaknesses are, and where it might be useful to seek further help.

Developing an effective writing style

Academic style

In everyday language the word 'academic' is sometimes used in a pejorative way to describe things that have no practical purpose or are divorced from practice. In the context of education and writing, academic style means something very specific and relates to a set of rules about how to deal with information and evidence. Although the pieces of coursework you are required to produce on your programme will probably have a variety of formats – essays, case studies, reports, critical incident analyses, reflections on competency achievement in practice – the principles in terms of writing style are similar. For example, in most cases it is important to justify and support the points you want to make with material that you have read. This does not mean, however, that you should cite ten authors to back up statements such as 'many women experience pain during childbirth' or 'maintaining patient/client dignity ought to be a high priority for nurses'. Make a clear distinction between what you know because you have read about it and what you know because of your own experience and reflections on those experiences. Being able to distinguish between different types of evidence is also important (see Chapter 8 for a further discussion about this).

It is vital to try to express yourself as clearly and as succinctly as possible by using short sentences and straightforward language.

Keep it simple. If you do not understand what you have written, it is unlikely that anyone else will.

For example, consider this clear and straightforward introduction to an article by Roe et al. (2008):

Falls and falling are common occurrences with increasing age (Tinetti et al., 1998). Older people are particularly likely to fall, and this can result in severe cases in injury, fractures, hospitalization and premature death (Rawsky, 1998; Cryer and Patel, 2001). Other consequences are repeat falls, fear of falling, impaired mobility, loss of independence, social isolation and significant costs to individuals, their families and public services (Gryfe et al., 1977; Morse et al., 1987; O'Loughlin et al., 1993; Rawsky, 1998; Cryer and Patel, 2001; Tinetti, 2003). Awareness of the costs and implications of falls in recent years has made falls prevention an important policy internationally for health and social services to address supported by initiatives in the voluntary sector (DH, 2003, 2004; Todd and Skelton, 2004). There has been little research investigating the consequences of falls from the perspectives of older people and their families. In this paper, we report the findings from qualitative research investigating older people's experiences of recent falls to analyse their understanding of these falls, and their autonomy. These findings could serve as the basis for service and practice development.

However clear and logical the argument, it is easy to get frustrated if you do not agree with what the author is saying. When reading, we are supposed to detach our thoughts from our feelings and put our own biases on one side to judge the validity of the author's arguments by their strength and soundness alone. This is practically impossible, because if we were able to do this absolutely we would not have a position from which to think about, or to judge and criticize, what we read. Eventually, we may or may not decide that the author has a point but we need to give ourselves the chance to find out what is on offer and so must try not to reject opposing points of view too quickly. Instead, we should use our feelings constructively by writing down our criticisms point by point.

Learning from others

A valuable aid to developing your own writing ability is to look critically at the work of others. You may find it particularly helpful to read other students' assignments and see what appears to work well and gets good marks. Similarly, when reading books and journal articles try to sort out why you prefer one author's work to another. Critically judging other people's writing in this way is a good way of increasing your understanding of what you are trying to aim for in your own writing.

Choose two journal articles that interest you. Read them thoroughly. Decide which is the better article and jot down the reasons why. You have probably picked the article that is well structured, clear and straightforward to read.

The subject

As a student, you may be given an essay title that specifies the subject you are to write about; for example, 'The public health role of the midwife'. The title might even identify the claim you are to defend or attack; for example, 'Time limits for the second stage of labour disempower women from achieving normal birth'. Alternatively, you may only be given broad guidelines; for example, 'Write a 3000-word essay on a contemporary professional issue'. In this instance, your first task will be to identify the subject for your essay.

 How might you go about identifying a subject?

Possible sources are:

- Your own experience of practice: are there issues that interest or concern you?
- Colleagues and managers: what are the current issues in your speciality, and in nursing and midwifery in general?
- Professional and specialist journals: what subjects are being written about?

The evidence

Chapters 3, 4 and 5 looked at the practical aspects of gathering information about a subject. Having found your information, you then need to analyse it to see what evidence there is relating to your assignment. Although you might start with a strong hunch, or with views already well developed in one direction, it is important to keep an open mind and consider all the evidence, not just that which supports your point of view.

Structure

All written work should include an introduction where you set the context and outline the 'map' of what is to follow. This map should include what you are going to cover, why you have decided on this particular approach and how your argument will develop.

If you have been given a formal title for an assignment, such as 'Discuss the evidence that distinguishes the differences between the responsibilities of a registered healthcare professional and a lay carer'. This title gives some clues about what the structure and content of your essay should be. The key words in this title are 'discuss', 'evidence', ' differences', 'responsibilities', 'registered healthcare professional' and 'lay carer':

- 'Discuss' suggests that there are arguments for and against and indicates that your assignment needs to consider both sides. The title thus can set down clear guidelines about the content that is expected.

- 'Evidence' indicates that you are expected to support your argument with research and other literature and not just provide your own unsupported opinion.
- 'Differences' asks for you to concentrate on what is different between a 'registered healthcare professional' such as a midwife and a 'lay carer' such as a family member.
- 'Responsibilities' highlights the area of difference which you need to focus on. So, for example, describing the different rates of pay for these two groups would not be relevant.

If, however, you have just been given a topic such as 'institutionalization' you will have to decide what you think the key points and issues are. For example, you might decide that you want to explore the effects of institutionalization on people with learning difficulties and put forward the case for community care in small group homes. First, you will need to define what institutionalization is. Then discuss the contribution of people such as Erving Goffman (1961) to our understanding of this concept, identify why people with learning difficulties might become institutionalized and consider the importance of small group homes integrated into the normal social life of local communities in preventing institutionalization.

You should outline the key themes and arguments in the main body of your assignment. So in our first example you might refer to the Nursing and Midwifery Council's 'The Code: Standards of conduct, performance and ethics for nurses and midwives' (2008) and 'Midwives rules and standards' (2004), as well as to the various policies (e.g. drug administration polices) put forward by different healthcare organizations. Then you would outline the arguments from the literature and your own experience of the difference between the two groups. This should take several paragraphs.

Finally, you should write a conclusion that pulls together and summarizes the key points you have made. The conclusion to 'Discuss the evidence that distinguishes the differences between the responsibilities of a registered healthcare professional and a lay carer', could be as follows:

> In this essay, I have used the literature and my own experience to show that the registered nurse's responsibilities for the care of a sick child are different from those of a parent, even though some of the activities they undertake may be very similar. A key responsibility for the registered nurse is to make sure that their expertise in care giving and familiarity with healthcare organizations, systems and other professionals does not result in the parents feeling disempowered and undermined.

Each sentence in your assignment should lead logically on to the next and there should be clear signposts to your reader when you are changing subject or introducing a new point of view. Paragraphs are collections of sentences on a particular theme. When you change tack, it is time for a new paragraph.

Clarity is crucial. There is often a tendency for students to use very long phrases and complicated sentences in an attempt to emulate what they read in heavyweight journals and specialist books. However, ease of reading and simplicity are far more likely to impress.

Never assume anything. Your reader has not necessarily read the same sources as you and certainly does not know what is inside your head, so you need to explain all your ideas fully and give examples to illustrate the points you are making.

The UK government is committed to ensuring that all NHS staff are information technology (IT) literate and so the ability to word-process your work is essential. You should print on only one side of the paper and leave a generous space between the lines – dense text is very hard on the eyes. Mistakes in spelling, punctuation and grammar do not lose you marks as such but can get in the way of the readability of your work and stop it making sense to others. Use the support that technology gives you, such as spell- and grammar-checking functions, but do make sure that these are set appropriately for the country you are writing in (e.g. UK English). You might be able to get help if you experience any of the difficulties listed in the box below.

Reading
- Slower than usual reading speed
- Difficulties with reading comprehension and therefore with summarizing
- Problems decoding new scientific words
- Loses place in a series or in reading

Memory
- A 'quick forgetter' rather than 'slow learner'
- Poor strategies for 'rehearsal' of information into long-term memory
- Difficulties memorizing facts and new terminology

Writing and spelling
- Handwriting problems
- Difficulties with listening and taking notes
- Difficulties in copying from the PowerPoint presentation
- Severe and persistent spelling problems
- Difficulties in getting ideas on paper, so that written work fails to adequately express student's understanding, ideas or vocabulary

Learning
- Difficulties with organization, e.g. work, assignments, projects, university life, notes and files
- Trouble generalizing and applying new rules, seems to or reports 'switching off'
- Problems working with background noise
- Short concentration span
- Needs to be told information more than once

(School of Health and Social Care, Oxford Brookes University, 2003)

Many organizations offer support to students with dyslexia and/or other learning difficulties. This can include providing access to staff with specific expertise in this area. If you are having difficulties, talk to your personal tutor, who will be able to put you in contact with the appropriate support. This confidential service should include supporting you through a formal assessment process and helping you to access specific equipment and funding to support your learning.

The following tips, hints and activities should help you develop and refine your academic style.

- Read the work of others: this will help you identify good and bad writing styles.
- Reading helps improve vocabulary and grammar: share your work with other students and colleagues and get feedback.
- Practice makes perfect: writing short sections can help polish writing skills and boost your confidence.

Compare the styles of argument and language used in the editorial columns of a range of newspapers; for example, the *Daily Mail* and *The Guardian*.

If you read something and find that you disagree with it, think about why this is. Do you think the author could have got the facts wrong? Or is the problem that the conclusion doesn't follow from the arguments given?

Developing an argument

The ability to construct an effective argument is vital in professional practice. The ability to offer a reasoned argument in support of an idea or belief is central to professional development and is a skill that you are expected to display in all forms of written work. For example, an essay should put forward an opinion and offer support for that opinion in the form of factual and rational evidence; and a protocol is a route map for practice based on an objective appraisal of the evidence.

'Argument' means something very specific in its academic sense and should be distinguished from the popular use of the term, which means a verbal fight or row. An academic argument is a claim or proposition put forward, with reasons or evidence supporting it.

Why argument is important

If you were proposing to introduce a new method of patient care it is unlikely that you would be allowed to do it merely on a whim. You would need to persuade managers and medical and other healthcare staff of the benefits of the proposed changes, and that these outweighed any costs involved. You would need to put forward your point of view in a structured way using evidence to persuade people that your point of view is the correct one.

Reflect on some situations from practice where your ability to put forward a good argument might be useful.

Identifying an argument

In your reading as well as in your writing, it is important to be able to distinguish an argument from other types of writing.

Read the two passages below. Which is an example of an argument?

1. All hospital-acquired infection would be prevented if nurses washed their hands properly.

2. Gould et al.'s work (2008) highlights that hand hygiene is the single most important procedure for preventing the spread of infection.

Now read the two paragraphs again. What does paragraph 1 offer, given that the facts in paragraph 2 are correct?

Paragraph 1 offers an explanation for the facts given in paragraph 2. It seems, on the face of it, a reasonable explanation but it is worth remembering that for any one set of circumstances there may be more than one explanation.

What could you do to test the truth of the explanation offered below?

A police officer arrives at a road junction and finds two dented cars and two angry drivers. The officer has no way of knowing who is at fault without looking at the physical evidence and taking statements from the drivers and any witnesses. Sometimes one explanation will seem more plausible than another, but this does not necessarily make it the correct one.

Description of facts and opinions is a necessary part of any argument: in fact, it is impossible to argue without describing various aspects of the subject you are arguing about. However, it is quite possible to describe without arguing.

When you present information that is relevant to the argument you are making, you must tell your reader or your listener why you are doing so and how you are using the facts.

Fact and opinion

When you are collecting the evidence that you will use to support your argument you must be careful to distinguish between objective facts and opinions.

In the passage below taken from a speech by the former General Secretary of the RCN, Beverley Malone, and reproduced in *The Independent* newspaper (Friday, 11 March 2005) what is fact and what opinion?

As nurses, we have to be clever, articulate and determined as well as caring. Strong and visible nursing leadership is part of effective nursing care. Patients still respect nurses and, more than ever, they expect us to speak up on behalf of patient care, wherever we work and whatever our role. The return of 'matron' – as a modern nurse – has been in large part due to pressure from the public. That is why I am so clear that the family of nursing will continue to be the backbone of the healthcare workforce. And why I believe that if nursing didn't already exist, people would be rushing to invent it.

How arguments work

Read the passage below. Can you spot any flaws in the argument? If you are not familiar with the studies cited, accept for the purposes of the exercise that they do demonstrate what the paragraph claims that they do. 'Preoperative visiting' is the term used for a system in which a theatre nurse sees surgical patients on the ward the afternoon or evening before surgery. During the visit they are given the opportunity to discuss what will happen to them – what they will see, hear, feel, where they will be when they wake up – and to ask questions.

Classic studies by Boore (1978) and Hayward (1975) reinforced by the findings of contemporary research (see, for example, McDonald et al., 2004; Schuldham et al., 2002) demonstrated that, if patients receive information about their treatment in advance, they recover more quickly, require less analgesia and are discharged earlier than those who do not receive this information. The information could be conveyed during a preoperative assessment visit from a member of the theatre team, who because of their specialist knowledge is well placed to describe what the patient will experience and answer any questions. Preoperative assessment therefore would bring benefits to the patient, and it is theatre nurses who should be carrying out such visits.

First, establish what the subject of the discussion is. In this case, it is preoperative assessment by nurses who work in the operating department.

The next thing to establish is the position that is being presented – the claim that is to be defended. Sometimes this is obvious, at other times less so, but you need to be clear about the claim made before you can judge the quality of the evidence provided in support.

What is the claim made in the passage above?

The author actually appears to make two claims. First, that 'preoperative assessment would bring benefits to the patient'; second, that 'theatre nurses should carry out preoperative assessments'. This is a mistake in itself: claims should be made singly, not bunched together. Claims need to be supported in some way.

What is the evidence presented in support of each claim?

Let us consider the first claim: that preoperative visiting benefits the patient. The author starts by citing two research studies that have demonstrated benefits to patients from preoperative information giving: the first sentence thus offers facts, the accuracy of which can easily be checked. The second sentence then puts forward a suggestion, namely that theatre staff could give this information during a preoperative visit. It therefore seems reasonable to conclude that, on the face of it, patients will benefit from preoperative visits. Note, however, that this makes the presumption that patients prefer, on the whole, to recover quickly and have short stays in hospital. Watch out for this kind of presumption and ask yourself 'is it reasonable to presume this?' For example, the argument that 'regular exercise makes you fit, slim and healthy: everybody should exercise' presumes that everybody wants to be these things: is this the case?

Let us turn to the second claim: that theatre nurses should be doing preoperative visits. Here the support offered for the claim is less obvious, but seems to be that theatre nurses have specialist knowledge. The chain of inference is therefore as in Figure 6.1.

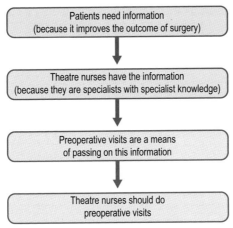

FIGURE 6.1 The chain of inference for whether theatre nurses should make preoperative visits.

 There are, however, a number of presumptions in this figure. Can you spot what they are?

First, is it reasonable to claim that theatre nurses have specialist knowledge? Some might well do, but not all. It might be better to say 'an experienced member of the theatre team' or 'a specially trained member of the team'. Second, is the theatre nurse well placed to answer questions? How about those that relate to the proposed surgery, or the anaesthetic to be used? Third, is a preoperative visit necessarily the best way of conveying the information that the patient might need?

Does the conclusion therefore follow from the evidence put forward? Should we accept that theatre nurses should be the ones to provide information? It would be perfectly possible to argue that ward-based nurses have more opportunity to develop the necessary rapport than a theatre nurse during a brief visit.

One final point to note is that the way in which the two claims – (1) that patients would benefit from preoperative visits; and (2) that theatre nurses should do preoperative visits – are put together at the end of the piece of writing suggests that the one implies the other, when they are, as we have seen, two separate ideas. This is called conflation.

Considering the evidence

Evidence can include fact, value statements or expert opinion. The simplest, most direct form is fact:

■ 'Approximately 670 000 practitioners are registered with the Nursing and Midwifery Council'.

- 'All NHS Trusts are required by statute to have a nurse on the Trust Board'.

Both these facts could be checked and verified. Certain value statements are also admissible evidence in argument:

- 'Human life is intrinsically valuable'.
- 'Nursing is a caring profession'.

Neither of these statements could be proved objectively but both express ideas that are almost universal and could thus be used to support an argument.

A third form of evidence is opinion. Opinion is not a prejudice or an unconsidered point of view but is arrived at by a logical thought process based on all available evidence. Evidence can also include the expert opinions of specialists in the topic under discussion: these usually come from books and journal articles. If you quote from these, you must remember to acknowledge your sources, using an accepted reference and citation system (see Chapter 8 for more details).

Note that one of the things that assignments are designed to test is your ability to select and use evidence appropriately in support of an argument.

Using argument appropriately in assignments

Like a lawyer in court, your task in an essay is to convince the jury (your reader) that your point of view is the correct one (or at least, one that is worth considering). Just as a lawyer uses evidence and statements by witnesses to build up the case, so you have to show how your evidence supports your argument.

Relatives should always be allowed to witness resuscitation within the Emergency Department because it helps them cope with the outcome for their relative.

The above example demonstrates one basic argument that could be used in favour of relatives witnessing resuscitation but is open to attack by anyone who believes that relatives may 'get in the way' of the work of the resuscitation team or that team members might make themselves vulnerable to litigation. As a general rule, it is a good idea to defend your overall argument (that relatives should always be allowed to witness resuscitation) with as many supporting arguments as you can develop in the time and space allowed.

What other arguments could be used to support the view that relatives should always be allowed to witness resuscitation?

You could approach the argument as follows.

Premise 1: family presence during resuscitation is beneficial.

- Supporting evidence: growing national and international research base (e.g. Critchell CD, Marik PE 2007 Should family members be present during cardiopulmonary resuscitation? A review of the literature. American Journal of Hospital and Palliative Care 24:311–317).

Premise 2: family members don't get in the way of the work resuscitation team.

- Supporting evidence: there have been no cases of interference with medical care by family members (O'Connell KJ, Farah MM, Spandorfer P, Zorc JJ 2007 Family presence during pediatric trauma team activation: an assessment of a structured program. Pediatrics 120: e565–e574).

Premise 3: written policies or guidelines for family presence during resuscitation and invasive procedures are recommended.

- Supporting evidence: expert testimony, publications by specialists in emergency care.

Premise 4: people want to be present.

- Supporting evidence: public opinion polls (*USA Today* 2000, NBC Dateline Poll 1999) have revealed that most people think that patients' family members would want to be, and should be allowed to be, present while emergency procedures were performed on the patients and at the time of death.

Premise 5: that there are multiple benefits to the practice of family presence during resuscitation.

- Supporting evidence: academic texts (e.g. Meyers TA, Eichhorn DJ, Guzzetta CE, et al 2000 Family presence during invasive procedures and resuscitation: the experiences of family members, nurses, and physicians. American Journal of Nursing 100:32–42) suggest that it reduces anxiety and fear (Robinson SM, Mackenzie-Ross S, Campbell-Hewson GL, et al 1998 Psychological effect of witnessed resuscitation on bereaved relatives. Lancet 352:614–617), engenders feelings of supporting and helping the patient (Doyle CJ, Post H, Burney RE, et al 1987 Family participation during resuscitation: an option. Annals of Emergency Medicine 16:673–675), provides a sense of closure on a life shared together (Hanson C, Strawser D 1992 Family presence during cardiopulmonary resuscitation: Foote Hospital emergency department's nine-year perspective. Journal of Emergency Nursing 18:104–106), facilitates the grief process (Belanger MA, Reed S 1997 A rural community hospital's experience with family-witnessed resuscitation. Journal of Emergency Nursing 23:238–239) and engenders feelings of being helpful to healthcare staff (Powers KS, Rubenstein JS 1999 Family presence during invasive procedures in the paediatric intensive care unit. Archives of Pediatric and Adolescent Medicine 153:955–958).

Conclusion: there are numerous evidence-based reasons for encouraging family members to witness resuscitation.

Note how each of the premises that support the main conclusion are in a sense the conclusions of supporting arguments.

How arguments go wrong

An argument can go wrong either because the premises are faulty and therefore the conclusion does not follow or because the premises are true but do not support the conclusion.

What is wrong with the argument below?

- All midwives are female.
- Chris is a midwife.
- Therefore Chris is female.

It can be easily shown that some midwives are male, therefore the first premise is untrue and the conclusion does not follow. Note, however, that the form of the argument is perfectly valid. If all midwives were indeed female, then the conclusion would be true.

What is wrong with this argument?

- All midwives are female.
- Chris is female.
- Therefore Chris is a midwife.

In this case, the problem is with the form of the argument. Even if it were true that all midwives are female, and that Chris is female, it does not follow that Chris is a midwife: she might be an engineer, an airline pilot or anything else. She might even be a midwife, but this argument does not prove it.

Consider the following statements/arguments, and try to identify the problems with them. The important thing is to be able to spot when and where an argument is going wrong.

1. Mr Lister married his sister.
2. You will meet a dark stranger and your financial affairs will be affected.

These statements are ambiguous: in the first, the word 'sister' can be understood in several different ways, as can the word 'married': did Mr Lister marry his biological sister and commit incest? Was Mr Lister the clergyman who officiated at his sister's wedding? (In fact, neither interpretation is correct. Joseph Lister, an eminent Victorian surgeon, married his theatre sister, in the best traditions of nurse–doctor romances!) In the second example, which might be found in the horoscope pages of a magazine, the whole statement could mean any number of different things.

3. Eight out of ten cats prefer Kat Din.

Here it is the information that is not supplied that is crucial. The statement sounds like the results of an experiment but how many cats were involved? 10? 100? 10 000? What were they offered as an alternative to Kat Din?

4. The argument for not wearing your uniform outside of work is supported by the works of many well-known nurse researchers, and also by several prominent politicians.

You might have wondered what special knowledge of infection control the people referred to possess. Certainly, they are well known, even famous, but are they qualified to comment on the subject of the infection risks posed by wearing uniforms outside of work? Using authorities is acceptable, but only to lend support in their area of expertise.

5. Nurses and doctors are always going on about the dangers of drinking alcohol, but lots of them drink alcohol, so it can't be that bad for you.

In this kind of fallacy, the argument is directed against the failings of individuals to discredit the argument put forward. However, in the example above, does the behaviour of some health professionals discredit the idea that drinking alcohol is bad for you, or does it simply illustrate that human beings are fallible and don't always live up to the ideals they express?

6. It's not worth treating smokers. They don't listen to advice and they won't stop smoking.

This example illustrates the same fallacy as the fifth statement. The problem is that there may be occasions when it seems acceptable to direct attention to the failings of an individual. The sixth example illustrates one aspect of a debate that is beginning to be heard more often nowadays. What do you think? (And why?).

7. The majority of midwives are confident that doctors regard them as fellow professionals.

We saw an example of this fallacy – the appeal to popular belief – in the fourth example above. The fact that a majority believes something to be true does not necessarily mean that it is true (although, of course, it might be). For this reason, the results of opinion polls on contentious issues should be treated with some caution.

8. I've never known using honey on pressure ulcers to do any harm, so it must be doing some good.

This is the appeal to ignorance, arguing that, because we don't know something is not true, it is true.

9. Fred Bloggs always tells the truth:
*   How do you know?
*   Fred Bloggs told me so.
*   How do you know he wasn't lying?
*   Because he always tells the truth.

This is the circular argument: the conclusion of the argument – that Fred Bloggs tells the truth – is used as one of the premises that supports the conclusion. You might have encountered it in your work in this form:

Question: 'Why do we do "it" (e.g. changing a dressing, dealing with patients/clients, organizing the off-duty rota) this way?'
Answer: 'Because we've always done it this way.'
Question: 'But why have we always done it this way?'
Answer: 'Because we always have.'

10. Nurses who use hoists to lift patients experience fewer back injuries than those who don't. If hoists are always used to lift patients no nurses will have bad backs.

This is a non sequitur (a Latin term meaning 'it does not follow'). The argument suggests that bad backs can only be caused by lifting patients.

Starting writing

When you have collected your resources together and organized your thoughts, you are ready to begin writing. Your work does not have to be perfect. Two or three drafts of any piece of work should be sufficient. Try not to write and edit at the same time: it is easy to lose your capacity to think clearly if you get bogged down in the intricacies of spelling and grammar. Also, avoid wasting time playing with fonts and formats.

- If you are working for a whole day, spend the morning writing and the afternoon editing.
- If you are working for part of the day, write for a couple of hours and edit for an hour.

Nothing is more off-putting than a blank page and, if you cannot think of a punchy opening sentence or introductory paragraph, start somewhere in the middle and work backwards. Do not try to complete your task in one go; approaching it in this way can make the task feel enormous and impossible. Instead, break the job down into manageable stages. If you get stuck at one part, try another and then go back to the first one once you have freed up your thoughts. Finally, it is important to trust your impressions and to have faith in yourself. There is usually no such thing as one right answer. You need to work out what your own thoughts are on the area. It is important to have your own opinion but it must be based on reasonable evidence rather than gut feeling or prejudice. Do not be constrained by fear of looking a fool or getting it wrong – have a go.

Before submitting a completed piece of work, check the following:

1. Is the right question/title at the head of your work?
2. Have you completed and included the relevant proforma specified in your assignment guidelines, for example:
   - Your name
   - Candidate/examination number
   - Course name
   - Lecturer's/marker's name?
3. Is your work legible and ordered:
   - Printed in an appropriate font size and type
   - Organized logically
   - Pages numbered?
4. Is the spelling and punctuation accurate: use spell checkers and dictionaries to help but remember that they will not pick up errors such as the misuse of 'their' and 'there', etc.
5. Have you submitted the correct number of copies?
6. Have you kept a back-up copy (on a memory stick or disk) in case the original is inadvertently lost or there is a problem with your computer?
7. Have you attributed your sources appropriately? Copying big chunks from a published or unpublished piece of work verbatim (i.e. using the same words as the original author, without adequate referencing to the source of the material) is a serious academic and professional offence (see Chapter 9 for a more in-depth discussion of this).

Handing in your work and receiving a mark and/or comments is not the end of the process. If you want to progress and improve, it is important to note the comments made by the marker and try to make constructive use of their feedback.

Accepting feedback

One of the most useful ways of developing yourself is to use your ability to listen to others and to make the most of constructive criticism. You will receive feedback on all types of assessment, achievement of practice competencies and coursework. It is important to take every opportunity you are offered for feedback and to try to learn from the feedback you are given, however painful this feels at first. It is always hard when you have spent a lot of time and energy on something not to get the mark you hoped for, or to receive pages and pages of feedback from the marker of your work or the editor of a journal. It is important to try to use this feedback as part of your development as a writer and not to take it personally.

As we suggested in the introduction to this chapter, there is no such thing as a born writer: practice is essential. Often, because we tend to compare our efforts with those of experienced writers rather than our peers, we can become very disillusioned. Nobody likes receiving negative comments about their work, particularly if these result in referral or failure of part of a course. When such things happen, we often tend to try to blame others: the marker didn't like us, the lecturer/our off-duty didn't give us sufficient time to do it properly. However, if we are to grow and develop, we need to acknowledge our own mistakes and take responsibility for our own performance. Look again at Chapter 2 for further discussion of the importance of taking responsibility for your own learning and development.

If you get a mark that you are not happy with or are referred on a piece of coursework, do not go and see your lecturer immediately. Give yourself time to adjust and get over the feelings of sadness, anger and disappointment. When you do go to see your lecturer, take along your assignment and any comments from the marker. The comments can act as a guide for the tutorial and can be useful prompts and pointers if you are required to re-submit the assignment.

One well known nurse researcher said 'I always keep a copy of the first essay I ever wrote for a professional course. If I ever feel disenchanted by feedback, I can read through and remind myself how my style and competence have developed.'

Conclusion

In this chapter, we have explored the process of developing an argument. You have been encouraged to be critical about what you read. The importance of clarity and structure in your preparation and your writing has been emphasized. In written work and discussion you need to be able to put forward your point of view clearly and effectively. This means telling your reader/audience exactly what the point you are making is, what evidence you are using in support and how that evidence supports what you are saying. Arguments go wrong either because the evidence is poorly presented and articulated or because it does not support the conclusion. Successful writing, as with so many other things in life, perfectly illustrates the truth of the old adage 'practice makes perfect'.

- Stick to the topic and follow the guidelines.
- The aim of an argument is to get the other person to accept that your point of view is the correct one, or is at least worth considering.
- When you argue, you must support your claims with evidence.
- The evidence must be of good quality, referenced, clearly stated and relevant to the argument.
- Succinct, straightforward, structured writing is the ideal.
- Use feedback positively to help you refine your skills.

CHAPTER RESOURCES

REFERENCES

Boore, J.R.P., 1978. Prescription for recovery: the effect of preoperative preparation of surgical patients on postoperative stress, recovery and infection (RCN research series). Royal College of Nursing, London.

Goffman, E., 1961. Asylums. Penguin, Harmondsworth, UK.

Gould, D., Drey, N. & Moralejo, D., et al., 2008. Interventions to improve hand hygiene compliance in patient care. Journal of Hospital Infection 68 (3), 193–202.

Hayward, J., 1975. Information – a prescription against pain (The study of nursing care project reports, series 2, no. 5). Royal College of Nursing, London.

Malone, B., 2005. Nursing is the backbone of the healthcare workforce. From a speech given at London's City University, *The Independent*, Friday, 11 March 2005.

McDonald, S., Hetrick, S.E., Green, S., 2004. Pre-operative education for hip or knee replacement. Cochrane Database of Systematic Reviews. Issue 1, Art. No.: CD003526. DOI: 10.1002/14651858.CD003526.pub2.

Nursing and Midwifery Council (NMC), 2004. Midwives rules and standards. NMC, London.

Nursing and Midwifery Council (NMC), 2008. The code: standards of conduct, performance and ethics for nurses and midwives. NMC, London.

Roe, B., Howell, F., Riniotis, K., et al., 2008. Older people's experience of falls: understanding, interpretation and autonomy. Journal of Advanced Nursing 63 (6), 586–596.

School of Health and Social Care, Oxford Brookes University, 2003. Support process for students with unconfirmed/confirmed dyslexia. QSH 24/2003. Oxford Brookes University, Oxford.

Schuldham, C.M., Fleming, S. & Goodman, H., 2002. The impact of pre-operative education on recovery following coronary artery bypass surgery. European Heart Journal 23, 666–674.

FURTHER READING

Bonnett, A., 2008. How to argue: essential skills for writing and speaking convincingly, 2nd edn. Pearson Education (US), Indiana.

Cottrell, S., 2005. Critical thinking skills: developing effective analysis and argument (Palgrave study guides). Palgrave Macmillan, Basingstoke, UK.

Greetham, B., 2008. How to write better essays, 2nd edn. Palgrave Macmillan, Basingstoke, UK.

Levin, P., 2004. Write great essays! Reading and essay writing for undergraduates and taught postgraduates. Open University Press, Buckingham, UK.

Examinations and revision

Heather Wharrad

Introduction

Examinations seem to create more anxiety for students than any other form of course assessment. In this chapter, you will learn strategies for preparing and revising for examinations and for optimizing your performance in the examination itself. Examinations are brief snap-shots of what you have learned from a period of study; by planning for them at the start of the course (and during it) you can minimize the stress you feel on the day of the examination. This cannot guarantee good results but it will give you the best chance of success.

Preparing for examinations

You will almost certainly have taken examinations before.

Think back to the last examination you took. How early in the course did you start to prepare for it? Did you feel confident on the day of the examination that you were fully prepared?

The chances are that you did not give much thought to the examination when you started your course – it probably seemed a long way off. When it came to the day of the examination you were probably wishing that you had been better prepared.

Be active not passive

Anxiety about an impending situation can lead people to be passive and 'just let it happen'. You should avoid leaving all your preparation to near the examination date. The more actively you plan and prepare for the examination at the beginning of (and throughout) the course, the more likely you are to succeed. Rhetorical comments such as 'Well, it's not in our hands' and 'What's in the exam's just a lottery' contribute to the feelings of helplessness experienced by students who feel that the lecturer is controlling the situation. Indeed, this principle applies equally to preparation for any type of assessment or placement: the more active and engaged you have been in preparing for the event, the more successful and rewarding it will be. One of the first tasks should be to check on the format of the examination paper(s) and the types of question you will be given.

Types of examination and question

Unseen examinations

Traditional unseen examinations (the student does not 'see' the question paper beforehand) are still the most common form of examination used, although the types of question on the papers can vary considerably. Some of the commonly used types of question are described in the box below.

Multiple-choice questions

These consist of a 'stem' (this is the question) and four or five branches (the answer choices). The student has to select one answer that, relative to the other choices, is correct.

Example
The normal number of pairs of human chromosomes in cells is:

| a. 48 | b. 47 | c. 46 | d. 23 |

Fill-in-the-gap questions

These questions require the student to enter the most appropriate word or phrase that fits into a gap in a statement. Sometimes students are given a list of responses to choose from.

Example
Fill the gap in the sentence below with the correct name of the procedure described.

A _____ is an artificial opening into the trachea at the level of the second or third cartilaginous ring, which is kept patent by the insertion of a metal or plastic tube.

[tracheonomy, tracheostomy, tracheotomy, bronchiostomy]

Short-answer questions

Students write short answers to a number of questions, the answers being anything up to one page in length. This type of question requires students to make concise, succinct points and they may be asked to draw a diagram to illustrate the answer. You should be clear about how many marks are allocated for these questions and obtain guidance from your lecturer about the length of answer expected, and whether bullet points, flow diagrams or illustrations are acceptable. Preferably, you should be given some 'model answers' as a guide.

Examples

1. Describe three criteria that promote wound healing.
2. Outline five factors that might cause an inaccurate measurement of oral body temperature.

Long-answer or essay questions

Essay questions require students to write at length about the questions posed. Marks are likely to be awarded on the structure of the essay – does it have an introduction and conclusion, does it flow logically – as well as on the content and inclusion of major points (see Chapter 9).

Open-book and seen examinations

Open-book (where you can use books during the examination) or seen examinations (where you see the questions before the examination and can therefore prepare your answers prior to the examination itself) are not as easy as they sound. In an open-book examination you will be penalized for copying down information word-for-word from the books; indeed, there are issues of plagiarism to consider too (see Chapter 5). You will need to be very familiar with the texts that you are expected to use so that you can go straight to relevant sections, otherwise you will spend a lot of time in the examination searching for the information.

In both these types of examination, you will be given marks for how you analyse the information and use it to develop a logical argument, and not for merely describing the information.

An open-book examination allows you to rely on the printed word for details; what it is testing is not your memory but how you can use the information to make a rational argument or analyse an issue.

A seen examination gives you time to gather relevant material and evidence and to think about the presentation and structure of your answer. Accordingly, the examination markers will expect you to present a more considered answer than in an unseen examination.

Practical examinations

Many nursing and midwifery courses now incorporate examinations of practical nursing skills into their assessments. The objective structured clinical examinations (OSCEs) are one type of practical assessment of nursing practice competence (Harden, 1988; Nicol and Bavin, 1999). During an OSCE, students rotate around a number of time-limited stations. These may comprise a patient scenario or situation devised to assess particular skills (e.g. taking blood pressure, assessing respiratory function or carrying out cardiopulmonary resuscitation), or the student might be required to complete a short, written assessment or interpret some clinical results. An examiner is present at each station, observing and scoring the performance according to predetermined objective criteria. The scoring systems used for OSCEs vary; an example scoring sheet indicating the criteria for a urine-testing station is shown in Figure 7.1.

Online examinations

Web-based course tools such as WebCT and Blackboard (http://www.blackboard.com) and software such as Questionmark (http://www.questionmark.com) enable examinations to be put online. The advantage of computerized examinations is that marking is done automatically within the computer application and a list of marks can be generated very quickly. Questions tend to be multiple-choice or fill-in-the-gap formats.

> ### *Viva voce* examinations
> *Viva voce* examinations are normally used to supplement other forms of assessment, such as dissertations. They normally take the form of interviews, in which students are questioned about selected sections of a piece of written work. Usually, a viva is used to convince examiners that a student is the 'owner' of a piece of work on the basis that the student can talk about it with familiarity and a certain amount of conviction. Vivas have often been used to help make decisions about borderline cases in degree award classifications and, less frequently, as a form of course assessment.

Examination preparation

At the start of the course

All students are supplied with course information, including learning outcomes or objectives, at the start of the course. You should also obtain information about the course assessments. Make sure you get as much information about the format of the examination (such as the number of papers, the length of the examinations and the types of question in the examination paper) as you can. This will help you to plan your revision and practise appropriate types of question when the time comes. It is also worth checking on the internet for web pages relating to the subject you are studying. More and more online nursing databases and sources of evidence for practice are being developed. Intute is a computer gateway to high-quality internet resources with a specific section related to health disciplines (http://www.intute.ac.uk/healthandlifesciences/nursing/). Intute provides only high-quality resources that have been through an academic review process. A number of open-access repositories contain free online resources and learning activities (sometimes called reusable learning objects or RLOs) to support your learning and revision (http://www.nottingham.ac.uk/nmp/sonet/rlos; http://openlearn.open.ac.uk/). Adding useful, high-quality web addresses to your list of favourites on your computer at this stage can save you time later when you are supplementing your notes, revising or looking for practice examination questions (see Chapter 5).

During the course

You will save time during your revision period if you follow the points listed below. Many students fall into the trap of thinking that they understood a teaching session until it comes to revising the material and then the concepts seem less clear. They then use their valuable revision time trying to make sense of the material, and they may have to seek assistance, perhaps from a lecturer – again, this can be very time consuming. By reviewing the lecture notes soon after the session you will ensure that you know whether you need to spend a little more time understanding the material and adding to your notes. A good test of your comprehension of the material is to try to write down a few key points to summarize the material covered in the session. You can then

Outline
The student will demonstrate the correct procedure for testing urine using labstix, identify any abnormal finding and give a possible cause and rationale for the abnormal finding.

Introduction
Greet the student and give the following information:
Assume two patients have provided a urine sample. The samples X and Y are here. Demonstrate how you would test the urine, identify any abnormal findings and state a possible cause with a brief rationale for the stated cause.

Time
8 minutes (1 min intro, 5 min practical, 2 min feedback).

Equipment
Urine sample, labstix, recording sheet.

Action	Score
Student identifies urine to be tested and prepares the record sheet	
Checks time	
Dips stick fully but briefly into the urine samples	
Taps excess urine back into the container	
Reads stick against reagent colours on the chart on bottle at approximately correct times	
Writes down findings on record	
Appropriately disposes of urine and used labstix and washes hands	
Identifies any abnormal finding(s)	
States a possible major cause of such abnormality	
Gives rationale for the stated cause	
TOTAL	

Key: Performs adequately – 1, Attempted but inadequate – 0.5, Not performed – 0

Signature: Student _____

Examiner _____

FIGURE 7.1 Example scoring sheet for an OSCE urine-testing station.

spend 5–10 minutes reading through these key points during the rest of the course. If you have had other coursework marked, use the lecturer's feedback to identify gaps in your knowledge or ways you need to improve your writing style.

- Make good notes and make sure they are complete (see Chapter 5)
- Review and summarize lecture notes as soon after the lecture as you can (see Chapter 5)
- Spend time understanding the material
- Read through summaries and key points regularly
- Learn from feedback from other assignments
- Underline and make marginal notes in your textbook or on handouts
- Link theory and practice components (see Chapters 10 and 11)

You will save yourself time during your revision period if you have underlined and made marginal notes in your textbooks or on handouts when you review and summarize your notes. This way, if there are points you need to check through again you will be able to go straight to the relevant sections of the textbook or handout. Even at this point you could give some thought to when you will begin your revision period. Some courses build a revision period into the timetable but you need to consider whether this is an appropriate length of time for you. At least provisionally planning your revision time at this stage means you are less likely to put off the revision planning as the course comes to an end, and you become more anxious about the impending examinations.

The final point in this section is about relating the theory and practice components of the course. Information is often much easier to remember when its use and relevance is seen in a 'real situation'. If you have a period of nursing or midwifery practice, look at your course notes to see where there are links with what you have practised and what you have seen in practice. Add marginal notes to remind you of these links (see Chapter 11).

At whatever stage you are at in your course, use the checklist below to find out how prepared you are for an impending examination. Have you:

- Read through the module objectives/learning outcomes?
- Checked the length and format of the examination?
- Got your notes up to date and complete?
- Supplemented notes using texts and websites?
- Made marginal notes about links with practice?
- Obtained practice examination papers?

Revision techniques

Your revision time is precious. It is a time for consolidating and organizing in your mind the material you have studied. You should not allow yourself to start looking at new information. Retaining a positive attitude at this stage is very important. Do not allow negative thoughts to enter your head; this will affect your concentration and reduce your efficiency.

There is no universal revision technique that suits everyone. The method you choose will depend on your personal preferences in the way you work and the type of course you are revising. You should also consider the format of the examination paper before you plan your revision strategy. A multiple-choice paper will cover a greater breadth of material than will a paper offering a choice of essay questions. This may influence whether you revise the whole course or focus on a number of key topics. If you have dyslexia the general rules for revising are no different to everybody else – you need to find the revision strategy that suits you best. The revision techniques will depend on whether dyslexia affects how you decode new words (dysphonetic dyslexia) or process visual information (dyseidetic dyslexia) and whether you have problems sequencing information. These will be addressed specifically in the following sections.

Planning your revision timetable

When planning your revision timetable, work out exactly how much time you have available – be realistic. You will not be able to work solidly for every hour of your waking day. Work out how long you will need for sleep, meals and recreation (see Chapter 1). It is important to allow yourself regular breaks in your revision time. Many students find it useful to draw a timetable grid like the one shown in Figure 7.2. Break down your study material into manageable chunks (the smaller the better, but this will obviously depend on the time you have available to revise) and place them into the time slots in the grid.

Adapt the grid shown to suit your own study style. For example, if you can only maintain your concentration for 40–60 minutes, have 1-hour time slots rather than the 2 hours shown. You might prefer to vary the topics from session to session within a day to retain your interest and concentration, or you may prefer to complete a whole topic before moving on to the next. If you find that your timetable slips, do not abandon it completely (and don't feel a failure either). Modify the timetable in whatever way is necessary to get you back on track.

Strategies for remembering information

The best strategy for remembering information is not to rely totally on short-term memory. Instead of soaking up the material like a sponge and regurgitating it during the examination, it is better to think it through and analyse it, make judgements about it and think how it relates to nursing and midwifery skills or practice settings. By performing these analytical and reflective processes, you are more likely to commit the

Week 1

	Monday	Tuesday	Wednesday	Thursday	Friday	Saturday
8.30 – 10.30	Anatomy	Microbiology	Revision group tutorial	Developmental psychology	Swimming	
11.00 – 13.00	Anatomy	Microbiology	Social policy	Developmental psychology	Health psychology	Health psychology
14.00 – 15.30	Play squash	Practise MCQs	Social policy	Developmental psychology	Health psychology	Shopping
16.00 – 17.30	Microbiology	Practise MCQs	Practise questions	Developmental psychology	Health psychology	Practise questions
19.00 – 20.30	Microbiology	Meet friends	Tennis	Practise questions	Club	Practise questions
21.00 – 23.00	Pub			Concert		Pub

Week 2

	Monday	Tuesday	Wednesday	Thursday	Friday	Saturday
8.30 – 10.30	Nursing theory	Nursing theory	Revision tutorial (lecturer)	Read revision notes	Exams	
11.00 – 13.00	Nursing theory	Nursing theory	Practise questions	Read revision notes	Exams	Relax
14.00 – 15.30	Play squash	Practise questions	Read revision notes	Practise questions	Exams	
16.00 – 17.30	Nursing theory	Practise questions	Read revision notes	Practise questions	Exams	
19.00 – 20.30	Nursing theory	Swimming	Tennis	Practise questions	Relax	
21.00 – 23.00	Pub			Meet friends		

FIGURE 7.2 A revision timetable.

information to your long-term memory, which is much more reliable than your short-term memory. There are, however, strategies you can use for remembering stages in a process, sequences of event or lists of items.

Association and visualization

If you have been making lists of key points or bullet points and have been reviewing them during the course, you will probably find that you can visualize the information on the page or card on which they are written. Processes or events can be drawn as flow charts, timelines or diagrams to explain a sequence of events or to link information. Mind maps are a useful way of remembering the relationships between concepts and ideas (Buzan and Buzan, 2000). Some examples of mind maps can be found at the Open University's 'Skills for OU Study' website (http://www.open.ac.uk/skillsforstudy/demo-creating-a-mind-map.php); the mind map shown in Figure 7.3 is taken from an article by Hendry and Farley (2003). Visualization approaches such as these can be a very powerful memory aid: we use them all the time in everyday situations such as visualizing what is in our wardrobe when choosing a new item of clothing or visualizing a room when choosing wallpaper or a new piece of furniture. Some examples of these ideas are given in Figure 7.4.

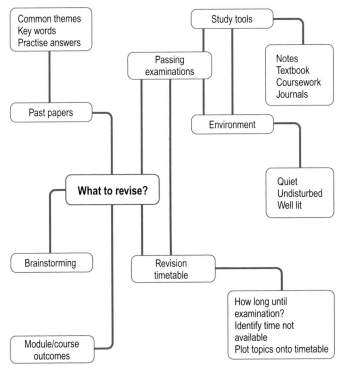

FIGURE 7.3 Example of a mind map (adapted from Hendry and Farley, 2003).

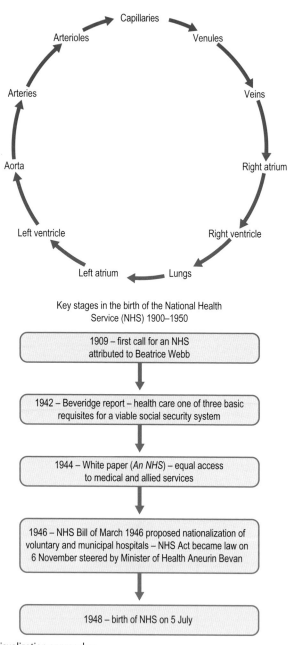

FIGURE 7.4 Visualization approaches.

Other ways of remembering your notes are to link topics with everyday objects or group things together verbally. Some people make up a story that incorporates the information they are trying to remember.

Using mnemonics; for example, the well-known mnemonic **R**ichard **O**f **Y**ork **G**ave **B**attle **I**n **V**ain, ensures that nobody forgets the colours of the rainbow and the order in which they appear (**R**ed, **O**range, **Y**ellow, **G**reen, **B**lue, **I**ndigo, **V**iolet).

Certain types of information can be remembered in the form of acronyms, for example NATO (North Atlantic Treaty Organization) or OMNI (Organizing Medical Networked Information) and rhymes (e.g. to remember the number of days in the months many people recite '30 days hath September, April, June and November...').

Can you think of a mnemonic to help you to remember the names of the different white blood cells in the body? These are basophils, eosinophils, lymphocytes, neutrophils and monocytes.

How about: 'Basil Eats Live Newts Mondays'.

During your course, you will be spending time in practice, or you may be learning practical skills in a skills laboratory. Students often find it easier to remember information if it is linked to practical skills or to other practical experiences. When you are in practice or learning these practical skills, think about the theory you have been doing in the classroom. The association you make between the theory and practice may help you to remember more of the information in an examination.

Repetition

Memory depends on repetition. Whether it is learning a technique or remembering certain facts, the more times you practise a technique or read through information the more likely you are to remember it. Try the following ways:

- write the information out a number of times
- repeat it out loud
- record it and replay
- read, recite then check.

Only the last of these needs some explanation: 'read, recite then check'. The best way of carrying out this exercise is to cover each set of key points in turn, then expose only the headings relating to your key points. Recite all the key points you can remember relating to that heading, uncover the key points to check how many you have remembered. If you are satisfied with your answers, move on to the next heading. If you missed out some important points, repeat the process until you get it right.

Try these repetition methods now with notes from a recent teaching session. Rather than relying on just one of the methods listed above, alternate between them, this will help to retain your interest.

Revision tips for students with dyslexia

- Dysphonetic dyslexia (problem with decoding new words): experiment with using spidergrams, mind maps or annotated drawings, also placing sticky labels in different places so that you revise as you walk round (kinaesthetic revision technique).
- Dyseidetic dyslexia (visual processing problems): experiment with auditory methods of revision such as mnemonics and the use of audio recordings.
- Sequencing problems: focus on association methods and using either auditory, visual or kinaesthetic approaches.
- Short-term memory problems: commit the material to the long-term memory by revising small chunks at a time and by giving yourself plenty of time to revise.

Self- and peer-testing

It is crucial to test yourself on what you have learned and revised; only then will you know how much you have understood and remembered.

- Write out half a dozen headings then jot down the key points under each sub-heading
- Make up some practice questions yourself or, better still, ask for some past papers or example questions from your lecturers
- Many textbooks now have self-test or self-assessment questions at the end of chapters; check your own textbooks

Self-testing requires self-discipline. Be strict with yourself – the more you test, the more you remember. Many students find great benefit in working with friends or groups, discussing topics and testing each other. This can create a very supportive environment in which to work.

Four key words underpin a successful revision strategy. Remember the first letters – PQRS – to remind you what they are:

- Planning
- Question practice
- Repetition
- Self- and peer-testing.

The P represents planning early and throughout the course. Q refers to question practice as often as you can. R is for repetition – the more times you practise a skill or go through the course material, the more likely you are to remember it. S is for self- and peer-testing. This will give you confidence in the coursework you do understand and will highlight any gaps in your understanding.

The night before and on the day of the examination

The night before the examination, check your timetable and organize pens, pencils and any other instruments you might need for the examination. Reading through your key points will not do any harm but cramming at this stage is probably not helpful. Check your timetable again when you wake up and give yourself plenty of time to eat a meal and travel to the examination. Try to fill the time before the examination with practical things rather than dwelling on what questions might come up on the paper. Arrive at the examination in good time, take some deep breaths and don't decide that everyone else looks far more confident than you do. Remember to switch off your mobile phone or leave it at home.

During the examination

General advice for all types of examination

Read right through the paper (for up to 5 minutes) and jot down any facts that occur to you as you read. This will help you to relax and give you confidence. Read through the instructions for candidates carefully and underline important instructions, such as the number of questions you have to answer in each section or that you have to write your answer on separate sheets.

Underline the key instructions on the front sheet of the exam paper below:

University of Trentham, School of Nursing and Midwifery

Semester 4 examination

Time allowed: 2 hours

Candidates should attempt to answer all questions in each of four sections. Answers should be written in the answer book provided.

Write each answer on a new page.

You should have underlined '2 hours', 'all questions', 'four sections', 'answer book' and 'new page' as the key instructions.

Spend a little time identifying what precisely each question is asking. Some of the 'action' words that might be used are shown in the box below, with brief definitions of what they mean. Underline these and other key words in the question.

- Analyse: explain the relationships between . . . (sometimes more vaguely stated as 'Comment on')
- Assess: determine the importance or value of . . . (sometimes more vaguely stated as 'Comment on')
- Compare: explain the commonalities (similarities) and differences between . . . (more emphasis on commonalities)
- Contrast: explain the commonalities and differences between . . . (more emphasis on differences)
- Critique/critically analyse: explain relationships and provide evidence for and against the relationships
- Define: state precisely and succinctly the meaning of . . .
- Describe: write what something is like, how something happens or what its main characteristics are
- Discuss: write a logical argument on . . . (may require you to analyse, critique, evaluate, explain . . .)
- Evaluate: for something that has already happened . . . use evidence to estimate its importance
- Explain: give reasons for . . . or say how something works
- Illustrate: use examples to demonstrate a point, e.g. statistics, diagrams, graphs
- Justify: say, giving valid evidence, why something is true
- List: provide a column or row of relevant items, with no description
- Outline: point out the main features of . . .
- Prove: use logical steps and evidence to establish the truth of . . .
- Review: look back over something and comment on its value
- State: write down the main points
- Summarize: write down the main points without all the detail
- Trace: follow the pathway of . . .

Underline the key action words in the exam question shown below.

Section 4 (25 marks)

Answer all the questions

1. Explain what is meant by immobility (2 marks)

2. Discuss the effects of immobility on three body systems (10 marks)

3. Describe, with rationale, measures that may be taken to prevent/alleviate the effects you identify (10 marks)

4. List three devices that might help a client who is immobile to carry out activities of daily living (3 marks)

You should have identified the key 'action' words as underlined below. Also, note carefully the number of marks allocated to each question, this determines how much time you should spend on each part:

<u>Section 4 (25 marks)</u>
Answer all the questions

1. <u>Explain</u> what is meant by immobility (<u>2 marks</u>)
2. <u>Discuss</u> the effects of immobility on three body systems (<u>10 marks</u>)
3. <u>Describe, with rationale</u>, measures that may be taken to <u>prevent/alleviate</u> the effects you identify (<u>10 marks</u>)
4. <u>List three</u> devices that might <u>help</u> a client who is immobile to carry out activities of daily living (<u>3 marks</u>)

Re-read the questions and answer your best question first. As you work through the paper, jot down any thoughts that come into your mind about answers to other questions. If you don't write ideas down immediately, the chances are you will forget them. If you miss out part of a question, meaning to return to it later, mark it clearly, so it stands out and you don't forget to answer it. Leave some space at the end of your answer in case you want to add another point later. Check your answers, and check that you have answered all the questions. If at the last minute you find you have forgotten to do a whole question, or you have run out of time, write an answer in note form with subheadings (similar to your revision key notes). You might gather a few extra marks this way.

Essay questions

Spend at least 5 minutes planning your answer before you start to write your essay. Jot down main ideas and important ideas as bullet points in rough. Write a brief introduction to your essay. In the introduction, refer to the question being asked. This will serve two purposes. First, it signposts the essay for the examiner and, second (and just as importantly), it will ensure that you focus on all parts of the question being asked. Many students make the error of writing a good examination answer on a similar but wrong topic and get no marks at all. After reading the question and recalling some of the key information in your mind, ask yourself 'Am I recalling the correct information for this question?' Don't allow yourself to waffle or over-answer – you won't get more marks and you might run out of time. You are likely to get more marks for two half-answered questions than for one answered and one unanswered. While you are writing your answers, think about the following points:

- Are you dealing with the major issues?
- Are you writing simply and directly to the point?
- Are you writing legibly, without misspellings and grammatical errors?
- Are you making drawings bold and clear?

Your plan should help you to write down the points you want to make in a logical order. You should always end your essay with a conclusion, drawing together all the points you have made in the main body of the answer.

Multiple-choice examinations

Multiple-choice examinations require as much revision preparation as any other type of examination. There is a tendency for some students to do less preparation and to rely on guesswork, rather than putting in the revision and practice time to allow them to make rational and logical judgements about the answers. You should remember that multiple-choice questions allow coverage of a greater breadth of material than other types of questions and require detailed knowledge and logical thought as well.

Multiple-choice examination papers are often marked mechanically and inappropriate pen marks could result in incorrect marking. Read the instructions carefully. Make sure that you don't mark two answers. If you mean to go back and decide on which you think is the correct response at the end of the examination – don't forget. Indicate these questions clearly to remind yourself.

Scoring systems in multiple-choice examinations vary. You should be clear about these before the examination and, ideally, you should have practised your technique. For example, if there is what is called 'negative marking' for incorrect answers, then you cannot make a guess at an answer you are unsure of. However, if there is no such penalty, it is reasonable to make a guess at the answer.

It is particularly important to read every multiple-choice question very carefully. Sometimes there may be a qualifying phrase that completely changes the meaning of the questions. You should also watch out for 'double negatives'. To clarify the meaning, try to translate double-negative statements into positive ones, for example 'not true' would become 'false', and 'not lacking' becomes 'having'. You can see in the examples in the box below how easy it is to be confused by a double negative and give a totally wrong answer.

Underline negative words, such as 'not', and qualifying phrases, in the questions below:

1. Which of the following is not an uncommon systemic symptom of inflammation?
   a. paralysis
   b. shock
   c. nausea
   d. fever

2. Uncontrolled type 1 diabetes is associated with which one of the following:
   a. a decreased urine output
   b. low blood glucose levels
   c. high blood glucose levels
   d. high levels of insulin in the bloodstream

3. Which of the following is false? Respiratory rate:
   a. in a newborn baby is faster than in an adult
   b. cannot be altered consciously
   c. is controlled by the medulla
   d. increases during exercise

You should have identified the words underlined below as those that are key to the meaning of the question. Misreading these words will totally change the meaning of the question and lead to you giving a wrong answer:

1. Which of the following is <u>not</u> an <u>uncommon</u> systemic symptom of inflammation?
   a. paralysis
   b. shock
   c. nausea
   d. fever

2. <u>Uncontrolled</u> diabetes mellitus is <u>associated</u> with which <u>one</u> of the following:
   a. a <u>decreased</u> urine output
   b. <u>low</u> blood glucose levels
   c. <u>high</u> blood glucose levels
   d. <u>high</u> levels of insulin in the bloodstream

3. Which of the following is <u>false</u>? Respiratory rate:
   a. in a newborn baby is <u>faster</u> than in an adult
   b. <u>cannot</u> be altered consciously
   c. <u>is</u> controlled by the medulla
   d. <u>increases</u> during exercise

Online computer delivery is becoming more commonplace for multiple-choice examinations. Computer packages (known as virtual learning environments) such as WebCT and Blackboard allow tutors to create tests and examinations relatively easily and have the advantage that marking is done quickly and automatically by the computer.

Preparation for these computerized examinations should be the same as for a paper-based examination. However, you should make sure you have used the computer package before the day of your examination so that you know how to log into it, have read the instructions about how to navigate around the package and understand the instructions about how to submit your answers.

Exam arrangements for students with dyslexia

If you have dyslexia, you are entitled to exam accommodations (special arrangements). Most commonly this is extra time (normally 15 minutes extra for a 1-hour examination). Other accommodations might include the use of a laptop computer or a separate room in which to sit the exam. You will need to visit your university or college special needs or learning support office to find out what exam accommodations you are entitled to. Make sure you do this in plenty of time before you are due to take the exam, preferably at the start of the term. There is a useful website with information for students with dyslexia at http://www.dyslexia-college.com/exam.html.

Coping with examination anxiety

It is perfectly natural to feel nervous and anxious about examinations. It is the nature of this type of assessment that creates this stress. Examinations are a one-off assessment requiring our best performance on the day. When you have worked hard throughout a course, you want to do yourself justice by performing well and achieving a high mark.

One of the physiological responses to stress is to produce more of the hormone adrenaline (epinephrine). Adrenaline puts us into 'fight or flight' mode – we can either face the challenge and give it our best shot, or we can run away from it. Whatever the challenge, be it public speaking, running a race, performing a solo or taking an examination, the extra 'nervous energy' can be used to enhance performance. By remaining focused and positive about the examination, you will find that your heightened state of anxiety will enable you to concentrate for longer periods and remain more focused on your work. During your period of revision, there will be a great temptation to use this energy for 'displacement' activities, such as tidying 'that' cupboard because you just can't put up with it any longer (even though it's been just as untidy for the last 6 months). You must try to avoid such displacement activity and focus on your revision. The other activity to avoid is panic conversation with your peers. This can waste a lot of time and will only serve to exaggerate negative thoughts. Remember, you have a revision timetable to stick to. If you feel you are getting over-anxious then talk to a lecturer or a student counsellor about it. They will be very experienced in dealing with these problems.

- Some anxiety is natural and will enhance your concentration and performance
- Channel your nervous energy into focusing on the task in hand
- Eliminate negative thoughts, remain positive and active
- Don't disrupt your normal eating, sleeping and recreational routine too much: this can worsen symptoms of stress

Support from social networking sites

Online chat rooms and discussion forums provide opportunities for students to seek help and support when preparing for OSCEs and examinations. For example, the StudentMidwife.NET (http://www.studentmidwife.net/) is an online education based community supporting student midwives; the site provides a range of discussion topics including an OSCEs and exams theme.

After the examination

Before the sense of relief you feel after the examination, you will naturally go over the paper in your mind and discuss your answers with your peers. Try not to dwell too long on these 'post-mortems', especially if you have other examinations to do. It is important to keep your morale high. You have probably done better than you think.

Ten tips for passing examinations:

1. Do some work regularly throughout the course
2. Be active and positive, not passive and negative
3. Start working towards the examination *now*
4. Manage your stress levels
5. Test yourself regularly
6. Ask for help sooner rather than later
7. Plan a timetable for study and revision
8. Don't stop all your recreational activities in the run up to the examination
9. Get an overview of the course material as well as the detail
10. Make links between theory and practice

Conclusion

This chapter has given you a range of strategies to help you to prepare for examinations. By building some of these strategies into your study plans, you will increase your chances of being successful and reduce the stress and workload in the days before the examination.

CHAPTER RESOURCES

REFERENCES

Buzan, T. & Buzan, B., 2000. The mind map book, revised edn. BBC Consumer Publishing, London.

Harden, R.M., 1988. What is an OSCE? Medical Teacher 10 (1), 19–22.

Hendry, C. & Farley, A., 2003. Examinations: a practical guide for students. Nursing Standard 17 (29), 48–53.

Nicol, M. & Bavin, C., 1999. Clinical skills learning: teaching and assessment strategies. In: Nicol, M. & Glen, S. (Eds.) Clinical skills in nursing: return of the practical room? Macmillan, Basingstoke, UK.

WEBSITES

The following links also provide some useful tips on coping with examinations and how to develop good revision techniques:

Bournemouth University Academic Support Study Support Exam Revision: http://www.bournemouth.ac.uk/study_support/exam_revision.html

Skills for OU Study Exams Revision and Assessment: http://www.open.ac.uk/skillsforstudy/revising-exams-and-assessment.php

StudentMidwife.NET: your student midwife support network: http://www.studentmidwife.net/osces-and-exams/

University of Manchester Faculty of Humanities Introduction to Exams and Revision: http://www.humanities.manchester.ac.uk/studyskills/exams/

FURTHER READING

You may find the following texts and articles helpful in developing your revision strategies and improving your examination technique:

Acres, D., 1994. How to pass exams without anxiety: every candidate's guide to success, 3rd edn. Northcote House, Plymouth.

Gibbs, G., 1994. Improving student learning: through assessment and evaluation. Oxford Brookes University, Oxford.

Hendry, C. & Farley, A., 2003. Examinations: a practical guide for students. Nursing Standard 17 (29), 48–53.

Information-seeking for assignments

Abigail Masterson and Netta Lloyd-Jones

KEY ISSUES

- Information-searching skills
- The internet
- Purposeful reading
- Evaluating different sources of information
- Primary and secondary sources

Introduction

As nurses and midwives, we must continually update ourselves professionally so that our practice is underpinned by the best knowledge available. To write meaningfully about a topic, you need to be able to identify the right sources of information and to review these in a systematic, organized and purposeful way. You can draw on many different information sources to inform your assignment preparation, including journal articles, books and research reports – available in libraries and from electronic sources – and expert opinion.

Information-seeking skills need to be learned and practised. Being able to evaluate what you read in journals, books and on the internet is fundamental to knowledge-based practice. Having read and worked through the activities in this chapter, you should be able to take appropriate notes and make decisions about the relevance and usefulness of different information sources.

The information-seeking principles we discuss apply to all types of assignments – essays, case studies, reports, dissertations or reflections on practice.

Preparation

It is important to start collecting information for assignments early. If you leave your preparation to the last minute, you will reduce your opportunities to secure the most appropriate information from the widest range of sources. Many web and intranet sites now offer full-text journal articles and research reports but often these require you to be registered with the appropriate company and/or to pay to download them. In 2008, a full-text article from the *Journal of Advanced Nursing* cost £30, although your higher education institution's (HEI) library and/or your professional association's library may offer some full-text journals online for free. Your placement organization or employer may have access too. Planning your time carefully and finding out about – and making the best use of – your local library facilities should be part of your preparation.

- Find out the opening times of the libraries that you will need to use. Remember that libraries may be closed or have reduced opening hours during holiday times. Most libraries allow free or cheap access to the internet but such sessions often have to be booked in advance.

- Find out which range of online journals your HEI subscribes to. You can search them by using the library catalogue. Most HEIs subscribe to Athens, which allows you to access full-text articles. This will require you to have a password and your course provider will provide you with details on how to access these systems.

- Identify how long you will allow yourself for getting together resources, how long for reading and how long for writing and editing. It is often tempting to be completely caught up in reading and gathering together more and more resources. Be sure to leave yourself time to actually read all the information you have collected properly and to write the assignment.

Making the best use of your resources

It is always worth taking some time to identify the most appropriate and relevant resources (see Chapter 3 for more details). Such resources should also include people who have a particular expertise in the area, or with whom it would be useful to talk through your ideas. For example, if you are working on an essay about the nursing care of a patient with diabetes, it might be useful to talk through your ideas with a patient who has this problem, a representative of an interest group such Diabetes UK and/or the local diabetes nurse specialist. If you are writing on a professional issue such as accountability and midwifery practice then you might find it helpful to seek the perspective of the Supervisor of Midwives in your practice area, and to contact the Nursing and Midwifery Council and/or your professional association/ trade union. If there are several of you all working on a similar topic or area, it might be helpful to share information-seeking strategies, pool your resources and try out your ideas on each other. Also, if you collaborate in this way you will not have to spend so much time individually in the library searching the literature, surfing the internet and photocopying articles.

Remember that your mentor and the other members of the team you are working in are important sources of information and ideas regarding resources available locally.

Planning

It is important to spend time thinking about your assignment before you start your literature search, and to talk to your patient/client if it is a case study. This thinking should involve clarifying the topic, jotting down your thoughts and listing all the questions and issues that occur to you. This type of approach should ensure that your reading becomes purposeful. It is crucial to focus on exactly what the assignment requires. It is often tempting to read things just because they are interesting rather than because you are absolutely clear that they are relevant. Equally, if you are not sure of your focus you may waste time going off on tangents and getting together loads of material that you do not end up using (see Chapter 5 for further tips and hints).

Imagine you have been asked to write a case study that demonstrates your understanding of theories of psychosocial development and their use in assessing the problems of a child within their family context and identifying appropriate interventions. Note down the key issues you would wish to include.

Your list might look something like this:

- Introduce Amy and her family. Explain your role in relation to Amy and her family. Explain why you have chosen to focus on them for this particular case study.
- Use a genogram to help explain Amy's family structure, the subsystems within her family, and the strength of relationships between different family members.
- Describe Amy's stage of psychosocial development, using Erikson's eight stages of psychosocial development.
- Use Carter and McGoldrick's (2005) family life-cycle stages to consider the family's current life-cycle stage(s).
- Use the Calgary Family Assessment Model (Wright and Leahey, 2001) to assess family functioning and to highlight family strengths and difficulties.
- Use evidence from your observations of and interactions with Amy and her family to support your assessment.
- Describe the key factors that have influenced the development of the presenting problem. Summarize the problem(s) as you now understand them (backing this up with relevant literature).
- Reflect on the appropriateness and effectiveness of interventions that you and other members of the multidisciplinary team were involved in implementing as part of your role with Amy and her family.

Information-seeking skills

Collecting material and resources for your assignment involves being systematic and organized. It is vital to record accurate details of what you are reading, however time consuming or irritating this may seem initially. When carrying out literature searches it is particularly important to note down the full reference, including the year of publication and the name and place of the publisher. In edited books it is necessary to record the names of the editors and the names of the authors, page numbers and titles of the individual chapters you wish to refer to. Some journals unfortunately do not include the details such as year of publication and volume and issue numbers on every page. Unless you write these on the copy of the article at the time, even though you have a photocopy of the article, you may waste valuable time finding these details again later.

Recording references

You should record each book, chapter, article and report that you read. The best way of recording and storing this type of information is by using a software package such as Reference Manager or EndNote. These allow you to type in details as you go, to insert references into the text of your assignment and to create a list of your references – in the style required by your education institution – either as a separate document or added to the end of your assignment. Most will also allow you to save references you have found on the internet. The end result is your own database of sources, which will provide a useful resource for life-long learning. Taking time to learn how to do use this type of software is extremely worthwhile (see Chapter 4 for a further discussion). For example, the information that should be recorded for a book is:

Andrew S 2008 Mixed methods research for nursing and the health sciences. Wiley-Blackwell, Oxford

For a journal article:

Lakeman R, Fitzgerald M 2008 How people live with or get over being suicidal: a review of qualitative studies. Journal of Advanced Nursing 64(2):114–126

For a chapter in an edited book:

Bennett J 2008 Supporting recovery: medication management in mental health care. In JE Lynch, S Trenoweth (eds) Contemporary issues in mental health nursing. Wiley, Chichester, pp 117–132

And for an internet resource:

Care Services Improvement Partnership (CSIP) and Valuing People Support Team (2008) Resources. Online. Available: http://valuingpeople.gov.uk/dynamic/valuingpeople59.jsp [last accessed 29 September 2008]

Some parts of the generic format are not always applicable to all electronic publications. With paper-based resources, it is often useful to note down where the reference is kept. For example, did it come from a particular library or did you borrow it from someone? Noting down the class number and accession number can also help speed things up if you need to find the same reference again. If you are using electronic resources be sure to note down the full internet/intranet address so that you can locate the reference again should you need to. The subject matter of the reference should be noted too, along with the key points of argument or information it contains.

For example, if you were writing an essay about disability and pregnancy, a useful reference, which you might come across in your literature search, is McKay-Moffatt (2008) Disability in pregnancy and childbirth. Churchill Livingstone/Elsevier, Oxford. Your card on McKay-Moffat (2008) might look something like this:

> Seems to be the only book on the subject. Notes that although an increasing number of women with disabilities are having children, their needs are not always effectively met. Explores the social construction of disability and motherhood. Offers some case-based material of the experiences of women with physical and/or learning disabilities using maternity services. Suggests how accessibility can be improved with appropriate signage, equipment and use of height-adjustable beds, cots and incubators, etc. Discusses how midwives' skills, knowledge and attitudes towards disability impact. Stresses the importance of the advocacy role of the midwife and the need for the midwife to liaise with other health professionals to ensure that women with disabilities receive appropriate care throughout pregnancy.

A review of research into the use of complementary therapies for symptom control in cancer nursing might lead you to the 2008 article in *Cancer Nursing* 'Reflexology for symptom relief in patients with cancer' by Wilkinson et al. The notes section in your Reference Manager entry might look like this:

> A systematic review – using Cochrane principles – which examines the research evidence base for the effectiveness of reflexology in cancer care. It aimed to identify whether reflexology:
>
> – reduced physical symptoms such as pain, nausea, fatigue, and constipation
>
> – reduced psychological symptoms such as anxiety, and
>
> – improved quality of life and produced any unwanted adverse effects.
>
> Concluded that because of the paucity of data in the five trials, no firm conclusions can be drawn about the effectiveness of reflexology for the relief of cancer treatment symptoms and comorbidities.

It is helpful to note down any direct quotes that you may want to use. For example, on page 359, Wilkinson et al. note that:

> The fact that there were no positive differences in favour of reflexology between sham and authentic reflexology is attributed to the non-specific effects of the intervention with both groups of patients benefiting from the opportunity to discuss their concerns and fears. The studies which showed that patients benefited almost as much or more from non-specific foot massage when provided by trained reflexologists than from genuine reflexology raise important questions about non-specific effects (common to all practitioner-based complementary therapies) about the active ingredient in reflexology and the relative cost-effectiveness of the use of trained reflexologists; these findings were not dependent on sample size or methodological quality.

The key is being succinct but informative. You might find it helpful to keep the question and your initial brainstormed plan close to you while you are reading to make sure that you extract only relevant information and do not get completely snowed under with notes.

The internet

The internet consists of millions of magazine-style pages containing text and images, plus multimedia elements such as sound samples, animations, video clips and learning objects. Most institutions and many individuals now have websites. Educational institutions provide information about their courses and often a range of interactive learning materials and resources, discussion boards and learning objects to guide reflection. You can access online bibliographic databases such as CINAHL, MEDLINE, the Midwives Information and Resource Service (MIDIRS), the British Nursing Index (BNI) and Athens. Some of these require you or your institution to be registered and can only be accessed using a password. There are also news services provided by organizations such as the BBC and CNN, online newspapers, such as *The Guardian* and *The Times*. Professional magazines such as the *Nursing Standard* and *Nursing Times* have an online version. Charities, support groups and pressure groups use websites to give details of how you can help them, what support is available for patients and families and information about the cause of the condition with which they are involved. Individuals with particular interests use websites to share their knowledge – this can range from obscure hobbies and interests to advances in cancer care (see also Chapters 3 and 4).

Wikipedia is an internet-based, free-content encyclopaedia project written collaboratively by volunteers. It was created in 2001 and is now one of the largest reference websites. Over 684 million people used Wikipedia in 2008. Every day, hundreds of thousands of visitors from around the world make tens of thousands of edits and create thousands of new articles to enhance the knowledge held by the Wikipedia encyclopaedia. Visitors do not need particular qualifications to contribute; this means that people of all ages and cultural and social backgrounds can, and do, write Wikipedia articles. Anyone can add information, cross-references or citations. As a result, concerns have been expressed about the quality and reliability of information available on Wikipedia; arguably, however, it is subject to more extensive scrutiny and review than more traditional sources of knowledge and inaccurate or disputed information is likely to be rapidly removed.

A great deal of information is devoted to health, nursing, midwifery and related topics on the internet. Much of this is American but the amount of information from the UK and other countries is growing rapidly. Pages are connected together by hypertext links, enabling you to move about by clicking on underlined text or highlighted images. For example, a page on human immunodeficiency virus (HIV) and acquired immune deficiency syndrome (AIDS) might have links to pages on drug treatments, complementary therapies and support services. You can also go directly to a particular page if you know its address.

Internet search tools

Searching the internet can be frustrating at first but, with a little practice, it is possible to locate information quickly and efficiently. Using search engines and subject gateways can help.

Search engines like Google gather websites automatically – there is no human intervention and no quality control. You will get lots of results but many might not be relevant to your needs. You have to create your own search terms and so it is always useful to look at the help pages provided, as each search engine works in a slightly different way and knowing how best to organize your search terms can save time and greatly improve your search results. Subject gateways provide access to evaluated websites so the quality is generally higher.

Try out the following internet search tools:

- Google: http://www.google.com
- Yahoo: http://www.yahoo.com
- Subject gateway to nursing, midwifery and the allied health professions: http://www.intute.ac.uk/healthandlifesciences/nursing/

Each offers different features. Follow their instructions on how to refine your search.

Discussion groups

Most internet service providers (ISPs) provide the means to subscribe to discussion groups. These are special-interest groups where you can follow or contribute to a discussion, ask questions and network. Many education providers also offer students discussion groups on their intranets.

Selecting sources and deciding relevance

It is much easier to read something if you have some idea about what it is going to be about and are sure that it is likely to be relevant or useful. To this end, research reports are usually prefaced with an abstract. This summarizes why the study was done, what it is about and what the main findings and conclusions were; it also includes a list of key words. In book chapters, this sort of information is usually included in the first paragraph or introduction. In this book, for example, the introduction states quite clearly what the contents of the book are, the order in which they are covered and who is likely to find the book helpful. In journal articles, this information might be included in the introduction and/or the abstract if there is one.

Well-constructed books will also have a list of contents and an index. It is useful to scan both of these to see whether or not there is any explicit reference made to the topic you are studying. Then turn to the relevant pages and scan them quickly, focusing particularly on headings and subheadings in order to see whether or not it contains anything useful.

Purposeful reading

To check the relevance and appropriateness, it is necessary to read the whole thing right through, carefully and thoroughly. This section builds on the reading skills that you worked on in Chapter 5. All the time you are reading keep stopping and reviewing what you have read. This will help you to weave new ideas and information into your own thinking in order to reach a new level of understanding about a subject or topic. It is often useful to mentally ask yourself questions as you read. Some examples are given in the box below.

'Is this an account of a research study or someone's views and opinions?'

There are many interesting, well-informed journal articles, web-based materials and books written by well-known authors but if your assignment asks you to review recent research then it would not be appropriate to include them. If, however, you are reviewing the literature to ascertain the current understanding of a phenomenon such as spiritual aspects of care, then such opinion articles, if well justified and referenced, would become relevant.

'How recent is the work/ideas being discussed?'

There is often a gap between writing and publishing of as much as 2–3 years. Journal articles tend to reach publication more quickly than books, although the work they report on may be a few years old. Articles can be published on the internet instantly. Some areas of nursing and midwifery are changing very quickly so the information in books may be almost out of date as soon as it is published. Or the recommendations may have been superseded by more up-to-date knowledge. This does not necessarily mean that it should be discarded; it depends on the question or topic area that you are trying to address. For some topics, an historical context might be very important. For example, if you were writing an historical account of changes in the education and preparation of nurses and midwives, or developments in nursing and midwifery interventions, then some quotes from original textbooks and journal articles would provide a rich source of examples.

'What country does the author come from and what country are they writing about?'

Increasingly, libraries stock books and journals from other English-speaking countries and many British journals contain articles from authors working in other countries. Although some aspects are common to all countries, others are not. Drug names, for example, are different in the USA and the UK, the length of education and the way nurses and midwives are taught differs in Australia, the law in Scotland and England is different. Depending on what you are writing about, these differences will be relevant or not. If you are writing about developments in the field of mental health nursing it may well be relevant to draw some cross-national comparisons. If, however, you are discussing the merits of different wound dressings, you need to be sure you are comparing like with like. Finally, a discussion of legal issues regarding the rights of people with a learning disability would need to be confined to a particular country.

'Why is the author/researcher writing this?'

A midwife researcher who has been sponsored by a baby-milk company to conduct research into patterns of breast feeding might have been encouraged to show bottle feeding in a positive light. Similarly, a patient/client education leaflet about the treatment of leg ulcers that has been sponsored by a wound-dressing manufacturer will probably suggest that the manufacturer's own products are particularly helpful.

'What are the points the writer/researcher is making? Are these points validated and justified by other literature or research?'

In some areas of nursing and midwifery practice there are differences of opinion about the 'right' way to intervene or support patients/clients with particular problems or the right way to organize things. For example, there is a lot of apparently contrary evidence in areas such as pressure-area care and wound healing; there is also a growing body of research and opinion articles supporting midwifery-led care (in which the same midwife sees the woman for all her care: antenatally, during labour and following birth), yet there are other reputable studies that advocate team midwifery.

'Do I agree with the inferences and conclusions the writer has made?'

In research studies in particular it is extremely important to read carefully all the titles or captions that accompany tables, charts and diagrams. Well-constructed work should flow logically and the foundations for the conclusions that are eventually drawn should be apparent throughout.

'Do I understand it?'

The unclear or overwhelming will usually make sense if you take the time to read what it says. It is helpful to be able to change your reading speed so that you can skim over the easy bits quickly but take your time during the difficult bits. How quickly you read also depends on *why* you are reading. For a key resource, it might be vital to spend a lot of time reading an article or book chapter to pick up every single point and nuance that it contains. Alternatively, if you are attempting to get a broad perspective on the range of opinion in a particular area then skim-reading several sources could be more beneficial.

Unfortunately, some of the academic writing in nursing and midwifery is very jargon ridden and is unnecessarily complicated, which can be very confusing, off-putting and frustrating at first. Specialists always develop their own language because it gives them extra power in analysing their subject in a detailed and systematic way. As you study subjects in greater depth and become a 'specialist' yourself, you will gradually find yourself using the same technical language without even noticing. For example, you may already find that you are beginning to talk about 'therapeutic relationships' and 'obs', 'MIs' instead of heart attacks and that you are comfortable using words such as 'symbolic interactionism' and 'dysphasia'. Using technical language helps develop new ideas and new words are part of the process of developing knowledge about a subject.

'How does this work fit with the rest of what I have read?'

It is important to be clear about the chronological order of developments. There is no point in rejecting someone's work because it does not allow for some development that occurred 10 years after it was written. Ideas are refined and developed over time. For example, good practice in care of the elderly settings in the 1970s in the UK involved a focus on maintaining safety and fostered dependence on nursing staff, whereas nowadays good care is seen as upholding the right of older people to be independent and to take risks. Similarly, some diversity of opinion is beneficial, and informed debate is healthy and necessary, but it is important to be clear about what the differing stances are and the merits or otherwise of a maverick opinion or finding.

'How does this work fit in with my own experience?'

It is often useful to think about occasions and events in which you have come across similar patients/clients or problems to those you are reading about and to consider how the author's point of view or description fits with your own.

'What are its strengths and limitations?'

Being able to evaluate the merit of a piece of work and the arguments or information that it contains is crucial. It is often useful to evaluate what you are reading in relation to your own practice and nursing as a whole.

Note taking

You might be wondering whether it is necessary to take notes, when you could just print off web pages and photocopy every text source you need. However, printing web pages can be very time consuming and expensive. If possible, download and save the information on to a memory stick (or disk) to read later. *Note*: some sites – particularly commercial ones – prevent you from doing this and public libraries don't always let you put your own disk into their computer drives. Photocopying is quick and is particularly useful for journal articles but can get very expensive. With books, there are restrictions about how much you are legally allowed to photocopy. Consequently, it is useful to learn how to take appropriate notes.

It can be useful to highlight key words, points and phrases on photocopies. However, if you are likely to use the same article again for something else then it may be better just to underline the salient bits in pencil, which can then be rubbed off when you are finished. If the book or article is your property, you might find it helpful to jot down in the margins comments, thoughts, questions and examples that came into your mind as you read it. When using e-journals, you can download the article and then use electronic tools to highlight particular sentences and paragraphs.

Note taking forces you to think as you read because you have to decide what to write down and clarify your interpretation of what you are reading. Notes should not merely summarize the text, they should identify the key words, points and phrases related to your purpose. The notes you require for a complex, key text will be very different from the notes you write to summarize an article that you just happened to read in passing. Different people acquire and store information in different ways but, generally, you need to think 'What is this about?' and 'What do I need to remember?'

Effective note taking depends on identifying and arranging key points to suit your own thought pattern and way of working. Some people find that drawing spider diagrams and flow charts is helpful; others develop their own shorthand (see Chapter 5 for further information on note taking.) The important thing is that your notes should make sense to you when you come back to read them several weeks or months later. You might not be able to borrow that particular book again, or get back to that library, so you need to make your approach as effective as possible so that one reading is enough. You do not need to take notes on everything that you read, as some reading should just be about broadening your knowledge base and familiarizing yourself with different ideas and different points of view.

You will need to develop a filing system for your notes so that you can find what you want when you need it. It is also useful to record which databases and libraries you have used, what you have already read, and any conversations with tutors/facilitators. Keep your notes safe – do not carry them all around with you or you might lose them and have to start all over again.

The infallible 'god' of print

There is a tendency to believe that if something is in print it must be true and the author's interpretation must be right. However, it is important to be slightly sceptical about everything that you read and to develop skills in evaluating the importance of a piece of work to your particular purpose, whether this is writing an academic essay or a research-based report. This is particularly important in relation to web-based material. Journal articles and books usually have to go through some form of review process prior to publication and there are therefore some safeguards about the quality of the material. Anyone who is prepared to pay a small fee for web space can publish on the internet.

Books and articles are written for different purposes and different audiences. Textbooks are intended to provide general introductions to specific areas of interest, such as the care of particular patient/client groups or subjects such as sociology and physiology. The intention of such books is to provide a straightforward, broad understanding. Specialist books aim to provide more depth and detailed analysis of defined areas.

The *Nursing Times* and *Nursing Standard* are the mainstream of popular nursing literature in the UK. They are written in an accessible style, have a huge circulation and are published weekly. They have panels of expert referees who review the articles submitted for publication to ensure that a particular standard is achieved, but the primary intention is to provide articles that are informative and readable rather than academic, scholarly work.

Specialisms within nursing – such as cancer nursing, services for older people, critical care and surgical nursing – also have their own journals, which aim to provide more in-depth discussion about particular areas of practice. For example, the October–December 2008 issue of *Critical Care Nursing Quarterly* included articles on renal replacement therapy in the critical care unit; gastrointestinal prophylaxis in critically ill patients; prevention of nosocomial infections in the intensive care unit; sleep in the intensive care unit setting; chronic obstructive pulmonary disease and cytokines; aspirin for the primary prevention of adverse cardiovascular events; and an exploratory examination of medical gas booms versus traditional headwalls in intensive care unit design.

The *Journal of Psychiatric and Mental Health Nursing* aims to focus on nursing innovation and the enhanced effectiveness of nursing practice within the area of mental health nursing. Potential contributions are sent to experts for review and the focus is on a high level of scholarship.

The *Journal of Advanced Nursing* aims to be an international medium for the publication of scholarly and research papers. It is available monthly on subscription only, is found in most healthcare libraries and is a valuable 'heavyweight' resource for students on pre- and post-registration courses, educators and researchers.

As mentioned earlier, an increasing number of journals are now produced in online formats; for example, the *Journal of Advanced Nursing*, *Journal of Neonatal Nursing*, *Nursing Standard* and *Worldviews on Evidence-based Nursing*. The exact format differs between publications but usually includes a list of contents and abstracts from the current issues, and some archived issues. Some allow you to print off full-text articles; others require payment for this service.

There is also a growing number of online-only journals, some of which would seem to be using the ideal publishing medium for their content; for example, the *Online Journal of Nursing Informatics*.

Midwives is a monthly journal that is sent free to all members of the Royal College of Midwifery (RCM). It is the official journal of the RCM and contains regular features on topics of interest to midwives, some research papers and review/opinion papers. A peer-reviewed scholarly supplement called *Evidence-based Midwifery* accompanies it twice yearly. The *British Journal of Midwifery* is a very readable, monthly, peer-reviewed journal with a very large circulation. It publishes topical papers from student midwives, midwives and other professionals, including doctors and legal experts. The *Practising Midwife* is another popular British journal, published monthly, which aims to address current clinical issues. For example, a recent issue included articles on pethidine as pain relief and improving the birthing environment.

The Association of Radical Midwives publishes a quarterly journal, *Midwifery Matters*, for its members. This offers a vehicle for its lay and midwifery members to discuss issues related to the values of the Association, which campaigns against the unnecessary medicalization of childbirth.

Two major international journals that are useful for UK midwives are *Midwifery* and the *Journal of Midwifery and Women's Health*. Both are available on subscription and are highly respected and peer reviewed. They aim to enhance quality of care for childbearing women and their families. *Midwifery* publishes research papers from all over the world on issues as wide ranging as preterm birth in Malawi, how much influence women have in Sweden on caesarean section and stress in pre-registration midwifery students in England. The September–October 2008 issue of *Journal of Midwifery and Women's Health* included articles on the effectiveness of the Edinburgh Postnatal Depression Scale and the links between breastfeeding and cognitive development in children.

Midwives also use the *Journal of Advanced Nursing*, general medical journals, obstetric journals and paediatric publications to supplement their knowledge for theory and for practice.

Whatever the source of the information you have collected, the following habits are recommended for purposeful and thoughtful reading.

Select one of the books or articles from your recommended reading list. As you read, ask yourself the following questions:

- Is the author providing me with the information I need?
- Who is writing (where do they work, what are their qualifications, do they know what they are writing about)?
- Who is the intended audience?
- Is the work published anywhere else?
- Is the topic dealt with in sufficient depth?

Compare your findings with a colleague.

You might find it helpful to use formal critical appraisal tools, particularly when reviewing research-based articles. A key resource is the Critical Appraisal Skills for Practice (CASP). CASP aims to enable individuals to develop the skills to find and make sense of research evidence, helping them to put knowledge into practice. For example, 'Making sense of evidence' provides ten questions to help you make sense of randomized controlled trials. You can access CASP tools from the following link: http://www.phru.nhs.uk/Pages/PHD/CASP.htm.

When reviewing the literature, it is usually sensible to start with the most recent article or book and then work backwards if more detail about original works or significant changes in thinking is required. Some authors will have written on the same topic in many different journals or books, in which case, even though you can access all of their publications, you should be able to extract their key thoughts on the subject by reading only one or two of them.

There is also a lot of repetition in the literature so you may find that, if you do a very detailed search, you keep coming up with essentially the same ideas. If the source you are reading does not appear to be stretching you or enabling you to get a better grasp on the subject, it might not be worth reading it any further. Often, it is best to restrict yourself to works that have been produced in the last 5 years. However, in most subjects, there are also 'classic' or 'seminal' works that need to be considered. For example, the work of Doreen Norton and others in developing a tool for the assessment of pressure sores in the 1960s was extremely significant in highlighting the importance of 'scientific' assessment in pressure-area care. Similarly, the work of Kurt Lewin in the 1950s on change theory has influenced much of the contemporary writings on planned organizational change. Such works are milestones in the development of our understanding about a particular subject or phenomenon.

Primary and secondary sources

Primary sources are articles and books written by the original authors; secondary sources are works that report on and critique the writings of others. For example, the book 'The emotional labour of nursing: its impact on interpersonal relations, management and the educational environment in nursing' (Smith, 1992) is an original report of a research study carried out by the author into the nature of nursing and caring that explored how nurses care and learn to care and the effects of emotional labour on the nurses themselves and the people they care for. This book is a primary source. It has been referred to or cited in many other pieces of work; for example, in Gray (2009), where it is noted that 'Smith (1992) identified the value of understanding care in nursing as "emotional labour"'.

Similarly, Bulman (2008) reports that the philosopher Donald Schon has had a great influence of the development of reflection in professional education and offers his definition of reflection in action:

'Thinking back on what we have done in order to discover how our knowing in action may have contributed to an unexpected outcome. We may do so after the fact, in tranquillity, or we may pause in the midst of action (stop and think).' (Schon, 1987, p. 26).

Whenever direct quotes are used, that is, the original authors' exact words are inserted into another piece of work, the full page numbers should also be supplied, as demonstrated above. This enables any reader of the secondary source to easily identify the primary source and to check for themselves whether or not the original author has been quoted correctly. Where possible, it is always preferable to go to primary sources. The information is likely to be more accurate and informative than a second-hand, paraphrased account or 'doctored' quote. Reviewing the original also enables you to make your own interpretations of the content and conclusions rather than relying on someone else's, which might or might not be accurate. However, if the primary sources are extremely complicated and difficult to read, it might be better to start off with a description of the original in the introductory text and then to follow it up with the original once you have some idea of the content and key issues.

Systematic reviews and meta-analyses

Organizations such as the Cochrane Collaboration and the NHS Centre for Reviews suggest that, because there is currently so much health-related information available to professionals, systematic reviews of this literature are required to efficiently integrate valid information and provide a basis for rational decision making. Systematic reviews use systematic methods to limit bias and reduce random errors, thus providing more reliable results from which to draw conclusions and make decisions. Meta-analysis – the use of statistical methods to summarize the results of independent studies – is thought to provide more precise estimates of the effects of health care than the results derived from individual studies.

The Cochrane Collaboration is an international organization that focuses particularly on systematic reviews of randomized controlled trials, because these are likely to provide more reliable information than other sources of evidence on the differential effects of alternative forms of health care. Cochrane Reviews have a standard format. This helps readers to find the results of research quickly and to assess the validity, applicability and implications of those results. The format is also suited to electronic publication and updating, and it generates reports that are informative and readable when viewed on a computer monitor or printed.

The NHS Centre for Reviews and Dissemination is funded by the four government health departments in the UK. It produces regular 'Effective Healthcare Bulletins' based on systematic review and synthesis of research on the clinical effectiveness and acceptability of health service interventions. This is carried out by a research team using established methodological guidelines with advice from expert consultants for each topic.

Before commencing any clinically focused assignment, it is useful to search the websites/databases of these organizations to see whether or not they have carried out reviews in the area you are studying.

Conclusion

Good researching for assignments depends on taking a systematic, organized and purposeful approach to accessing relevant and appropriate resources. The key to a successful literature review is the ability to evaluate critically the work of others. You need to know what is asserted to be good practice and to be able to judge whether the arguments that are being put forward are grounded in research-based evidence and whether the research itself has been properly carried out. Evaluating the work of others is a difficult skill to learn. It involves deciding what are valid and invalid arguments, telling the difference between a good source and a bad source, seeing gaps in the literature and developing good analytical skills.

Points to remember:
- Work with your peers
- Keep a good filing system
- Take clear, relevant, appropriate notes
- Read with a purpose

CHAPTER RESOURCES

REFERENCES

Bulman, C., 2008. An introduction to reflection. In: Bulman, C. & Schutz, S. (Eds.) Reflective practice in nursing, 4th edn. Wiley-Blackwell, Chichester, UK, pp. 1–24.

Carter, B. & McGoldrick, M. (Eds.), 2005. The expanded family life cycle, 3rd edn. Allyn and Bacon, Boston.

Gray, B., 2009. The emotional labour of nursing – defining and managing emotions in nursing work. Nurse Education Today 29 (2), 168–175.

Smith, P., 1992. The emotional labour of nursing: its impact on interpersonal relations, management and the educational environment in nursing. Macmillan, Basingstoke, UK.

Wright, L.M. & Leahey, M., 2001. Calgary Family Assessment Model: how to apply in clinical practice. MDI Videos, Calgary, Canada. Online. Available: http://www.eFamilyNursing.com

WEBSITES

British Nursing Index: http://www.bni.org.uk

Centre for Evidence Based Nursing and Midwifery: http://www. joannabriggs.tvu.ac.uk/joannabriggs/

Centre for Reviews and Dissemination: http://www.york.ac.uk/inst/crd

Cochrane Collaboration: http://www.cochrane.org

Critical Appraisal Skills Programme: http://www.phru.nhs.uk/Pages/PHD/CASP.htm

Kings Fund: http://www.kingsfund.org.uk

Midwives Information and Resource Service: http://www.midirs.org/

Midwives On-line: http://midwivesonline.com

Nursing Standard: http://www.nursing-standard.co.uk

Nursing Times: http://www.nursingtimes.net

Open University: http://www.open.ac.uk/skillsforstudy/

Royal College of Midwifery: http://www.rcm.org.uk

Royal College of Nursing: http://www.rcn.org.uk

FURTHER READING

Most HEIs now offer information-seeking skills advice on their intranets. Listed below are some books on researching information, including Internet resources, that you may find useful in your studies.

Cottrell, S., 2008. The study skills handbook, 3rd edn. Palgrave Macmillan, Basingstoke, UK.

Greetham, B., 2008. How to write better essays, 2nd edn. Palgrave Macmillan, Basingstoke, UK.

O'Dochartaigh, N., 2007. Internet research skills: how to do your literature search and find research on line. Sage Publications, Los Angeles.

Presentation of written material

Sian Maslin-Prothero

- Different styles of writing
- How to prepare a project
- Report writing
- Presentation of written material
- Reviewing a book/article
- Non-discriminatory language
- Copyright and plagiarism
- Writing for publication
- Different styles of referencing

Introduction

The aim of this chapter is to assist you in preparing and presenting material either for oral or written presentations. The first part of the chapter looks at different styles of writing and the remainder looks at the presentation of written material. This will provide you with a framework, which you can adapt to meet your requirements.

Being asked to write something – be it an essay, a report or an article – can be a daunting task. If you are undertaking any course of study, completing a written assignment is still the most common form of assessing student learning. How to write an essay is covered in Chapters 6 and 8; this chapter examines other ways of presenting written material.

You will already have considerable experience of writing and presenting material for others; for example, completing assignments as part of coursework in school or college or, in practice areas, writing care plans and reports to colleagues in handover or ward rounds. This allows you to link theory with practice. In each of these scenarios, you have to identify what is the most important information; that is, what needs to be communicated and what is not essential. You then provide the essential information in the most appropriate format and style. This will be different according to whether you are providing a presentation (to an audience) or a written piece of work.

Different styles of writing

In Chapter 6, you looked at writing skills and developing an argument. There will be other forms of writing that you will need to do as part of your course or as a daily activity. These will include some of the following:

- letters to friends and family
- job and course applications

- lecture notes
- reports on patients and clients
- projects
- memos
- essays
- examinations
- reviews of books or articles.

Each one of the above has special features that need to be considered prior to preparation and before actually writing.

- What is the material for?
- Who is going to read it?
- How long should it be?
- Should it be written in the first or third person?

Writing for different purposes

The style and content you adopt for writing will vary depending on the task. A letter to a member of your family or to a friend is likely to be very different from a memo sent to a colleague. A memo or memorandum is a communication used in businesses; they are more informal than letters, and do not require a signature or closing statement. They are usually written as a reminder or to present some basic information. A memo format is generally short, consisting of between one and four sentences (Figure 9.1).

MEMORANDUM

To: Sue Ashby

From: Sian Maslin-Prothero

Date: 7 January 2009

Subject: Book chapter

Thank you for email of 4 January 2009 reminding me about the deadline for submitting our changes for the 'Primary Care' chapter for Alan.
I have read the editor's comments and responded to his queries. I have used a combination of track changes and comment, and sent this electronically to you and Sarah.
Can you confirm that you are still available to meet with me on 14 January 2009? We'll meet at my office on campus at 15.00hrs.

FIGURE 9.1 An office memorandum.

Tips for writing a memo
- How much information do you need to convey?
- Who do you need to communicate with?
- Include:
  - times, dates and places to meet
  - reminders
  - new basic information
  - requests for confirmation, information or feedback

How to prepare a project

You are likely to have to undertake a project as part of a course or in your work environment. This can seem a frightening prospect, although it can also be a satisfying experience. The key to success is preparation; this involves developing a plan. Before embarking on this, you need to consider the following questions.

What have I got to do?

Use the assignment guidelines to help you decide:
- the subject
- the word limit
- the date for submission.

How much time do I have to complete the project?

Be realistic. You need to structure and plan your time. Remember to include some extra time to allow for events such as lost data or computer breakdown. Once you have drawn up a timetable, try to stick to it.

Drawing on Chapter 1, which discussed planning and organizing your time, completing a project is similar to writing an essay (see Chapters 6 and 8). The flow diagram shown in Figure 9.2 can help you organize your work effectively. Your aims and objectives (see Chapter 1 for definition) will be the basis for deciding what information you require to complete the project.

Do use headings and sub-headings to help guide the reader.

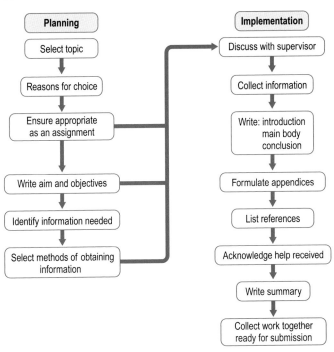

FIGURE 9.2 Planning and implementing project work.

How to prepare a report

The structure of a report is different from an essay or a letter. Reports are written because there is a need for specific information; for instance, where a problem has been identified and requires investigation. Reports are written for a purpose and target a specific audience. They are statements presented in a logical sequence leading to conclusions and possible recommendations for future action. A good report is characterized by its objectivity and systematic presentation. Reports have a format that leads the reader quickly to the main themes and findings.

Content of a report

All information contained in the report must be relevant, concise and substantiated, and it must be presented in a clear, logical sequence. The report should have an introduction in which the terms of reference are defined. The terms of reference include: who has commissioned the report; why they have asked for the report to be written; the purpose of the report; who the report is for; and who is going to read the final report. Essential background material may be included, or you can put details in the appendices. Some or all of the following may be included in the report. The method is where you tell the reader how you went about obtaining the information or analysed the information for the report. The results are where you present your findings. The discussion is where you discuss the implications of your findings. The summary is where you summarize the results. The recommendations are based on your findings.

The writing style should be clear and specific. Aim to use short and simple sentences, so that the reader easily understands the report. The report should be coherent and non-anecdotal. All sections, sub-sections and points must have headings and must be numbered and indented. This is so that the report flows logically and information can be easily retrieved. The box below illustrates the layout of a report.

Abstract

1   Introduction

   1.1   Style

      1.1.1   Ensure that the writing style, language and level are appropriate for the intended audience.

   1.2   Report writing is formal; reports are usually written in the third person.

   1.3   Who am I writing for?

   1.4   What is their knowledge of the subject?

2   Structure

   2.1   Reports often need to be read quickly, so ensure that the reader can find their way around the document easily.

      2.1.1   Sections and sub-sections should be numbered appropriately.

   2.2   Your introduction places the report in context. The conclusion draws the argument together and makes recommendations where appropriate.

   2.3   The abstract should be a précis of the introduction and conclusion.

3   Material

   3.1   Be selective and stick to the point.

   3.2   Report writing is a review of all the evidence, rather than a personal view.

   3.3   Start with the most important things first, then add the necessary detail.

   3.4   Avoid repeating yourself. You may find you need to rearrange the material.

4   Conclusion

   4.1   Use clear, simple language and stick to the point. Break the report into sections and sub-sections, with headings to guide the reader.

   4.2   Number the pages.

   4.3   If there is a specific word length, stick to it.

Your report will need an abstract, an introduction, a main body, a conclusion, recommendations and appendices. Any diagrams must be appropriate, numbered and clearly labelled. Include diagrams only if they are relevant and referred to in the report, otherwise there is no point in including them. If you have a word processing package, look under the 'Help' section; most packages have a system for report writing.

To summarize, to achieve effective communication you should use clear, simple language with well laid out sections and appropriate use of headings and summaries that will guide the reader through the report.

Reviewing a book or article

The ability to critically evaluate the work of others is important for a number of reasons: preparation for any assignment or project necessitates the individual critically evaluating the work of others in the area – not all research or reports have been reviewed by referees or peers. Critical evaluation is about being able to evaluate other people's work, both positively and negatively, thus judging the quality of the work. This is a valuable and useful skill to develop, and should be used when you read papers, reports and books (see Chapters 5, 6 and 8).

You might be asked to review a published book either as part of your course or for a journal. You will be provided with specific guidelines on what is expected in the review. This usually includes:

- A specified word limit for the review.
- Details of the book to be reviewed: author(s), title, place of publication, publisher, date of publication, number of pages, ISBN number and the price of the book.

The review is expected to provide a clear idea of the content of the book, and should be an interesting and critical appraisal of the work and its place in the existing literature, as well as providing an insight to current thinking and trends in nursing. For further information on writing a book review see Johnson (1995), Watson (1998, 1999) and Hartley (2008).

Non-discriminatory language

The aim of language is to communicate. Our use of language reflects our own attitudes. Therefore, if the language we use leads to misunderstanding or offends individuals, we will experience problems with communicating.

When using language, whether written or the spoken word, you need to be sure that you are not excluding people or discriminating against them. The way we speak and the language we use can reinforce inaccurate stereotypes. For example, the term 'mother and toddler group' insinuates that only mothers are responsible for childcare, and this is not the case. The term playgroup actually describes what is available and includes all carers.

Non-sexist language

The term 'man' should not be used to refer to both sexes. Non-sexist alternatives are available (Table 9.1).

TABLE 9.1 Sexist and non-sexist terminology

SEXIST	NON-SEXIST
Chairman	Chair
Mankind	People, humanity
Manpower	Workforce
Forefathers	Ancestors
Fireman	Fire fighter
Headmaster	Head teacher
Dear Sirs	Dear Sir/Madam

- He/him/his are not universal terms for men and women. Use titles and modes of address consistently for men and for women.
- Use similar terms when describing the same characteristics in women and men. Very few occupations or roles are exclusive to either males or females – the language used should reflect the job or task being performed.
- Avoid unnecessary reference to the gender and/or sexual orientation of a person or a group.
- Avoid terms that denigrate a person or a group on the basis of gender and/or sexual orientation.
- Avoid unnecessary reference to the relationship and/or parenting status of a person or a group.

The most important thing is to think, and to avoid discriminatory language in your written and spoken words. This is most likely to occur when using pronouns. A pronoun is a word used instead of a proper or other noun to indicate a person or thing already mentioned. For example: I, me, she, her, he, him, it, you, they, them, are all pronouns.

There are several ways to avoid discriminatory language.

- Avoid the pronoun altogether by using 'a', 'an', 'the' instead. For example: 'A nurse has his special patient' could be written: 'A nurse has a special patient'.
- Use 'they': 'Once a nurse has registered to practise, he knows in what area he wants to work' could be written: 'Once nurses have registered to practise, they know in what area they want to work'. Be careful not to mix singular and plural: 'Once a nurse has registered to practise, they know in what area they want to work'.
- Use both pronouns 'he/she' or 'his/her'. For example: 'A nurse has her/his special patient'. However, this can be clumsy. Use a second-person pronoun, 'you': 'As a nurse, you have your special patient'.
- Use the first-person plural, 'we': 'We nurses have our special patients'.
- Use 'one' (with caution, as it also has class connotations): 'As a nurse, one has a special patient'.
- Use a plural pronoun with a singular antecedent (e.g. everyone, every, etc.): 'Every nurse has their special patient' or 'Everyone has their special patient'.

Remember … think before you write or speak.

The use of non-discriminatory language might seem difficult but, with practice, it becomes natural to use terms that do not discriminate against people because of their gender, sexuality, race or other attributes.

Copyright and plagiarism

It is unclear how frequently plagiarism occurs because the aim tends to be to deceive, so many cases go undetected. It is important that you reference all material used. If you include other people's ideas or work without acknowledging their contribution then you are plagiarizing and risk failing your course or losing your job (see Chapter 5). People plagiarize for different reasons: ignorantly, innocently and deliberately.

If you copy a quotation from a book or article, you must credit the author, i.e. reference their work including name, date of publication and page number. Referencing other people's work is very important for a number of reasons: it enables readers to refer to the original work and check the authenticity of the quotation if they wish to; it enables readers to use the source for their own research; and it helps readers to distinguish between other people's ideas and your own. The safest way of avoiding plagiarism is to acknowledge the sources you have used. When preparing an assignment, make notes using the following 'avoiding plagiarism' guide.

Avoiding plagiarism

Separate direct quotations from your own work by using quotation marks. Always cite the precise source in your reference list. List all sources used in the bibliography. When paraphrasing another's work, identify the original source, including the author and date of publication.

You can refer to another person's work by paraphrasing in your own words. In this situation you must still reference the original work using the author and date. This is referred to as the primary source. In the case where an author you are reading refers to another author and their work, and you do not access the original work, you may cite this work. This is sometimes referred to as secondary source, for example 'Gough (1994, cited in Maslin-Prothero, 2008)'.

To successfully avoid the pitfall of plagiarism consider the following points.

- Don't attempt the question until you understand it.
- Do consult your lecturer and colleagues.
- Check your university or college website for its plagiarism policy and guidelines. There might be software that you can use to check your work before submitting it, such as Turnitin (see http://turnitin.com/static/index.html).
- Plan your time carefully.
- Reference your notes and sources as you go along. Don't wait until you have completed the essay and then try to remember where they came from.

Reference and citation systems

It is an essential requirement when researching and producing a written project that all sources used are properly acknowledged. It is important that you employ and become used to a standardized reference system.

These guidelines describe the Harvard and the Vancouver systems of referencing, which are the most commonly used. You may use another system, but bear in mind that it is important to keep to a standard form throughout your written contribution.

Definitions

- Annotated bibliography: a bibliography where each reference is accompanied by a critical or explanatory note.
- Bibliography: a list of other relevant material used but not referred to in the text.
- Reference list: a bibliographic list of items referred to in the text.
- Reference: a bibliographic description including author(s), date, title, publisher and place of publication.

The Harvard system of referencing

The box below shows how to cite a reference in the text and create an alphabetically compiled list of references at the end of the text.

Doctors who make the diagnosis are in a powerful position. Access to such power is controlled by professional associations with their own vested interests to protect (Naidoo and Wills, 1994). The 1858 Medical Act established the General Medical Council, which was authorized to regulate doctors, oversee medical education and keep a register of qualified practitioners (Hart, 1994).

Medical colleges resisted the entry of women to the profession for many years. In 1901 there were 36 000 medical practitioners, of whom 212 were women. There is evidence that Black and Asian doctors face discrimination in their medical careers (Tschudin, 1994a). This implies that ability is not the sole criterion for gaining a place to train in medicine or in subsequent career progression. Special counselling is a good idea in such cases (Tschudin, 1994b).

References

Hart C (1994) Behind the mask: nurses, their unions and nursing policy. Baillière Tindall, London

Naidoo J and Wills J (1994) Health promotion: foundation for practice. Baillière Tindall, London

Tschudin V (1994a) Deciding ethically: a practical approach to nursing challenges. Baillière Tindall, London

Tschudin V (1994b) Counselling. Baillière Tindall, London

At every point where the text refers to a particular document, insert the author(s) last name, first name initial(s) and year of publication. Use lower case letters after the year if referring to more than one piece of work published in the same year by the same author.

Book references

Give the following facts, in this order:

- name of the author(s), editor(s) or the institution responsible for writing the book
- year of publication in brackets
- title and subtitle, underlined (or in italic type)
- volume and individual issue number (if any)
- edition, if not the first
- publisher
- place of publication, if known.

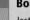

Book reference

Jester R (2007) *Advancing Practice in Rehabilitation Nursing.* Blackwell, Oxford

Journal references

A reference to an article in a journal contains the following information, in the order listed below:

- author(s)
- year of publication in brackets
- title of article
- title of journal (in italic type)
- volume number
- issue number in brackets
- specific date (for a weekly journal)
- inclusive pages.

> ### Journal reference
> Read S and Bowler C (2007) Life story work and bereavement: Shared reflections on its usefulness. *Learning Disability Practice* 10(4): 10–14

References to contributions in books

Enter under the name of contributing author and include the relevant page numbers.

> ### Reference to a book chapter
> Toward S and Maslin-Prothero S (2007) 'The impact of health and social policy on the planning & delivery of nursing care' In: J Brown and P Libberton (eds) Principles of Professional Studies in Nursing. Palgrave Macmillan, Basingstoke, Chapter 7, pp. 113–134

Handbooks, directories in single or several volumes

> ### Reference to handbook or directory
> Cambridge Information and Research Services Limited (1986) Industrial Development Guide 1986, 8th edn. Longman, Harlow, UK

Theses and dissertations

Include the details of level and awarding institution.

> ### Reference to a thesis
> Wrigley M (2008) Engaging Families with a Premature Family History of Heart Disease: Primary Prevention for Coronary Heart Disease. Unpublished PhD thesis. University of Southampton, Southampton

Quotes

This is where you refer to an author's work. You can have direct and indirect quotes.

> ### Example of direct quote
> 'There is a need for nurse and midwifery managers to have an understanding of devolution and post-devolution structures and how they operate in order to work effectively, as well as to learn from the experiences of other parts of the UK' (Maslin-Prothero, Masterson and Jones, 2008, p. 662).

When using direct quotes, you should also include the relevant page number(s). This allows the reader to find the original source.

Example of an indirect quote

Maslin-Prothero et al. (2008) suggested that midwives and nurses needed to understand devolution and its impact on systems if they were to work efficiently.

In both these examples, the authors would be listed in alphabetical order in the reference list.

Secondary references

Wherever possible, you should always attempt to use readily available or recent primary sources; that is, the original publication. However, this is not always possible and you might also want to refer to a classic piece of writing that has been quoted by another author. In this case, you use the term 'cited by' (a secondary reference) and the name of the author and the date of the text actually accessed.

The role of pressure groups was outlined by Masterson (1994, cited by Maslin-Prothero, 1996).

For a secondary reference only the details of the publication accessed – Maslin-Prothero (1996) – should appear in the reference list.

The Vancouver system of referencing

The Vancouver system of referencing is widely used in journals and some books. All references are identified in the text by numbers, either in brackets or as superscript. The philosophy behind this system of referencing is that the use of numbers in the text does not distract the reader by interrupting the text.

Reference to the same author and publication uses the same number. The references are then listed in numerical order.

EXAMPLE OF THE VANCOUVER SYSTEM OF REFERENCING

While there have always been variations in structure, devolution has increased the level of diversity,[1] because of changes in political leadership; for example, in Scotland the shift of power from Labour to the Scottish National Party (SNP), and in Wales the increasing influence of Plaid Cymru. There is evidence of policy inconsistencies within the UK; for example, charging older people for personal and social care.[2]

References

1. McClelland S & Johnson K (2007) NHS Structure: The Impact of Devolution. Online. Available at: http://www.library.nhs.uk/healthmanagement/ViewResource.aspx?resID=29577 [accessed 1 December 2007].

2. Pollock AM (2001) Scotland's decision on long-term care challenges a centralised NHS and treasury. BMJ 322: 311-312. (10 February). Online. Available at: http://www.bmj.com/cgi/content/full/322/7282/311?ck=nck [accessed 2 December 2007].

The style of reference for material from a book or journal is the same for Vancouver and Harvard referencing; the difference is the use of numbers in the Vancouver system.

A number of other referencing systems are available. Each individual and institution has their preferred system of referencing. It is important that you identify the method preferred prior to submitting work, and use this method when compiling. You should check your references to make sure they are accurate, so that should you or anyone else want to find the original source, they can.

If you are undertaking a piece of work that requires a lot of references you could choose to keep track of your references using a database. Reference Manager and EndNote are packages specifically designed for this purpose. They allow you to search internet databases, such as PubMed or ISI Web of Science®, and build your own personal reference collection. In addition, you can save abstracts, pdf files and share your references with other users. There are other packages, such as NVivo, which is a database manager and a program for analysing qualitative data.

Writing for publication

Writing for publication provides an opportunity to share your ideas with a wider audience and is crucial if nursing is to develop and improve patient care. For those working in academic institutions, it is a fundamental requirement. If you examine the nursing press you will find that only a small number of the total nursing workforce are submitting work for publication. Masterson (1994) identified that the majority of publications and awards go to either nurses in management or nurse educators. If there is to be a more representative, balanced view of nursing then you need to contribute your thoughts and ideas to the nursing press. Learning to write is straightforward as long as you prepare and follow some simple guidelines.

Learning to write

- Identify your audience (and journal)
- Write about what you know
- Do background reading and preparation
- Use the guidelines for contributors and follow the 'house style'.

From personal experience, it is worthwhile approaching the intended journal editor or publisher with your idea. Read a variety of journals and decide whether what you want to write about is suitable for that particular journal. There might be a journal that is more appropriate. For example, an article on the experience of part-time, mature midwifery/nursing students would be more suitable in *Nurse Education Today* than in the *Journal of Clinical Nursing*. Then, prepare a detailed plan of what you intend to cover and write to the editor. This will save you time because the editor can express an interest (or otherwise) in your intended published work.

Having identified the journal, use its most recent contributor guidelines when preparing the script. This will help create a favourable impression with the editor and reviewers when submitting the completed script. The guidelines for contributors include the following details: number of words, presentation issues (word processed, double spacing, width of margins, style of referencing) copyright and payment. There are a number of stages you need to follow:

- the desire to write
- decide on a subject
- define your subject
- know your target journal
- approach the editor
- plan the article
- write the article.

Proofread your work prior to submitting it, or ask someone else to, for typographical errors and content. Make use of a critical friend – someone who will read, critique, ask pertinent questions and provide constructive criticism. You can make changes in light of this person's suggestions and submit it to the chosen journal for consideration. Each journal has its own rules and guidelines for submission; the journal's individual guide for authors provides instructions for submission. Many journals use online submission, where you go to the journal's website and load your article online. For an example, have a look at the *Nurse Education Today* website (http://ees.elsevier.com/net/default.asp) – look at 'Main menu' and 'Submit paper'.

The editor will decide whether your manuscript is appropriate for publication and will have your article reviewed. The reviewers will comment and advise on the standard and quality of your manuscript, and give feedback using a framework, usually devised by the journal editor. The reviewer will make recommendations such as: accept, minor revision, major revision or reject. The journal editor will contact you electronically and let you know if your work has been accepted for publication. If the editor recommends making some changes, and you are willing to do these, then make the changes and return the article; there is usually a time limit of 6–9 weeks. Once your article has been accepted, the process to publication follows the path summarized in Figure 9.3.

Be prepared for a wait of up to a year before seeing your work in hard copy; although if the journal is online, once it has been accepted and prepared for publication it can be found electronically on the journal website and will have a unique Digital Object Identifier (DOI).

Don't get despondent if your article is not accepted for publication. I have, and continue to have, works rejected – you need to persevere.

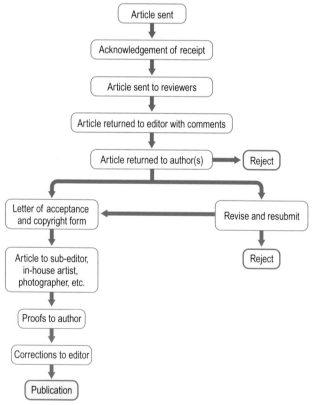

FIGURE 9.3 The process from submission to publication (adapted with permission from Cook, 2000).

Conclusion

This chapter has looked at presentation of written material. The main aim has been to provide you with a framework that you can use when preparing written material. This can be used in conjunction with information from other chapters for presentation of assignments, and so on. It is useful to gain feedback on any written or verbal presentations you give; this will enable you to develop your skills further. You will gain in confidence and learn each time you have to submit written work.

Identify an assignment for which you have received positive feedback from your assessor. Using guidelines from a nursing journal, make necessary changes and submit it for publication.

CHAPTER RESOURCES

REFERENCES

Cook, R., 2000. The writer's manual: a step-by-step guide for nurses and other health professionals. Radcliffe Medical Press, Oxford.

Hartley, J., 2008. How to…write e book review. Online. Available: http://info.emeraldinsight.com/authors/guides/book_review.htm [accessed 9 January 2009].

Johnson, M., 1995. Writing a book review: towards a more critical approach. Nurse Education Today 15, 228–231.

Masterson, A.H.R., 1994. Explaining the values of British nursing and the values enshrined in United Kingdom health policy: a research proposal. Unpublished Master of Nursing Thesis. University of Wales College of Medicine, Cardiff.

Watson, R., 1998. A message from the book review editor. Journal of Advanced Nursing 27, 1103.

Watson, R., 1999. Another message from the book review editor. Journal of Advanced Nursing 29, 1283–1284.

WEBSITES

EndNote (2009): http://www.endnote.com/ [accessed 13 January 2009]. *EndNote is a tool that integrates bibliographic database searches on the internet; organizes references, images, pdfs and other files; and collaborates using the web-based research tool.*

NVivo (2009): http://www.qsrinternational.com/ [accessed 13 January 2009]. *NVivo is a software package that can help people to manage and make sense of qualitative data. The package has tools for classifying, sorting and arranging information. It can also be used as a database.*

Reference Manager (2009): http://www.refman.com/rminfo.asp [accessed 13 January 2009]. *Reference Manager is another tool that combines: online reference searching, database manager, web publisher, bibliography builder, and reference sharing.*

Turnitin (2008): http://turnitin.com/static/index.html [accessed January 2009]. *Turnitin UK is a software package that can be used by staff and students to assess coursework, assessments and publications. The software can identify the original source of material included within work by searching a database of reference material gathered from professional publications, student essay websites and other student works.*

FURTHER READING

Doyle, M., 1995. The A–Z of non-sexist language. Women's Press, London. *This book is an interesting and useful read. It includes a complete listing of sexist terms and their non-sexist alternatives.*

SECTION 2
LEARNING FROM PRACTICE

SECTION CONTENTS

Clinical skills

Andrew Finney

- The clinical-skills laboratory
- Building confidence
- Demonstration and practising
- Addressing your learning needs
- Skills acquisition

- Practical skills for pre-registration
- The importance of understanding
- Practical skills for post-registration
- Clinical simulations
- Revisiting clinical skills
- Assessment

Nursing and Midwifery training must fulfil the educational requirements of the current 'Fitness for Practice' curriculum (Peach Report, 1999). A weakness highlighted in previous nursing and midwifery curricula was the over-emphasis on theory, which was too big a shift from traditional training methods, leaving a void in students' practical skills and questioning whether students were fit for purpose (Platt, 2002). It was felt that students were inadequately prepared for everyday work in clinical practice and had insufficient expertise in practical skills. This situation had arisen for a number of reasons: the academic belief that clinical skills were best learned in clinical settings; the clinical assumption that students would enter placement with the necessary skills established and thus the purpose of the placement was to provide opportunities to practise those skills; the shortage of registered practitioners to teach students in clinical settings; the increased efficiency-demands of hospitals, leading to rapid turnover of patients and a shorter length of patient stay. As a result students did not receive the high level of professional training and supervision that they needed to become competent technically and fit for practice (Lauder et al., 2008).

The re-introduction and funding of clinical-skills laboratories by universities and their recent support by the Nursing and Midwifery Council (NMC) has placed skills development at the forefront of professional development. To ensure nursing students develop the necessary clinical skills, the NMC (2007) has mandated that students successfully demonstrate specific skills known as 'essential skills clusters' as a condition of professional registration. By the end of their programme, students have to be verified as being 'fit for practice'. A level of competency in clinical skills is a course requirement. Competency in clinical skills is achieved through the ability to problem-solve insightfully and apply underpinning theory to practical skills. With increasing technology and the changing role of the midwife and nurse, there is an ever-increasing number of clinical skills required upon qualification and beyond, requiring life-long learning.

This chapter aims to help you develop professional skills so that you can benefit from practical skills teaching in the skills laboratory and subsequently in your practice setting, irrespective of whether you are a pre- or post-registration nursing or midwifery student.

The clinical-skills laboratory

Busier clinical-practice areas, the high expectations of patients/clients and an increased awareness of legal and professional issues means that it is essential that students have a safe level of technical skill and professional awareness commensurate with their stage in training and the clinical placement. Equally, the opportunistic nature of practice placements and the move to patient-centred care (rather than task-orientated care) means that there might not always be the chance for repetitive practice of clinical skills to become competent. Although a skills laboratory can never replace direct patient care, it is an important environment for the development of technical competence for placement practice. So it is vital that you use the skills laboratory as much as possible to develop technical competence and confidence.

Professional clinical skills are very complex and frequently entail a range of different component activities. Some of these components are:

- knowledge of the procedure and required equipment
- technical dexterity
- management skills
- psychosocial skills
- professional knowledge (such as legal and ethical issues, anatomy and physiology, psychology, health and safety)
- evidence base (such as bacteriology, pharmacology, advances in technique).

Learning how to deliver an apparently simple element of care, such as moving and handling or meeting personal-hygiene needs, requires elements of all these components, as demonstrated in the case study below.

 CASE STUDY: MARK

Mark is a child-branch student in his first placement area, which is a trauma/orthopaedic unit for children. He is carrying out some fundamental care for Toby, an 8-year-old boy who has a fracture of his femur. Despite the simple task of helping Toby to maintain his hygiene needs, Mark realizes that Toby is currently in traction and in quite a lot of pain. Mark asks for help from his mentor to care for Toby. Mark's mentor makes him aware that for Toby there is a need to manage his pain, and be aware of his cognitive development by informing Toby of what they are doing, whilst also carrying out safe and approved manual handling for both themselves and Toby according to the Manual Handling Operations Regulations (1992). At the age of eight, Toby has body weight substantial enough for him to be seen as an 'unstable load' if he is uncooperative during the manual handling procedure: he, Mark and the mentor could be at risk. Following the procedure, Mark is encouraged by his mentor to do a manual handling risk assessment for Toby for all his hygiene and sanitary needs.

In most cases, skills laboratories are built to replicate the layout of clinical settings, simulating hospital layouts such as bedded wards, and utilizing medical equipment that you will see in practice placement settings. As a student nurse/midwife or as a qualified health professional perhaps utilizing a clinical-skills laboratory as part of a course, you should consider it to be a safe, controlled environment where learning takes place through practice and perseverance. There should be no fear of failure, as you are not compromising patient safety or welfare (Cioffi, 2001). Nobody is perfect, and getting a skill wrong or practising incorrectly is anticipated in the laboratory setting. These mistakes, when supervised by your clinical skills lecturer, can be 'ironed out' and corrected. A skills laboratory is often equipped with life-size manikins that allow you to practise invasive procedures and use specialist equipment through simulation (Figure 10.1), thus enabling you to improve your skills and techniques safely.

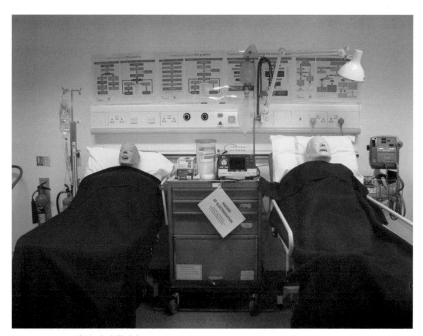

FIGURE 10.1 Clinical-skills laboratory.

Building confidence

Practising clinical skills in the laboratory setting is aimed at embodying the physical actions into your repertoire of skills and so building your confidence and ability to practise these skills on patients in clinical settings. However, due to an often natural lack of confidence, many people find practising in the laboratory setting to be a daunting experience due to:

- finding demonstrations too fast and confusing
- being watched whilst practising
- needing to learn the different stages of the technique and their sequencing
- specific/individual learning needs, such as dyslexia.

These four points can influence your confidence when practising skills in the laboratory.

Demonstration and practising

Clinical skills demonstrations can be difficult to follow; you can help yourself by arriving at the skills session on time and pre-prepared. You may have received a lecture prior to the demonstration, but it is important that you take some responsibility for your learning needs for clinical skills. Consider textbooks that are solely aimed at clinical procedures, such as the Royal Marsden Hospital's *Manual of Clinical Nursing Procedures* (Dougherty and Lister, 2008). Does your university library have any DVDs of clinical skills that you could watch? Has the university created any online videos that demonstrate clinical skills that you could familiarize yourself with before the session? Once in the skills laboratory, you should find a suitable place to stand and make sure you can clearly see what is being demonstrated and also hear any commentary or instructions that you are being given. The clinical skills lecturer will talk you through the process step by step and provide an opportunity to practise with a colleague, and maybe even have it video recorded so that you can watch your own performance, as this is a useful way to see where you need to improve. It is a good idea to try to talk yourself through the procedure as you undertake the activity; this might seem strange and difficult initially, until you have got the hang of the different stages in the task. Don't be afraid to ask your colleagues to talk you through (this will also help them to learn the sequence of stages). Consider the work of Ausubel (1968) and follow the stages of skill acquisition in the box below.

AUSUBEL'S STAGES OF SKILL ACQUISITION (1968)

Ausubel's four stages consist of:

Stage 1: the skill is demonstrated to you in real time
You are not distracted by words, you simply observe the experienced competent mentor or skills lecturer, who provides you with strong visual images to learn from.

Stage 2: the skill is demonstrated again slowly, with dialogue
The skill is demonstrated again with the mentor or skills lecturer providing you with an explanation and reasoning for any actions. This is your opportunity to ask relevant questions.

Stage 3: you now guide the demonstrator
This time you should aim to talk your mentor through the skill. The purpose of this is to allow you to gather and organize information. This engages your understanding of the skill, the transition from theory to practise and an opportunity to see the skill again.

Stage 4: you now perform the skill
This completes the learning process. You now practise the skill, demonstrating your understanding, facilitated by your mentor.

Could you use Ausubel's approach when learning a skill such as drug administration? It is also essential to recognize the need for good numeracy skills with skills such as drug administration. Check whether you have access to an internet software package that can help you with numeracy and drug calculations. Many universities now utilize a software package called 'Authentic World' (Authentic World, 2008: www.authenticworld.co.uk). Founded in 2004, Authentic World Ltd is a spin-out company of Glamorgan and Cardiff universities, whose mission is to improve patient safety by reducing medication error through the development of innovative educational software solutions. Their medication dosage calculation products are being used by higher education institutions and NHS Trusts across the UK.

The skill of drug administration has many stages. If the demonstrator has performed the skill along the lines of Ausubel's stages 1 and 2, then think of stage 3 as a chance for you to talk the skill through with a colleague.

The stages you could divide the skill of drug administration into might be:

- check the patient's details against those of the prescription chart
- check for allergies
- identify the drug name on prescription chart
- check the prescribed dose
- identify the date and time for administration
- check the route of administration
- check the prescriber's signature
- check the drug has not already been given
- locate the medication
- check the expiry date
- correctly calculate the dose (see www.authenticworld.co.uk for guidance)
- decant the medication.

What may have seemed a simple skill has many separate tasks. If we were to now adopt Ausubel's final stage, you would work through these tasks unaided to safely administer a placebo medication to a colleague or lecturer.

Many students feel vulnerable and nervous when being watched performing a clinical skill by a demonstrator or colleague. Being the first person to practise following a demonstration means that the pressure is on you; what seemed to be straightforward and easy often becomes impossible as your memory of the sequence of the skill fades and you suddenly feel that you cannot possibly perform the skill as competently as the demonstrator while your friends and peers are watching. This sort of fear is common and it is important that you acknowledge them by talking to the demonstrator (who may be a tutor or clinical skills lecturer) before the start of the scheduled session. You might want to practise later in the session or after watching others. The opportunity to watch others and provide constructive criticism will help those around you and raise your self-confidence.

Addressing your learning needs

If you have specific learning needs, such as dyslexia, you need to discuss these prior to the session with the person leading the session. Extra time is usually allocated to dyslexic students in the clinical-skills laboratory for assessment purposes such as objective, structured, clinical examinations (OSCE; see Chapter 7, p. 143, for more details). The need to practise skills in addition to allocated skills laboratory activities is important. Students can use memory or prompt sheets to aid learning needs; breaking clinical skills down into smaller parts is often easier to practise and remember. An example of skills broken down into stages is provided through algorithms used by the Resuscitation Council UK (2005b) to guide people through basic and advanced life support. These algorithms act as a flow chart that prompts the next stage of the technique and justifies your next action (Table 10.1).

The opportunity to visualize a sequence and action together aids understanding, and adding your own comments gives you the opportunity to pinpoint questions or reminders for future reference. It is useful to consider textbooks and journal articles that help you to practise clinical skills this way. The use of DVDs and online videos can also help as they offer the opportunity to re-watch skills demonstrations as many times as you wish.

When you are in a practice setting, try to work closely with your mentor and other experienced staff. Your mentor is required to establish an effective working relationship with you that facilitates your learning (NMC, 2006). You should be able to consider your mentor a role model; someone with competence and knowledge that you wish to gain and they wish to share. Billet (2001) used the term 'modelling' when considering the training undertaken by nurses as a 'cognitive apprenticeship'. Modelling involves the mentor as expert demonstrating skills in order for you to observe and build a conceptual model of the processes required to accomplish them.

TABLE 10.1 Paediatric Basic Life Support (based on the Resuscitation Council UK 2005b guidelines)

	SEQUENCE	ACTION	COMMENTS
1.	Safe approach	Checked	
2.	Responsiveness	Shake gently and shout	
3.	Call for help	Shout 'Help'	
4.	ABC: assess airway	Check mouth Neutral position or head tilt, chin lift	
5.	ABC: Breathing	Look, listen, feel for 10 seconds	
6.	Effective breaths	Up to 5 attempts 1–1.5 seconds Note any gag or cough response	
7.	ABC: Circulation	Movement/breathing/coughing Child: carotid pulse for 10 seconds Infant: brachial pulse for 10 seconds	
8.	Compressions	Correct position, either fingers, thumbs or one hand: – lower third of the sternum – one finger breadth above the xiphisternum – depth one-third of the chest Rate 100 per minute	
10.	Ratio	15 compressions to 2 breaths (15 : 2) Lay person (30 : 2)	
11.	Emergency call	After 1 minute	
12.	Unconscious	Assess ABC Assess for injuries Turn into recovery position Get help	

Skills acquisition

Acquiring clinical skills by practising through simulation or through direct patient care can help to build your confidence and maintain safety when supervised by a tutor or mentor. To retain a skill, you need to practise: remember that repetition leads to retention. The more exposure you get to that skill the easier it is to retain the knowledge and technique required.

Most professionals will aim to become the expert in their own field. Some educational theorists have provided a tool or model to understand and develop expertise; for example, Patricia Benner whose guidance on presiding as a novice and working towards expertise can be applied to the context of the health professional. Benner considered the path taken by student nurses and midwives to qualified nurses and midwives as 'novice to expert', and adapted the Dreyfus Model of skills acquisition (Dreyfus and Dreyfus, 1980) to the health professions. This model suggested five stages of proficiency that you must pass through to develop expertise (see the box below).

FROM NOVICE TO EXPERT

Stage 1: novice

The novice stage suggests that you as a beginner have no experience of the situation in which you are expected to perform. As a student, you will enter a new clinical area as a novice. Benner also believed that all nurses and midwives entering into new working environments can be initially limited to novice level (Benner, 2001).

Stage 2: advanced beginner

As an advanced beginner, you can demonstrate an acceptable performance. You have experienced similar situations or skills before. You can now dictate actions and understand the need for required skills.

Stage 3: competent

Benner thought that competence was typified by a nurse or midwife with 2–3 years experience. To be competent you must have the ability to plan, coordinate and deliver complex clinical skills.

Stage 4: proficient

Proficient nurses or midwives fully understand the clinical skills and the situations in which they present themselves. This allows for experience that provides them with the skills not only to cope with situations but also to modify skills and respond to a change of events.

Stage 5: expert

An expert nurse or midwife has a wealth of experience and an intuitive grasp of nursing or midwifery skills. The expert does not waste time considering wasteful alternatives to what is actually required but has the ability to act accordingly, immediately. Experts are often found in management and leadership roles because they are highly skilled and experienced.

Reflect on your current levels of competency or proficiency – where do you think you are on this path?

Despite its age, the Ausubel approach (see the box on pp. 200–201) is still relevant and is an easy and straightforward way of understanding the process of acquiring a skill, with an opportunity to observe the skill before demonstrating it yourself. This tool can be used in the skills laboratory setting and transferred to practice when being shown an isolated skill. Benner's theory shows the transition required for expertise, and makes it clear that, as a student, you are likely to reach a level of competency, but that expertise requires experience.

When practising a skill on a patient/client for the first time, aim to see the skill performed by your mentor directly before performing the skill yourself on the next patient. For example, it is better to give your first subcutaneous injection to a patient after just seeing the same injection given to a different patient/client. Watching an injection being given to a patient/client and then offering to perform that same injection the next day, will mean that you might have forgotten what you observed and may be less confident because of the time that has passed since you observed the skill. It is the simple process of 'see one, do one' under the direct supervision of your mentor.

Practical skills for pre-registration

As an undergraduate, pre-registration student undertaking a nursing/midwifery diploma or degree, you will be aware that practical clinical skills are a large feature of the 3-year duration of your chosen course. You should consider the practical skills taught to be simply the beginning of a life-long learning need to provide an evidence-based care. Your chosen university or school of nursing and midwifery will have selected a number of attainable clinical skills for you to be taught throughout the course. These clinical skills will be very simple to start with, leading to more advanced and acute skills as the course progresses. The skills that you are taught will become more complex, meeting the learning needs of your course and practice placements.

The most important thing to consider when you start the journey of acquiring practical clinical skills is that no clinical skills should be deemed 'basic', as this often gives the impression that such skills will eventually be beneath the qualified nurse or midwife and no longer required. All clinical skills are essential for safe practice and high standards of patient care. The first clinical skills you are taught should be deemed 'fundamental', as they are the actual building blocks to everything else in your practice. These skills are the foundations of your knowledge and performance; if we were using the analogy of a building, if you removed the foundations of a building, the building would come tumbling down!

The fundamental, practical, clinical skills that may be taught in your foundation or first year will be skills such as communication, making a bed, maintaining hygiene, feeding and drinking, and manual handling. Each of these skills is crucial to effective care and, for this reason, skills laboratories offer the opportunity to practise them over and over again. There will never be a time when these skills are not required, and these should be the skills that you are not only competent at but also master of. When you have mastered the fundamental skills of nursing or midwifery, you will be able to develop your professional knowledge to generate other skills and actions. For example, making a bed can alert you to infection-control issues: if the linen were soiled or your patient has haemorrhaged or got excessive discharge coming from a wound. It should also prompt you to be aware of tissue viability issues for your patient/client, as a poorly made hospital bed could cause damage to pressure areas. In addition, making patients' beds gives you time to observe and communicate with them while they are sat out at the side of the bed or in bed. This important time spent communicating can alert you to new problems or concerns that can then be addressed.

Learning how to meet hygiene and nutritional needs can provide opportunities for a huge source of information when performed as a skill with your patient/client. The opportunity to help a patient/client with hygiene needs provides the nurse or midwife with the chance to visually inspect the patient/client for weight loss, weight gain, skin problems such as rashes and infections, as well as checking for pressure area damage. The same can be said of feeding a patient, as this allows for interaction and an opportunity to assess appetite, swallowing ability, nutritional intake and general ability to eat.

CASE STUDY: KATIE

Katie was a third-year student midwife who had been alerted to a patient (Liz) not eating on one of the maternity wards. This was a concern to the midwifery team because both Liz and her baby were about to go home; they were concerned because poor appetite can be an early sign of a post-natal problem. In addition, staff noticed that Liz seemed reluctant to hold her baby. Katie noticed that Liz was a 35-year-old woman diagnosed with rheumatoid arthritis. At the start of her course she had worked on a Rheumatology ward and remembered the difficulty people sometimes had with handling cutlery or performing simple actions, such as cutting food. Katie discovered that Liz had had to stop taking a lot of her medication for the condition during her pregnancy due to harmful effects on the unborn child, and that she felt she was suffering from an arthritic flare because of this. Katie talked to Liz and discovered that she had excruciatingly painful hands and shoulders, which put her off eating but also meant that picking up and holding her baby was very painful. Liz had not said anything because she just wanted to go home, where she would get help. Due to her awareness and insight, Katie was able to find adapted cutlery for Liz, and a comfortable position in which she could hold her baby before discharge home.

The importance of understanding

When learning new practical clinical skills during time in the skills laboratory or in the practice placement setting, you need to understand not just what the skill involves but why it is required. Higgs (1992) argued that clinical simulations promote learning for understanding and meaning rather than just the learning of facts and principles. The foundation year or first year of the course is a time when there are many new things to see and discover and you may feel like you just cannot take all of the information in. This is normal: most students feel this way.

As you begin to feel more confident and established with clinical skills, it is important to ask why. Theory will inform practice throughout your course, but practice should also inform theory. An important step to helping you learn and to becoming a professional is developing an attitude that each skills laboratory session provides a stimulus for further reading. Finding out about different skills, why you need to perform them and when there are variations on policies or delivery of the skill, such as those listed below, is important.

The kinds of questions you might wish to ask about diabetic patients are:

- What type of diabetes do they have?
- How do they manage their diabetes: medication, diet, exercise?
- Why is it necessary to take blood glucose readings?
- How many kinds of blood glucose tests are there, and to what extent are they accurate?
- What kinds of person might have their blood glucose taken?
- What preparation needs to be taken prior to a blood glucose test?
- What is the normal range of blood glucose and what causes any changes to the range in values?
- If the person has diabetes what are the possible indications of the disease?
- What special nursing observations might they require – to their skin? or their diet?

Consider a list of questions for a different procedure or condition. Draw a spider diagram; this will help you to plan for the care needs of patients/clients prior to your next clinical placement.

Practical skills for post-registration

It is crucial to understand that on qualifying as a registered nurse or midwife you find yourself at the beginning of a career that will require life-long learning (Gopee, 2005). On your journey, you will be equipped with certain skills, knowledge and experience gained throughout the 3-year course. On qualification and beyond you must be prepared to learn new skills, develop yourself and others so that you meet the needs of your clients and that the care you provide is evidence based.

Speak to an experienced colleague who has seen changes in nursing or midwifery. Think of a clinical skill that you perform and ask them how that has changed since they were in your position as a recently qualified nurse or midwife. This may give you an indication of the advances in nursing/midwifery and how skills change.

Meeting the NMC (2008) requirements to be a responsive reflective practitioner means you need to find ways to keep your skills and knowledge current and evidence based. The NMC states that:

- You must have knowledge and skills for safe and effective practice when working without direct supervision.
- You must recognize and work within the limits of your competence.

- You must take part in appropriate learning and practice activities that maintain and develop your competence and performance.

Practising within the guidelines provided by the NMC is often challenging. Both you and your employer have a responsibility to facilitate you keeping your skills up to date and this is often done by providing and attending training for mandatory skills such as basic life support (BLS), manual handling, infection control, and so on. Very often, you will find that new skills require you to build on your existing knowledge and ability in order to perform more advanced skills. Table 10.2 shows the sequences and action for the skill of automated external defibrillation (AED). You can clearly see that the first sequence and action suggest starting with BLS, presuming you are at least competent with this skill.

Table 10.1 is a guide for learning BLS and Table 10.2 requires prior knowledge of BLS for you to even begin participating in the practice of the advanced skill of AED. Reflect on Benner's work (Benner, 2001); you will have advanced from the 'novice' stage in order to perform AED. The stage you find yourself at will be based on previous exposure to the skill. You may be 'proficient' or even 'expert' when performing BLS; however, AED may find you back at 'novice' stage because this is a new skill.

Just as important is the need to know when skills must change and advance because of patient safety. The case study below will help you to recognize why this is so important.

CASE STUDY: NICK

Nick is a newly qualified learning-disabilities nurse and has just started to work at a local Trust bungalow for four clients with differing learning difficulties. Nick is the key worker for Terry, a 63-year-old man who is being temporarily fed using a nasogastric (NG) tube after having an infection around the site of his percutaneous endoscopic gastrostomy (PEG). At the start of his shift, Nick is informed that Terry has removed his NG tube and a new one will need re-siting before he can be fed. The staff tell Nick that they have located some blue litmus paper to aspirate from the new NG tube to check its position on re-siting. They also suggest a 'whoosh test' so that they can be sure that it is positioned correctly by forcing 5 ml of air from a syringe down the tube; which will allow them to use a stethoscope to hear if the tube is in Terry's stomach. Nick is immediately concerned because when he was a student nurse he was made aware that both of these methods of positioning an NG tube were no longer used because of the inaccuracy of the technique and the dangers of the NG tube being in the wrong place. Nick tells the staff of this change in practice for this skill, thereby making them aware of the National Patient Safety Agency (NPSA) safety-alert bulletin (2008; Figure 10.2). Nick was able to get a pack of pH indicator strips from the pharmacist and teach other members of staff how to use them. This action prevented a potential clinical incident and informed the practice of other staff members due to the rigorous evidence provided by the NPSA.

TABLE 10.2 Automated external defibrillator (AED) assessment (based on the Resuscitation Council UK 2005a guidelines)

	SEQUENCE	ACTION	COMMENTS
1.	Start BLS if defibrillator not immediately available	Follow BLS protocols	
2.	Safe approach	Check environment: – water – metal – oxygen Check patient: – moisture – jewellery – chest hair – patches – pacemaker	
3.	Attach pads and switch on defibrillator	Turn energy select to AED on Follow spoken/visual prompts	
4.	'Analysing rhythm'	Tell everyone to stand clear Ensure everyone is standing clear!	
5.	If shock is advised	Ensure safety, observe area Press shock button when directed and state shock is being delivered	
6.	CPR	Immediately provide 2 minutes of CPR Repeat analysis as directed	
7.	If no shock advised	Immediately resume CPR for 2 minutes Repeat analysis as directed	
8.	If circulation present	Monitor in manual mode Leave pads attached to patient	
BLS, basic life support; CPR, cardiopulmonary resuscitation.			

The NPSA provides an online website that strives to maintain patient safety. Their 'Patient Safety Division' seeks to establish why clinical errors occur and aims to prevent similar accidents from re-occurring. The bulletin-broadcast alert system that they utilize, will inform you of changes in practice that can go as far as abolishing techniques in order to maintain patient safety. You can find bulletins like the one in Figure 10.2 and other health-related information by visiting www.npsa.nhs.uk.

When considering the advances in the nursing role, such as that of 'night-nurse practitioner' and 'advanced-nurse practitioner', along with the ever-present need for midwives to work as autonomous practitioners, it is clear that the practical clinical skills that are required are much more advanced and sophisticated than ever before. Clinical skills that are performed repetitively are usually retained. Where repetition does not take place it is necessary to update by reading or researching and where required, attending courses to keep knowledge and skills evidence based and primarily aimed at improving patient care.

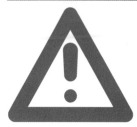

Patient safety alert

NHS

National Patient Safety Agency

05

Alert

21 February 2005

Immediate action	☑
Action	☐
Update	☐
Information request	☐

Reducing the harm caused by misplaced nasogastric feeding tubes

Nasogastric tube feeding is common practice in all age groups, from neonates to older people. Thousands of feeding tubes are inserted daily without incident. However, there is a small risk that the nasogastric feeding tube can be misplaced into the lungs during insertion, or move out of the stomach at a later stage. Although misplacement can be recognised at an early stage, i.e. before the tube is used, studies have shown that conventional methods used to check the placement of nasogastric feeding tubes can be inaccurate.

The NPSA is aware of 11 deaths and one case of serious harm due to misplaced nasogastric feeding tubes over a two-year period.

Action for the NHS

NHS acute trusts, primary care organisations and local health boards in England and Wales should take the following steps immediately.

1 Provide staff, carers and patients in the community with information on correct and incorrect testing methods:

- measuring the pH of aspirate using pH indicator strips/paper is recommended;

- radiography is recommended but should not be used 'routinely'. Local policies are recommended for particular groups of patients e.g. those in intensive care units and neonates. Fully radio-opaque tubes with markings to enable accurate measurement, identification and documentation of their position should be used;

- DO NOT use the 'whoosh' test – this practice must cease immediately;

- DO NOT test acidity/alkalinity of aspirate using blue litmus paper;

- DO NOT interpret absence of respiratory distress as an indicator of correct positioning.

2 Carry out individual risk assessment prior to nasogastric tube feeding.
3 Review and agree local action required.
4 Report misplacement incidents via their local risk management reporting systems.

For response by:
- NHS acute trusts (including foundation trusts), primary care organisations and local health boards in England and Wales

For action by:
- Directors of Nursing in England and Wales

We recommend you also inform:
- Medical Directors
  Clinical governance leads and risk managers
- Medical staff (including radiologists, neonatal staff and intensive care staff)
  Nursing staff (including community nurses)
  Nutritional nurse specialists

- Speech and language therapists, physiotherapists, dieticians
- General practitioners
- Chief pharmacists/pharmaceutical advisers
- Patient advice and liaison service staff in England
- Procurement and managers

The NPSA has informed:
- Chief executives of acute trusts, primary care organisations and local health boards in England and Wales
- Chief executives/regional directors and clinical governance leads of strategic

health authorities (England) and regional offices (Wales)
- Healthcare Commission
- Healthcare Inspectorate Wales
- NHS Purchasing and Supply Agency
- Welsh Health Supplies
- Royal Colleges and societies
- NHS Direct
- Relevant patient organisations and community health councils in Wales
- Independent Healthcare Forum
- Commission for Social Care Inspection

FIGURE 10.2 NPSA bulletin broadcast alert (from NPSA, 2008, with permission).

Clinical simulations

Simulations can facilitate a learning process that is active and mimics clinical reality. (Cioffi, 2001)

One method of developing competency in clinical skills is through the educational strategy known as simulation. Simulation allows you to move away from prescriptive skills teaching methods, allowing you to learn using an experimental approach that will aid your communication skills and confidence; all clinical skills require social skills. Once you have mastered the sequence of activities and the technique as a whole, the next stage is to learn how to use your interpersonal skills at the same time. Taking time to practise your social approach to the skill, such as talking to your simulated patient, is just as important as practising the psychomotor elements. Most students find this difficult because it feels so artificial, but if you can overcome this, you are more likely to be able to act confidently when working with a patient. Research by Murray et al. (2008) suggests you are more likely to engage in simulation as a method of teaching through an artificial or hypothetical experience if it engages you – the student – in an activity that reflects real-life conditions, without the consequences or the risk taking of actual situations. Simulating practice aims to mirror situations in real practice placement settings. However, simulation will not replace direct patient/client care. Its aim is to complement and improve on other teaching methods by preparing you for your role in providing quality patient/client care (Maran and Glavin, 2003).

An example of the successful use of simulations in training is provided by the aviation industry. Trainee pilots can prepare for both normal and abnormal situations (Murray et al., 2008), such as errors and emergency situations. Such examples can equally benefit nursing and midwifery. Consider the simulated cardiac arrest for an adult nurse or the simulated patient in labour for a midwife. Using simulation in either of these examples allows the student to learn how to manage a potentially dangerous situation for the client, without causing risk. The simulation can be made more complex by adding increasing risk, such as that the patient who is arresting might have an existing respiratory condition or be HIV positive, or obstruction to the labour. Simulation can deliver a correct or an incorrect outcome. This allows you to gain experience of your role in both the positive and negative scenarios. Simulation allows you to ask the questions of a skill that may not be appropriate whilst practising on a patient/client.

In the case study below, Alana is in the clinical setting experiencing venepuncture following simulation of a technique. You will notice how she is beginning to make connections between the practical experience, her skills-laboratory experience and her reading on and around the procedure. However, like many students she is facing a conflict because of the different techniques used for the same procedure, which is confusing.

CASE STUDY: ALANA

Alana was in her third year as a student nurse on the pre-registration programme and was excited by the prospect of her next clinical skills session, which was on the skill of venepuncture. Taking blood from patients had been one of the skills she had been looking forward to practising since starting her nurse training, as it was a crucial part of the nursing role. However, Alana had become quite concerned at the different ways that many of her mentors had approached this; some of her older colleagues had used a syringe and needle, whereas in another setting all the nurses had used a small butterfly-type needle. Her most recent placement was in an acute medical setting where a technique that required a device called a Vacutainer had been used. Alana had been told by her mentor that when she returned to this most recent placement she would be allocated a full day working with a phlebotomist, as this would help to build on the venepuncture training day she had received at the school of nursing. This could have been a good opportunity for Alana; however, she became concerned that the method she was shown in the skills laboratory would be different to that of the phlebotomist, not enabling her to practise with the technique and equipment used in practice.

To Alana's great relief the clinical skills day was a success and reassured her. A theory session in the morning covered all techniques to the skill with a rationale for each. The session covered the evidence base for each technique and stated according to research what was 'best practice'. The theory was then related to the practice as Alana observed a clear and accurate demonstration of the skill using different techniques before allowing Alana sufficient time for simulated practice. Alana felt that the session had not just allowed her to relate theory to practice, but also relate practice to theory; therefore when spending the day with the phlebotomist, she will be able to make independent decisions on the technique she uses and the site and selection of a vein, and so on. Most crucial to Alana's confidence were the psychomotor aspects of the skill she had practised, such as how she held the Vacutainer or butterfly needle, which position she found most comfortable to take the blood, where she would like the patient's/client's arm positioned and where she placed the blood sample bottles and sharps box for easy access. These were things she realized that she did not want to practise for the first time on a real patient/client.

Revisiting clinical skills

This chapter has focused on the importance of practical clinical skills and the ways to acquire them. It has stated that retained skills are those that are performed repeatedly. However, it might not always be possible to retain your knowledge of clinical skills and, when this is so, you should consider some refreshment training before performing skills without direct supervision and support. If you were used to performing a clinical skill regularly – for example, urinary catheterization – then you might have reached a level of competency or mastery to perform this skill indirectly supervised by your mentor. As a qualified nurse or midwife you would find yourself performing this skill independently and perhaps considering yourself at a level of expertise; you would instinctively know what was required of you. You would be aware of the infection-control elements of the skill and be able to identify all the equipment required without too much conscious thought. The skill itself would be something you could adapt to while maintaining the patient's/client's privacy and dignity. This level of mastery or expertise has to be maintained. If you do not have an opportunity to perform the clinical skill regularly you may need to think more carefully about your actions.

CASE STUDY: JUDY

Judy is a registered adult nurse and has been qualified for 8 years. Following a career break, Judy decided to retrain to become a nurse in the mental-health branch of nursing, as she felt that, despite enjoying her previous role, she had always wondered if she had chosen the right branch. After enrolling on a programme to train in her new chosen branch, Judy found herself on a ward placement for the elderly mentally ill (EMI). On realizing that Judy was an experienced adult nurse, the staff asked her to catheterize an elderly man during her shift. She was also approached by a student nurse who enquired whether it would be possible for her to observe the skill. Judy quickly stated that it would be, only to realize that, because of her career break, she had not performed the skill of catheterization in a long time. Judy discovered that what was once a skill she performed regularly without too much conscious thought was now something she actually had to stop and think about. She explained this to the student nurse, who suggested that she could update Judy on the technique as she had recently performed the skill in a skills laboratory. Together, Judy and the student safely and correctly catheterized the man. Judy performed the skill in a controlled manner while being assisted by the student nurse. The student nurse helped Judy to familiarize herself with the skill again while also benefiting herself from seeing the technique performed by Judy.

The example in the case study related to the skill of urinary catheterization, which is a situation that can reflect problems encountered when nursing patients of different sexes. Working in a setting that has always had female patients can make you an expert at female catheterization, but when the patient is male you could find yourself outside your comfort zone. In this situation, you are aware of the purpose of the skill but you now have to put conscious thought into the equipment required, as the catheter size will be different. You also remember that when you last catheterized a male you used an anaesthetic gel and you had to be aware of the difficulty of by-passing the prostate when passing the catheter.

When having to consciously revisit a skill you feel that you have been unable to retain a suitable knowledge of, consider the work of Vygotsky (1978, cited in Tharp and Gallimore, 1988). Lev Vygotsky, a Russian psychologist, considered four stages of development, the last of which he named the 'zone of proximal development' (ZPD). Adapted to fit the context of nursing, the ZPD can be seen as what you can do independently and what you can do with the help of others, such as your peers. Based on the needs of a child's development, Vygotsky considered three key stages to be necessary for a skill to become 'fossilized'. We could

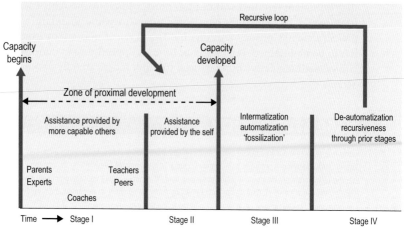

FIGURE 10.3 Zone of proximal development (from Tharp and Gallimore, 1988, with permission).

consider fossilization to be competency or mastery in our chosen skill when related to nursing or midwifery. Crucial to the work of Vygotsky is the fourth stage, or the ZPD. If you are no longer competent at the required skill, you are required to consider a 'recursive loop' (see Figure 10.3). This is your acknowledgement that you need the help of others to regain competency or mastery of the skill.

Continuing to use the example of catheterization, we need to consider where the recursive loop should take us. Do we go back to stage I and ask someone to perform the skill of male catheterization for us so that we can observe it, or do we not need to go back that far? Could we consider stage II, and consciously think about the skill again before performing it. Using the ZPD to consider your level of competency in clinical skills will remind you of the need to problem-solve and reflect when trying to retain skills, but – more importantly – it should help you to understand that sometimes recognizing when you need help is a sufficient way to perform clinical skills competently and safely.

Assessment

Clinical skills acquired in the practice placement setting are often subject to simple observational assessments by your mentor. These assessments are usually documented in a learning contract or evidence of achievement document, which provides evidence of your levels of competence at clinical skills.

The majority of assessment carried out in the educational institution has predominantly been theory-based assessment, such as written assignments and exams. The increasing use of simulated practice and the ever-increasing number of clinical-skills laboratories, as alluded to in this chapter, has resulted in much clinical-skills assessment being completed in the simulated setting. Perhaps the most widely acknowledged form of skills assessment in the simulated setting is objective, structured, clinical examinations (OSCE; see Chapter 7). Foster and Hawkins (2004) suggested that in the case of nursing and midwifery education, a move away from the traditional, academic forms of assessment to a more creative and innovative assessment procedure for both individuals and groups is clearly needed. Not only does simulation of practice offer students the opportunity to learn and practise their clinical skills in a realistic, meaningful and non-threatening environment, it also enables the assessment of students' clinical competence in simulated situations without risk to patients and minimal risk to themselves (McCallum, 2006).

OSCEs usually comprise a number of stations where you demonstrate clinical competency through a simulated assessment. Stations usually have a required time for you to complete the assessment in front of an examiner. The stations may have a theoretical element as well as the practical skill for you to complete. Alinier (2003) suggests that OSCEs are a positive form of assessment favoured by students. OSCEs can help students to determine their own weaknesses (Sloan et al., 1995) while informing tutors of students' abilities.

When preparing for OSCEs consider:

- What will be the format of the examination?
- Are there practice sessions that you can attend?
- Is there a checklist of procedures for possible skills?
- What might the examiner be looking for?
- Will you be timed?
- Can you practise techniques in the placement area?

This form of assessment often requires formal learning as you strive to understand what is required to pass the assessment. On the whole, the requirement to acquire clinical skills can be achieved through informal learning, 'learning on the job' and practising informally in the laboratory setting. Dornan and O'Neil (2000) suggest you take a far-sighted view of OSCEs and don't try to cram in information at the last minute. Building skills over time will grow confidence and competence, allowing you to take clinical exams in your stride.

Prepare yourself for the OSCE. Your lecturer may provide a checklist of criteria required in the OSCE; study this and try to work through it in the practice placement setting (your mentor may help). Notify your tutor if you feel there are weaknesses in some of your skills; these are problems better identified before rather than after the OSCE. Approach your fellow students, have they completed an OSCE? Can they offer you any advice?

Conclusion

Through the re-introduction of clinical-skills laboratories, the ever-developing possibilities of simulation and a need to meet NMC skill requirements in the practice setting, clinical skills have never been more evident in nursing and midwifery curricula. This chapter has offered case studies and tips to inform you of the need not only to acquire practical clinical skills but also to understand the underpinning theory behind these skills. It is essential that you understand the importance of retaining your clinical skills, while always being aware of the need for change through life-long learning, enabling evidence-based practice to be the focus of patient-centred care. The theory you are taught will inform your practice and your practice can inform the theory. Competency in practical clinical skills will bring you a belief and confidence not just in the practical elements of your role but in the many other multi-faceted skills you will require as you strive to become an expert in your field, through the transition from student to expert practitioner.

 CHAPTER RESOURCES

REFERENCES

Alinier, G., 2003. Nursing students' and lecturers' perspectives of objective structured clinical examination incorporating simulation. Nurse Education Today 23, 419–426.

Ausubel, D.P., 1968. Educational psychology: a cognitive view. Holt, Rhinehart and Winston, New York.

Authentic World, 2008. Safety in numbers. Innovative solutions for reducing medication errors. Online. Available: www.authenticworld .co.uk/index.php [accessed 22 July 2008]

Benner, P., 2001. From novice to expert, excellence and power in clinical nursing practice, commemorative edition. Prentice Hall, New Jersey, USA.

Billet, S., 2001. Learning in the workplace: effective strategies for practice. Allen Unwin, Singapore.

Cioffi, J., 2001. Clinical simulations: development and validation. Nurse Education Today 21, 477–486.

Dougherty, L. & Lister, S., 2008. The Royal Marsden Hospital manual of clinical nursing procedures, 7th edn. Blackwell Publishing, London.

Dreyfus, S.E. & Dreyfus, H.L., 1980. A five-stage model of the mental activities involved in direct skills acquisition. In: Dornan, T. & O'Neil, P. (Eds.) 2000 Core clinical skills for OSCEs in medicine. Churchill Livingstone, London.

Foster, T. & Hawkins, J., 2004. Performance of understanding: a new model of assessment. Nurse Education Today 24, 333–336.

Gopee, N., 2005. Facilitating the implementation of lifelong learning in nursing. British Journal of Nursing 14 (14), 761–767.

Higgs, J., 1992. Developing clinical reasoning competencies. Physiotherapy 78, 575–578.

Lauder, W., Watson, R., Topping, K., et al., 2008. An evaluation of fitness for practice curricula: self-efficacy, support and self reported competence in pre-registration student nurses and midwives. Journal of Clinical Nursing 17 (14), 1858–1867.

Manual Handling Operations Regulations, 1992. (updated 2002) I: Manual handling; guidance on regulations. HSE Books, Norwich

Maran, N.J. & Glavin, R.J., 2003. Low-to high-fidelity simulation – a continuum of medical education?. Medical Education 37, 22–28.

McCallum, J., 2006. The debate in favour of using simulation education in pre-registration adult nursing. Nurse Education Today 27, 825–831.

Murray, C., Grant, M.J., Howarth, M.L. & Leigh, J., 2008. The use of simulation as a teaching and learning approach to support practice learning. Nurse Education in Practice 8, 5–8.

National Patient Safety Agency (NPSA), 2008. Advice to the NHS on reducing harm caused by misplacement of nasogastric feeding tubes. Online. Available: www.npsa.nhs.uk [accessed 8 July 2008].

Nursing and Midwifery Council (NMC), 2006. Standards to support learning and assessment in practice. NMC standards for mentors, practice teachers and teachers. NMC, London.

Nursing and Midwifery Council (NMC), 2007. Advance information regarding essential skills clusters for pre-registration nursing programmes. Online. Available: www.nmc.org [accessed 25 March 2008].

Nursing and Midwifery Council (NMC), 2008. The code. NMC, London.

Peach Report, 1999. UKCC commission for nursing and midwifery education. Fitness for Practice. UKCC, London.

Platt, C., 2002. Nurses 'fit for purpose': using a task-centred group to help students learn from experience. Teaching in Higher Education 7 (1), 33–43.

Resuscitation Council UK (RCUK), 2005a. Automated external defibrillation. RCUK, London.

Resuscitation Council UK (RCUK), 2005b. Basic life support. RCUK, London.

Sloan, D.A., Donnelley, M.B., Stewards, R.W. & Stoilid, W.E., 1995. The objective structured clinical examination. The new gold standard for evaluating postgraduate clinical performance. Annals of Surgery 222 (6), 735–742.

Tharp, R.G. & Gallimore, R., 1988. Rousing minds to life. Cambridge University Press, Cambridge.

WEBSITES

http://www.authenticworld.co.uk

http://www.learndirect.co.uk

http://www.npsa.nhs.uk
http://www.sciencedirect.com

FURTHER READING

Billet, S., 2001. Learning in the workplace: effective strategies for practice. Allen Unwin, Singapore.

Dougherty, L. & Lister, S. 2008. The Royal Marsden Hospital manual of clinical nursing procedures, 7th edn. Blackwell Publishing, London.

Tollefson, J., 2004. Clinical psychomotor skills: assessment tool for nursing students, 2nd edn. Social Science Press, Australia.

Learning in practice settings

Jenny Spouse

KEY ISSUES

- Getting to know your practice setting and your supervisor
- Planning your placement experience
- Working and learning as a collaborator with your supervisor
- Working and learning in and from practice
- Emotional labour in practice: dealing with emotions
- Professional and ethical issues
- Integrating theory with practice

Introduction

Irrespective of whether you are a newly qualified practitioner, a healthcare worker starting your first appointment, an experienced clinician providing temporary relief or a student on a new placement, you will share the sense of being an outsider to the 'resident' team or the community of practitioners who normally work and interact in the setting. Finding someone to take you under their wing, to sponsor you or simply to befriend you will be the most important predictor of your experience in the setting, as well as the length of time you are likely to stay there (Nicholson, 1987). Without such support, most newcomers adopt a low profile, out of the way of the general hurley-burley of everyday events and becoming increasingly marginalized and disenfranchised until they either leave or suffer high levels of sickness or absence (Fuhrer, 1993). Learning to become an insider is vital if you are to become a member of the community of practice and if you are to develop the language and skills of the resident experts. In this chapter, you will be introduced to some of the ways that will help you to become an insider and some strategies that will help you to develop your professional expertise in the clinical field.

Research by Spouse (1998a, 2003) indicated that pre-registration students are concerned to develop their professional knowledge in seven specific areas of clinical practice. These are:

- relating to patients and their carers
- developing technical knowledge

- learning to bundle activities together (management skills)
- developing professional craft or finger-tip knowledge
- relating to, and functioning within a clinical team (the community of practice)
- managing feelings and emotions appropriately (both their own and those of patients and relatives)
- developing the essence of practice, which promotes therapeutic action.

The research investigated how nursing students from adult, mental-health and children's nursing developed their professional knowledge and found these seven areas of personal and professional development to be core to their development as nurses. It is possible that practitioners entering an unfamiliar clinical setting will have similar learning needs relating to the unfamiliar clinical speciality but their learning is faster because of their existing foundations of professional knowledge.

This chapter introduces you to the six principles of successful learning in and from practice experiences, and you will find detailed examples of each of them as they relate to the seven areas of professional development mentioned above.

The six principles of learning in and from clinical practice are as follows:

1. Getting to know your supervisor.
2. Developing and documenting a plan for your learning experiences.
3. Implementing and evaluating your success in achieving the plan.
4. Working as a collaborator with healthcare practitioners.
5. Flying solo: working under distant supervision.
6. Making connections between practice and theory.

Getting to know your practice setting and your supervisor

Entering an unfamiliar practice setting can be daunting and many new-comers worry about how they will be accepted by the resident team of practitioners. These teams are often a tightly knit community of people who have shared expertise in the clinical speciality and are committed to providing high standards of care. You can make your first few days successful by some good preparation and detective work.

Making contact with the practice-setting manager before your first day gives you a chance to introduce yourself (and for them to meet you) before starting work in the placement; to know the hours of working and any other important requirements, such as dress code. It also gives you time to find out about clinical activities that are practised in the setting and thus an opportunity to arrive better informed. Healthcare students who change placements fairly regularly can arrive knowing something about the kinds of patients cared for in the setting, having an understanding of the different routines of the placement and knowing a little about the clinical speciality. You will be equipped with some of the vocabulary that might otherwise be completely unfamiliar and this will boost your confidence.

Most healthcare organizations (such as a voluntary, private or charitable organization, an NHS Trust or a Foundation Trust) have dedicated websites with information about the clinical specialities on offer. In addition, there is usually an intranet website with photographs or names of key personnel for each of the different departments, wards, units or health centres. Studying the dedicated website (perhaps through the library or study room) of your new practice setting will help you to find out about the place, to know the names of key staff and perhaps even to recognize some of the staff when you first start working. Making a good entrance by appearing on time, smartly dressed according to the local uniform and dress code, being serious about your learning and respectful of the staff, as well as having some knowledge of the setting, will normally earn you respect and thus the support of the staff. If you have the opportunity, it is often worth spending some time working through a toolkit of activities that you will find on http://evolve.elsevier.com – these are designed to help you learn about your new workplace and the healthcare needs of your clients.

Establish contact with your placement manager at least 1 week before you are due to start and learn as much as you can about the placement and the clinical specialisms, so you start with a good foundation of knowledge.

Sponsorship

Having got off to a successful start, how do you fit in? Your placement manager should have arranged for you to be attached to a sponsor; this may be a mentor, a preceptor, supervisor or a member of staff who has responsibility for looking after new staff or students on arrival. Arrangements should also have been made for you to be supervised during your placement. The person in this supervisory role will normally be someone who is in the same profession as you and who is knowledgeable about your potential needs (especially if you are studying for an academic or professional award). If you are a newly qualified nurse then you should have a staff member who will be your preceptor for at least your first 6 months.

Your sponsor has responsibility for inducting you to the setting. This means that he or she must ensure that you understand your responsibilities, the boundaries of your role, how to implement your role and where to find help. Below is a case study of a first-year nursing student, David, who is on the first day of his third clinical placement.

CASE STUDY: DAVID

This was my first day in the community centre, and everything was so different to my earlier placements. The pace seemed slower but everyone seemed very focused on their jobs. The telephone was ringing all the time. I felt so out on a limb. Fortunately, I had popped into the centre a couple of weeks before and had met the deputy manager who was working that day. It was a relief to see a familiar face. She introduced me to Sasha, who was to be my mentor during the 10-week placement. Sasha was very friendly and told me she had a reduced workload that morning so she could look after me. We went and sat down in the staff coffee room and had a chat for about 40 minutes. This was great as I ended up feeling she was really listening to what I wanted to achieve during my placement. It also reassured me to know that she had a lot of experience of working here and also of supporting students. I showed her all my assessment documents and my placement passport with the comments from my earlier mentors. After we had had a coffee, Sasha gave me a tour of the centre, showed me where the different policy and procedure books were stored and gave me a general overview of the place. As I was going to be shadowing her for the rest of the week I felt quite reassured that I was not going to be thrown into the deep end and left on my own.

During his first week, David worked alongside Sasha and assisted her when she was conducting an examination or a procedure. The kind of activities Sasha asked David to do were tailored so that she could observe his communication and technical skills. These might have been simply holding the client's hand and helping her to relax, fetching pieces of equipment or dealing with samples. However mundane the activity that Sasha gave David, it helped him to learn new things about the centre and to meet different people. It also gave David the opportunity to observe a skilled practitioner deliver care, thus providing opportunities for him to develop new knowledge. Working as a legitimate member of the team and undertaking essential activities or tasks in this way, David gained quite a high profile within the centre and by the end of his first week he also felt at home with almost all the members of staff. Working together also gave Sasha opportunities to monitor David's conduct and assess his strengths and areas where he needed or wanted to develop further. It gave her the opportunity to decide how much she could safely delegate to David and where he needed to work under close supervision:

- Sasha was consequently able to honour her commitment to her professional Code of Conduct and client safety by ensuring David only undertook activities that he was safe to deliver.
- David made a good start to his placement by taking responsibility for his own learning, by his preparation and willingness to share his aspirations, his learning history and his programme documents with his new mentor.

If you find that no one has been designated as your supervisor, or they are not on duty when you arrive, alert your placement manager as soon as possible and no later than the end of your first week so that suitable arrangements can be made.

Planning your placement experience

The second principle of working and learning in practice is to develop an appropriate learning plan, or a learning agenda. Over his first week, David and Sasha developed a good working relationship and also a sense of what learning David was capable of.

At the end of the first week, Sasha and David had a private meeting in a quiet place and discussed David's learning plan for the first part of his placement. This they agreed could be used to structure his mid-way assessment and they could then plan his learning for the second half of his placement. By documenting this agreement both David and Sasha were clear about what had been agreed and could monitor his progress.

Agreeing goals

David was preparing for registration as a nurse and his programme is structured around the requirements of the professional statutory body (the Nursing and Midwifery Council; NMC). Clinical placements constitute 50% of all approved nursing and midwifery programmes. By the end of each placement period, students are expected to achieve pre-specified learning outcomes. These learning outcomes are deliberately generalized so that students can be placed in a wide range of placements and still achieve the outcomes as they relate to the clinical speciality of the setting. The clinical speciality in David's placement was community care, including a day centre for older people and children with chronic healthcare needs. During his placement, David would be exposed to a wide range of healthcare situations, but would still be able to learn how to plan and deliver care and to evaluate its effectiveness.

David's mentor, Sasha, was able to advise David on the range of services and staff he could learn about. Sasha had also assessed David's capability and knew that he would develop his skills quickly by spending some of his time in the different clinics and on home visits. She gave David a menu of the kinds of experiences he could have throughout his placement and they agreed what would be most suitable for the first 5 weeks. They agreed that if all went well and he made good progress, he would have the opportunity to conduct a clinic under distant supervision and spend more time visiting clients in their homes, either assisting the community nurses or under their more distant supervision. Together they compiled a learning plan for weeks 2–5 (Table 11.1).

TABLE 11.1 David's learning plan for weeks 2–5 of community placement

GOAL	CLINICAL ACTIVITY	ACHIEVEMENT CRITERION
Understand the community services for older, mentally frail adults	Participate in the respite clinic for older, mentally frail adults and enjoy effective relationships with the clients	Able to contribute to the daily work of the team, by knowing and following the routines, procedures and policies of the unit Able to deliver safe and effective care with distant supervision
Understand the role of members of the multidisciplinary team (MDT)	Work with physiotherapist, occupational therapist, podiatrist, nurses, healthcare assistants, geriatrician	Able to communicate sensitively and effectively with the clients Able to discuss knowledgeably the different contributions of the MDT to the health and wellbeing of clients and their carers
Develop knowledge and understanding of care planning and care delivery	Admit 2–3 older persons to the clinic Make a routine assessment of existing clients' condition, to develop assessment skills, communication skills, documentation skills Talk with clients' carers to understand their experiences	Can document an accurate and comprehensive assessment of a new client and provide a full verbal handover to the client's key worker Able to recognize and document accurately changes in clients' condition; communicate such changes promptly and accurately to the nurse in charge Where necessary, be able to take prompt and effective remedial action Have a comprehensive understanding of the everyday experiences of carers and the client in their homes
Understand the role of the community nurse	Attend 3 home visits	Be able to dress and conduct self in an appropriate manner whilst visiting clients' homes Be able to document the care provided accurately Discuss the pros and cons of home care provision and clinic provision for the client and the service
Understand the community services for children (and their carers) with chronic disorders	Participate in the clinic for children with chronic disorders and enjoy effective relationships with them and their carers	Able to contribute to the daily work of the team, by knowing and following the routines, procedures and policies of the unit. Able to deliver safe and effective care with distant supervision. Able to communicate sensitively and effectively with the children and their carers
Understand the role of members of the MDT	Work with physiotherapist, occupational therapist, dietician, nurse, healthcare assistant, paediatrician	Able to discuss knowledgeably the different contributions of the MDT to the health and wellbeing of clients and their carers
Develop knowledge and understanding of care planning and care delivery	Make a routine assessment of existing clients' condition, to develop assessment skills, communication skills, documentation skills Talk with children and their carers to understand their experiences	Able to recognize and document accurately changes in clients' condition and to communicate such changes promptly and accurately to the nurse in charge Where necessary, be able to take prompt and effective remedial action Have a comprehensive understanding of the everyday experiences of children and their carers in their everyday life

Assessing David's progress

David's learning plan covers a wide range of skills and an even wider range of knowledge that David hopes to achieve by the mid-point of his placement. He has already practised some of these skills in his earlier placements, but using them in an unfamiliar setting is more difficult and takes some rehearsal. Similarly, he has probably had taught sessions and read about caring for the different client groups that he will be meeting on this placement. However, research (Spouse, 1998a) suggests that this knowledge is not recognized as being salient until students feel part of the team and able to perform many of the local skills and techniques that they see being used in the setting.

David knows that Sasha and her colleagues will be monitoring and assessing his development throughout this next 4-week period. They have some minimum expectations of David's achievement by the end of this first period that can be identified under four headings.

1. Safety of the clients: in addition to knowing the normal safety procedures, David should also be able to recognize the common situations that can arise when working with vulnerable adults and children. He should be taking steps to identify and prevent incidents such as slips, trips and falls by older clients; ensuring they have sufficient nutrition and hydration and that they remain continent during their stay at the centre.

2. Communication skills: David is expected to be able to recognize regular clients and call them by their preferred name, to communicate effectively with them and their carers; to make newcomers feel welcome. He is also expected to seek help if he is unsure about anything. Most practitioners are reassured if their student discusses their actions (potential and actual) as it implies that the student is aware of their boundaries and can be trusted.

3. Wellbeing of the clients: David is expected to demonstrate that he has the interests of the clients foremost in his mind and that he is willing to take trouble and effort to meet their needs appropriately. He should also be prompt and thorough in responding to requests for help and to comply with the Trust procedures and best practice when delivering care.

4. Understanding of the routines, policies and procedures of the unit: David needs to have sufficient knowledge of the two clinics to help with preparing for the day, to anticipate the routines and to know where equipment is stored, and to carry out the policies and procedures effectively.

These are the minimum standards that David is expected to achieve, and he will be encouraged and supported to develop beyond that minimum. If David showed signs of struggling, Sasha has a duty of care – both to her clients and to David – to give him prompt feedback and to revise the action plan into smaller 'steps', and to ensure that he has closer supervision and support until he makes progress. Sasha will also be required to document his progress and any change of learning plan so David's record is an honest and accurate reflection of his performance during his placement.

Towards the end of this 4-week period, Sasha and David met to review and document his progress. Then they developed another plan for his remaining 6 weeks in the placement, which would help him to achieve all his required learning outcomes and to learn additional skills and knowledge as he had made such good progress.

So how can a student or a newcomer develop this knowledge and understanding?

Working and learning as a collaborator with your supervisor, mentor or preceptor

Why collaboration as the 'junior' partner is a helpful learning opportunity

Working alongside experienced practitioners provides opportunities to observe and listen to how situations and techniques are managed by different people. It also helps novices to develop their professional knowledge both in terms of the technical skills required and the vocabulary used, as indicated by the following extracts taken from research into nursing students' experiences of learning in clinical placements.

 CASE STUDY: HELEN

My mentor really helps as well and it makes a big difference. It's like having a personal tutor there all the time. If you need something you can just go and ask her and she talks about it. In addition, the other people in the team, the associate nurse is really helpful to me ... I was more listening to her [the mentor's] instructions and helping her, but I didn't feel under pressure at all because she was showing me how to do it. When she goes through it, she reflects on things that you might think in your head but wouldn't necessarily say. I felt at ease with her because she was helping me, as opposed to watching and criticizing me. (From Spouse, 2003, p. 40.)

Helen describes how she was able to ask questions and receive explanations, suggesting that she recognized that she noticed something unfamiliar and that there was a question to ask. It takes some time for novices to notice and to have the necessary language to frame questions. The advantages of being the novice assistant or observer are described by Nicola, a mental-health nursing student.

 CASE STUDY: NICOLA

Veronica's been really good this term, because we'll do something together and she'll turn round and say, 'What do you think of that?' I'll tell her [how] I thought it went and we'll have a bit of discussion about it. She does quite a bit of CBT [cognitive behavioural therapy], that's her speciality. So I sit in on her several times when she's doing that with patients. And she's been quite good talking me through what's she's doing while she does it. I suppose I'm learning all the time, but it doesn't seem like learning. It's like I've opened my pores up to being receptive to everything that's there. (From Spouse, 2003, p. 196.)

An important aspect of your learning plan must include times when you and your mentor work together in partnership, sharing in providing care to the same client at the same time. Sometimes it is more appropriate that you work in a more menial or low-key way, but as you gain in confidence and understanding you need to negotiate with your mentor to take the lead in a procedure, with your mentor or supervisor coaching you through the process as illustrated in the two extracts below.

CASE STUDY: RUTH

It was quite a technical placement, so we were doing things [together]. The drugs, techniques, and she would go through it all: 'This is the drug chart, this is what it means'. We might look up a drug because neither of us knew what it did. It struck me as much more a learning situation. I really felt I was not a burden on her. I was working with her. I was helping her. (From Spouse, 2003, p. 190.)

CASE STUDY: MARIE

[I] changed dressings. My mentor would be there and helping me and helping me to think about how it should be done and saying, 'Yes you are doing it right. The padding needs to be a bit thicker there, or don't do the padding so thick.' I've seen my mentor do it before. She never said 'Well you're doing it totally wrong'. So it'd be more me talking myself through the stages, telling her what I was going to do and she'd say 'Yes that's OK'. (From Spouse, 1996, p. 128.)

In both situations the students enjoyed a trusting relationship with their mentor and could be honest about their concerns and their learning. In Marie's narrative, she describes how leading a specific task with the help and guidance of her mentor gave her confidence, especially if things did not go smoothly. Talking aloud as she practised the technique helped Marie to learn the procedure. This collaborative process meant their patient was receiving safe care of a high standard and Marie's mentor could assess her progress and give her feedback immediately.

As a healthcare student, you should have opportunities to work alongside your supervisor or mentor for 40% of your placement hours (NMC, 2008a) and during the remaining time be supervised – either directly or indirectly – by another registered practitioner. The following example from a different setting illustrates the importance of this.

CASE STUDY: RUTH

Some things are so obvious and you don't think. Like doing post-operative checks for the first few hours. You concentrate on the blood pressure, fine; and [my mentor] said, 'Did you check the wound site?' I didn't look at that. He'd had major abdominal surgery and I suddenly thought how obvious it was. She'd say 'What I do Ruth, for post-op is the observation per the chart, but more than just the chart. This man has had a big operation on his leg, so look at his leg. His temperature might be fine for the next 5 minutes but he might be bleeding profusely the whole time'. That's so obvious and I didn't think of it! (From Spouse, 2003, p. 171.)

Receiving this kind of support is vital to your own professional development as well as to the safety of your clients. Ruth's inexperience is not unusual, and without her supervisor's presence and support during her placement (irrespective of the stage in her programme), she would not have learned this very simple piece of nursing care. Here Gilles is describing the learning he achieved in a children's ward by watching his mentor Robyn.

CASE STUDY: GILLES

In some ways, seeing how Robyn dealt with the little lad was how I dealt with the [child] … plus experience at the children's hospital and the children's ward. Pooling your knowledge together, not remembering one bit of it. We were certainly looking at that, how they are and giving them reassurance and telling them what's happening. A lot of the wards I've worked on are very busy. You don't have time to stand still. Whereas Robyn almost made time, even if we were busy she had time. (From Spouse, 1999.)

Learning by watching more experienced practitioners is sometimes described as role modelling (Bandura, 1977) or social–cultural learning (Vygotsky and Luria, 1970; Vygotsky, 1978), where learning is achieved through a social relationship with an expert. The process of participating in activities that contribute to the overall workload of the team is known as legitimate peripheral participation (Lave and Wenger, 1991; Spouse, 1998b). It provides an important opportunity for newcomers to learn by watching others while contributing to the immediate process in hand. Once newcomers can demonstrate understanding and can conduct the same processes safely, then they can work on their own with distant supervision and thus contribute to the overall workload of the team.

Working and learning in and from practice: flying solo

Agreeing an achievable workload and support availability

Working without direct supervision implies trust and capability as well as awareness of personal limitations. If at any time you feel that you are being asked to undertake an activity for which you feel unprepared or unsafe then, for the protection of your clients (and yourself and colleagues) you must insist that you are given the necessary training and support. You also have a responsibility for preparing yourself to work independently, as Marie describes below.

 CASE STUDY: MARIE

Last night there were seven children and I read up on all their conditions and I could quite happily nurse [any] one of those children today. Just looking up so many different books I can get the complete picture, because I know one book is not going to be enough. (From Spouse, 2003, p. 58.)

Being included in the work team provides a sense of being respected and valued as well as being part of the team. If you have been supported by collaborating with your supervisor and other members of staff while engaged in clinical routine, you should be ready to embark on practising those techniques on suitable clients, selected because of their overall condition and care needs. You will need to know who is the named registered practitioner or principal carer responsible for the clients' treatment and from whom you can obtain support and report to.

Planning your workload, doing a nursing round and assessing priorities

When working under more distant supervision you need to plan how you are going to manage your workload. This is important for the smallest and simplest of tasks as well as managing a caseload of several clients. The principles are similar. The problem is that normally you have less time to think about planning. Considering how you manage your own everyday life activities often provides a good starting point.

 For example, when preparing for a shower, what preparations do you make?

Do you for example make sure:

- there is sufficient hot water
- no one else is wanting to use the shower room
- you have all the necessary bathing equipment: shower gel, shaving equipment, shampoo, face cloth or gloves, a dry towel, a bath mat to protect you from slipping on the floor and anything else you might need
- you have fresh clothes to wear after your shower and they are at hand.

You can probably recognize that these preparations are the same as those needed when assisting a patient to have a wash or bath. Using a routine to plan care helps it to go smoothly and you will find with repeated practice that you no longer have to think about planning. The same principles apply to preparing materials for drug administration, such as injections. Some basic questions and answers to think through might be those in Table 11.2.

Even if you have never given an injection before, it is helpful to go through the above procedure with your mentor and observe how an injection is carried out on a patient. If possible, it is good for learning if you can give any other pre-medications during the same shift, under your mentor's supervision, so you can develop your confidence, as Jack describes below.

 CASE STUDY: JACK

If you do it once (and it doesn't hurt), you think maybe it's just a one-off. But to do it 20 times, and for everyone to say 'Have you finished? Oh that didn't hurt'; then you realize that you can do it. (From Spouse, 2003, p. 82.)

Irrespective of which part of the professional register you are preparing for, you will need opportunities to practise different techniques many times before you gain your self-confidence. This often means making clinical staff aware that you want the opportunity, and reminding them several times. Some techniques are best practised in unexpected settings, such as community centres and GP clinics where there are clinics for travellers or children needing vaccinations. Some outpatient departments have routine clinics for patients requiring surgical dressings. As a midwifery student, you can learn how to palpate a mother's abdomen

TABLE 11.2   Points to ponder before a procedure

QUESTIONS TO ASK	POSSIBLE ANSWERS
What procedure will you be using?	Intramuscular injection of pre-medication (location?)
What equipment will you need?	Sterile syringe, needle (size?), container, file, swab
What charts will you need?	Patient's drug chart, controlled drug book
Should anyone else be present when you do the procedure?	Key registered practitioner (midwife/ nurse) for the patient, or deputy
What preparation must you give the patient?	Check that the patient is appropriately prepared for the operation. If the patient needs to go to the toilet, this can be done while the medication is being prepared
	Check the patient is wearing the correct identity band
	Warn the patient not to get out of bed after the medication has been administered

or conduct vaginal examinations in antenatal clinics or community centres. It is always a good idea to arrange to attend such clinics as an additional part of your programme. They also provide opportunities to observe and listen to experts discussing with their clients their health-care needs.

Caring for a group of clients

Planning to care for a group of clients over one shift is an important part of the process. By first reading through your patient's case notes and care plans, you will learn about their medical or obstetric history and thus their care requirements. You should be alerted to any planned interventions, such as physiotherapy or off-the-ward investigations, which might necessitate some preparation (such as fasting) that, if unnoticed, could cause disruption to the plan and the patient's treatment. Different settings have different priorities and for example working on a busy surgical ward is different on an operation day to non-operating days. Effective planning becomes even more critical when surgery relies on effective preoperative management and patient safety relies on their safe transfer back into the ward by ward staff. As a student you might find it bewildering when you first start because you are unfamiliar with the routine and the overall plan. Here is Ruth describing what she was able to achieve after a few weeks on such a ward.

 CASE STUDY: RUTH

I could actually see someone from admission through to going to surgery without constantly having to ask what to do next. I could virtually do the pre-med, but I just needed the countersign and I could fill in forms and would just double check … I spent the first few times with my mentor and then I'd take the easier cases on my own. That would be a case of us both saying hello to the patients and I'd come back and she'd say: 'What are you going to do this morning for this person?' and we'd go through it, agree it and then I'd go off … It was nerve-wracking and I wondered what I was getting nervous about. (From Spouse, 2003, p. 170.)

As Ruth indicates, an essential part of good planning is a preliminary nursing or midwifery round of patients to assess their condition and also introduce yourself and your mentor as their carers for the shift. This is in addition to the formal handover from the previous shift staff. By visiting each of your patients and assessing their physical and mental condition, you can ensure that their treatments are up-to-date and note any interventions that are planned for the shift. You can also work with your patient to plan when to provide their care and thus avoid disruptions later. It reassures patients that you are taking care of them efficiently and that you are being supported by your supervisor. Ruth's assessment of her patients' immediate, short- and long-term needs enabled her to set her priorities and plan her time. She could negotiate with her patients when they received their treatment and deal immediately with the urgent matters, such as pain relief or drug administration, while her mentor was available. A second advantage of conducting a round of her patients and setting priorities meant that both her patients and any members of the multidisciplinary team could also plan their day, leaving Ruth free to implement her plan without interruptions and delay. Initially, Ruth and her mentor worked through her plan for the shift, but as Ruth got more familiar and thus confident with the process, she was able to get on with less supervision from her mentor. Her plan for the shift is shown in Table 11.3.

By writing up her work plan, Ruth is getting a stronger sense of her priorities and so is less likely to be taken by surprise, such as finding that Miss Mobberley has no outpatient's appointment or her take-home drugs have not arrived, just as she is about to leave the ward. Ruth might not be able to stick to the detail of the plan but at least she has a sense of the order in which she wants to do her work and, just as importantly, her patients know when she is coming to give them their care. Being able to look after one high-dependency patient and two low-dependency patients is quite challenging in an unfamiliar setting and a good way to start learning how to plan your workload.

TABLE 11.3   Ruth's management plan for the morning shift

NAME OF PATIENT	CARE NEED	TIME	OTHER ISSUES
Mrs Jones	IVI antibiotics & analgesia Post-operative care: full hygiene needs 4-hourly obs Physiotherapy: sit out of bed with physio × 10 minutes + help back Analgesia	8.30 a.m. 9.30–10.15 a.m. 10.30 a.m 11 a.m. 12.30 p.m.	Check wound and behind wound for bleeding Give hourly breathing and leg exercises Help to change position
Mrs Ahmet	Drugs & analgesia – oral Self-care for hygiene, help with legs and back Physiotherapy Dress wound Make sure she gets Hallal diet, drugs and analgesia	8.0 a.m. 9 a.m. 9.30 a.m. 10.30 a.m. Lunchtime	Check fluid balance and that she drinks 1.4 L this morning
Miss Mobberley	Analgesia Check she can manage self-care Going home – relative collecting at 11 a.m. Ensure take-home drugs are ordered and on ward ready; has an appointment for outpatients Help with packing up belongings and get valuables signed off	8.0 a.m. 8.15 a.m. 10.15 a.m.	Ask ward clerk to make outpatient appointment; get house officer to write up TTAs and ask pharmacist to ensure the TTAs are on the ward for 10.30 a.m.
TTA, to take away.			

You might find it helpful to practise writing up some work plans for different groupings of patients on your placement, varying their level of dependency, the different kinds of care they need and the number of patients you have.

After practice at writing work plans, you will be more able to identify your priorities and learn how much can be reasonably achieved in the time span. It is a good idea to discuss a work plan with your mentor and see what modifications can be suggested. With experience you will be able to do the same kind of planning in your head and to know what can be done in the time available.

The advantage that Ruth had was that she recognized and dealt with the challenges – getting the support of key people such as her mentor and the ward clerk early in the shift, thus preventing delays. By checking her patients' drug charts early in the shift, Ruth could see which patients needed their medications and pain relief. With her mentor on-hand, she was able to get these administered at once and, as a result, her patients were able to mobilize and to participate in their treatments effectively, thus reducing the risk of post-operative complications as well as making it possible for her most dependent patient, Mrs Jones, to participate in her bath and to respond to her physiotherapy while the analgesia was at its maximum potential. By planning her morning, Ruth made the whole experience of caring and being cared for more satisfying.

Towards the end of her shift Ruth needs to do another round of her patients. This time to ensure that they are comfortable and that their needs have been met. For example, Mrs Jones will be ready for more analgesia and this will help her to sleep while the ward is quieter and for her to be ready for the afternoon's treatments. Making this second nursing round helps Ruth to assess the effectiveness of her care delivery and the analgesia she has given, all of which she will document in writing in the nursing notes. This provides staff of the next shift with a record of her activities and informs their own care planning. As a learning tool, the process of report writing helps Ruth to consolidate her actions and in the debriefing time with her mentor, she can ask questions and clarify her knowledge.

Another way of planning your work is to develop a map of the different activities. These are called either a spidergram or a mind map (Buzan and Buzan, 1996). Figure 11.1 is an example of a mind map that Miranda likes to create when she is planning her shift.

Miranda's mind map provides a quick visual plan of the important activities she needs to remember that shift. You may notice that there are some activities missing, such as ensuring that the mother whose baby is

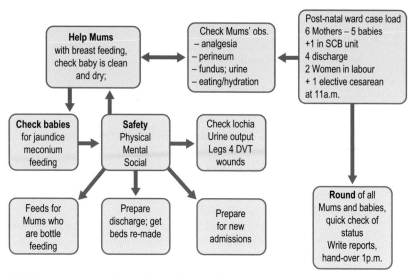

FIGURE 11.1 Example of Miranda's mind map to plan her workload on a busy post-natal unit.

in the special care baby unit (SCBU) goes to visit her baby; perhaps she will need help when she expresses her milk for the baby's feeds, and so on. If Miranda had discussed her mind map with her supervisor, she would have noticed such discrepancies and suggested some additional activities to be included. Inevitably, there will be incidental activities that Miranda will undertake during the shift as well as when she helps women to get ready to go home and admits new mothers following their delivery.

Writing to learn

Some students find it helpful to write up their shift for their own learning. Nicola, a mental-health student, found this was helpful for an assignment she was preparing.

 CASE STUDY: NICOLA

This time I've made more of an effort to write down everything that happens on the shift and I've been using a spider diagram. I'll put something down and draw my points from it. There's been so much I can put in that, I don't think it's going to be a big problem writing what's happened. (From Spouse, 2003, p. 173.)

If you learn by using visual images you may like to use the technique that either Miranda or Nicola found helpful. Nicola liked keeping a record of her practical experiences by creating mind maps, such as the one in Figure 11.2. Developing the habit of making records such as this helps you to not only remember what you have done and thus what you have learned, but also to notice what is happening in your workplace. As a novice, it is often difficult to 'see' what is taking place, or at least to recognize the significance of what you are seeing. Keeping such a simple record helps you to notice things and learn their significance.

Using this form of record keeping Nicola found that she was also learning the vocabulary of her placement. This made it easier to ask questions both of her placement colleagues or when she was sitting in on case conferences and also to prepare questions for the texts she was reading, such as clients' case notes. She got into the habit of regarding her placement time not as only a practical learning opportunity but also as an opportunity to make links between what she saw and her reading. She would take time out to check the disorders or procedures that she wanted to know more about in the books and journals in her placement (or, if none was available, the intranet, worldwide web or the library) and make notes linking these into her mind map, remembering to include the reference details.

Other people find it easier to learn if they keep an audio diary and use a small dictaphone to record conversations with their mentor and to take verbal notes, which they can then review later and write up for assignments. These activities show a willingness to learn and to record personal progress, which helps you to prepare for assignments.

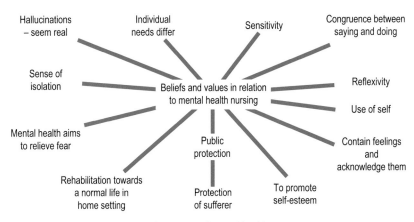

FIGURE 11.2 Nicola's mind map of an aspect of mental health.

Emotional labour in practice: dealing with emotions

Managing personal feelings

Working in healthcare settings frequently presents challenges that are outside your normal everyday experience. Many students are unfamiliar about how to respond emotionally to some of these challenges. One of the most fearful challenges that all midwives and nurses face is having to perform an invasive procedure such as giving an injection, an enema or doing a sterile wound dressing. Other activities that can become routine but are nonetheless challenging in many ways are providing physical hygiene care to a stranger, removing a bedpan of faecal material, encountering abnormality or responding to bizarre behaviour. For most people, their first experience of such events incurs sensations of nausea, revulsion, fear or embarrassment.

CASE STUDY: JACK

I know at first I was quite frightened, … I don't like the smell of vomit, but if someone is vomiting I have to do something, so I am usually so busy and absorbed in making sure they're OK that I haven't got time to think that I either want to vomit or don't feel well. I wouldn't want the patient to feel that they're so bad that it makes nurses throw up as well. (From Spouse, 2003, p. 84.)

Jack was able to handle his own discomfort by keeping his patient's needs foremost in his mind and devoting himself to making sure that the patient's needs were addressed. It is not an easy step to take but often works when facing similar situations.

Witnessing events that stir strong emotions, such as a baby being born or being present while a patient is dying or receives bad news about their terminal illness, is equally disturbing. Many students feel uncertain whether they should share their own feelings. They often wonder if they are being 'unprofessional'. The skilful practitioner is able to share the happiness or grief, while at the same time provide the patient with emotional support and comfort. Sometimes, the conditions of a death can be traumatic for all who witness it, such as following an unsuccessful resuscitation event or a stillbirth, or when death is unexpected, such as a child dying while undergoing investigations:

CASE STUDY: MARIE

I knew a child was going to die at some point in my career … it had such an impact that I went away the following weekend and I started wondering, where I wanted to go in life, … Maybe it's because of my own personal beliefs, but I think she (the patient) is in a better place now anyway. It's the parents I feel sad for more than anything else, and her brothers and sisters. (From Spouse, 2003, p. 61.)

Marie's experience caused her to face her own mortality and beliefs. Many students have strong spiritual beliefs about death and dying, and often these can be a great comfort and support. Others who do not have this background might find that their experience of death triggers a desire to learn more from different spiritual sources so that they can formulate their own philosophy. This is an important process in which to engage and enables you to support patients who are uncertain and frightened, as many are when facing the unknown. Smith and Lorentzen (2008) have researched and written extensively about emotional labour in healthcare settings and nursing particularly, and found that this aspect of professional practice is often unsupported by senior managers. However, in some high-dependency settings, such as oncology units and intensive care units, staff have group support sessions where they can discuss and make sense of issues that are distressing them. With this kind of support, staff are less likely to suffer from emotional burn-out and high levels of sickness and absence.

Knowing how to respond when a patient who is suffering from a mental-health problem or who has a learning disability and who behaves inappropriately, for example with as sexual disinhibition, can be challenging and disturbing to a novice. Here, Grace describes an incident where she was working in a community home for people with learning disability.

 ## CASE STUDY: GRACE

One of the residents kept trying to look up our tops and he'd become a bit (too) friendly. But Pam [mentor] said 'You mustn't look up Grace's top'. And he'd get annoyed or try to look up her top, but she said it wasn't acceptable, and so they knew the boundaries and they just didn't cross them. He tried to get away with it with me, but Pam told him not to by saying, 'Other people wouldn't look up Grace's top so you mustn't either'. (From Spouse, 2003, p. 99.)

Encountering this kind of situation can be frightening as well as embarrassing if you do not know how to handle it effectively. Fortunately, Grace's mentor witnessed the situation and was able to provide an example of how to talk to the resident in a firm but straightforward manner that helped him to accept her admonition. It also provided Grace with a strategy for dealing with such a situation should it happen again.

In the past, nurses and midwives were taught that it was unprofessional to get emotionally involved with patients (Smith and

Lorentzen, 2008). This view had historical origins when patients often endured months of hospitalization and strong, sometimes romantic, relationships developed, possibly to everyone's detriment. Most patients will argue that the practitioners who helped them the most were the ones who engaged with them as people and who did form a caring but professional relationship. Jourard (1971) describes such a relationship as a 'special case of loving'. Developing relationships that have this therapeutic effect takes great skill and self-knowledge. Sometimes, patients, who are in a dependent and vulnerable position, which might feel like a familiar parent–child relationship, respond by projecting the same kinds of feelings that they had in their original relationship. These feelings could be of love or anger, which are projected onto the carer. Learning how to prescribe clear professional boundaries that protect you as the practitioner and the patient takes time and skill.

 CASE STUDY: NICOLA

Thinking about me as a nursing student and me as Nicola, a lot of them over-link. But definitely the way you talk to people is different from the way you do at home, and that's healthy and good. You have to be professional about it and do your job. I'm not trying to sound callous, but you've got to be very careful to make some boundaries and keep them separate, otherwise you just take everything home with you, and that's not good. It's not good for the client either … I'm trying to get more in touch with my feelings, like 'Hell I found that really hard'. So therefore I need to take some time out for a few minutes just to get my head around it. I've got to know what's work … (From Spouse, 2003, p. 179.)

Nicola's personal development helped her to develop a form of emotional membrane so that she could witness the distress of her patients without feeling personally damaged by the experience. This freed her to work therapeutically with them, to cope with their emotional trauma or mental illness.

Using humour in care delivery

The skilful use of humour by a practitioner can sometimes lighten the tension of a situation, such as when a client is becoming despondent or frustrated by their circumstances. Research by Åstedt-Kurki and Liukkonen (1994) found that nearly 50% of nurses used humour in their practice as a strategy to help patients overcome particular difficulties and that male patients were more likely to use it to relieve stress. Humour of course must only be used to ridicule the situation in which the nurse and the patient find themselves as Jack describes.

CASE STUDY: JACK

At first it sometimes seemed inappropriate but it broke the ice and clients seemed to like it. The jokes were aimed at getting the client to laugh, not laugh at the clients … It seemed to work, especially with Peter who was a wheelchair user and has a similar sense of humour to me. (Jack in Spouse, 2003, p. 85.)

Other researchers, such as Goody (1977), found that jokey behaviour is often used in relationships when there is a risk of a loss of face, such as in Jack's situation where he was trying to help Peter forget about his helplessness, thus relieving the tension and facilitating his mobility and independence.

Therapeutic nursing

As you have been reading in the above scenarios and quotations, learning to nurse and to become a midwife can be very challenging, and knowing how to behave in a professional manner that is firm, but courteous, is difficult. Whaites (2008) describes students discussing their clinical experiences in the context of the professional code of conduct and thus learning how to behave in an ethical manner.

If you have a group of friends that you can meet up with on a regular basis to discuss your practice experiences (anonymizing any identities) in private, it is a helpful way of developing your understanding and monitoring your progress. Being able to articulate your experiences and to engage in discussion allows you to remember and consolidate your learning thus making it easier to discuss your practice experiences at important events such as clinical case conferences, ward rounds or handover reports as well as classroom discussions and assignments.

Hochschild (1983), writing about how airline cabin crew and debt collectors develop an emotional shield, called the process 'emotional labour'. Developing an empathetic relationship where you have understanding and insight into the 'other' is part of the process but there is the aspect of how you manage your own feelings without denying them or becoming 'hard hearted' (which many students fear). Being able to become detached from your feelings, or to compartmentalize your own emotions when dealing with an emotionally difficult situation, takes courage and a willingness to develop insight into the other's behaviour. Savage (1995), writing about nurses' practical handling of intimate relationships, found that nurses were more willing to engage in therapeutic relationships when they were supported by colleagues and their senior managers. She also found that clinicians, patients and their carers valued such relationships. Working and learning in a supportive environment is essential for you to learn how to conduct personally challenging relationships effectively and safely for both yourself and your patients.

It is important to be able to debrief from emotionally challenging situations, preferably with someone you trust and who will understand the situation, such as your mentor or another student. If that is not feasible, then writing it up in a journal perhaps using a reflective model as a framework is a helpful strategy to learn from the experience.

Ethical and moral challenges

You will engage in discussions about ethical practice throughout your academic programme. As science enables medicine to become increasingly radical, so healthcare practitioners will have their spiritual and ethical beliefs challenged. Drawing on your professional code of conduct (see, for example, www.nmc-uk.org) and your interpretation of ethical principles, you can engage in a systematic analysis of the presenting situation and thus develop an understanding of your own feelings and dilemmas to develop best practice. You will find some useful texts for further reading at the end of this chapter. Most students find it helpful to discuss such dilemmas with their peers so they can develop their own thinking and understanding. You may find it helpful to make some written notes (such as a mind map) if you are facing a dilemma that has an ethical or spiritual challenge. You can then recognize the strengths and weaknesses of your arguments and where you need to learn more. This process helps you to talk about the dilemma, especially if you are going to have a classroom discussion or if you find an opportunity to discuss the matter with your mentor or another clinical colleague.

Another form of emotional challenge can be when the practitioner is confronted with a situation that they find offensive or shocking; their response can jeopardize the professional relationship, as Katie describes in the scenario below. Going to placements in community settings often raises personal challenges as the experience exposes you to different styles of living and cultural values that you may not otherwise encounter when working in an institutional setting.

CASE STUDY: KATIE

Katie is on her community placement with senior midwife Ferzana. She is visiting three mothers this morning. One is Mrs Ahmed, a woman from Somalia, who is having her third child and the first to be born in Britain. She has a 5-year-old daughter and a 7-year-old son. Katie's midwife suspects that the daughter has recently been circumcised while visiting her grandmother in Somalia; Mrs Ahmed had been circumcised at the same age. Ferzana is pleased that Mrs Ahmed has come for antenatal care and is aware that scarring and the effects of female circumcision make her ability to pass urine or to engage in sexual intercourse very painful. It will also have implications for her delivery. During labour, the adhesions holding her labia together will need to be cut and later re-sutured post-natally. Katie and Ferzana discussed their own emotional response to the practice of female circumcision, which is illegal in the UK and prohibited by the World Health Organization. Katie realized that her anger could affect her relationship with Mrs Ahmed and that she is as much a victim of her own culture as her daughter. Katie accepted that it was more important that she provided the best care she could to Mrs Ahmed in the hope that through a trusting relationship Mrs Ahmed would take a more informed approach to this cultural practice.

By discussing her feelings with her supervisor, Katie developed a different perspective that helped her to care for Mrs Ahmed appropriately. Spires (2008) discusses in some detail how to support clients with different religious and cultural needs, but emphasizes the importance of self-awareness as the practitioner is the medium through which understanding and cooperation can be achieved when wishing to respect a patient's cultural values while delivering effective care.

Dealing with doubt and uncertainty: reporting unprofessional practice

 CASE STUDY: RUTH

I did the injection with someone else and I didn't really like it. I was actually copying how my mentor does it and this person does it differently. That got me in a complete tizzy about what we were doing. It was 'Don't do that'. That was in front of the patient. 'Why are you doing it that way?' She talked to me as if I was an idiot … unfortunately at this stage I don't have much experience. (From Spouse, 2003, p. 167.)

Ruth describes a situation where she was being criticized by another registered nurse for following a procedure she had learned from her mentor. It is not unusual for practitioners to have different approaches to the same technique and, providing the principles of causing the patient no harm are met – physical, social, spiritual or emotional – then the differences do not matter. It is sometimes very helpful to be able to deliver the same kinds of care in different ways to meet individual needs. It is the mark of an expert to be able to adjust the method to suit the moment. However, in the situation described above, Ruth was humiliated in front of the patient, which is bad practice and embarrassing for the patient as well as being disempowering for Ruth. As Ruth mentions, she did not have enough experience to know who was right. She needed to discuss the experience with her mentor and also go away and read the relevant literature on giving injections.

Reporting unsafe practice

It might have been that Ruth believed she was witnessing unsafe practice and needed to go through more formal procedures to make her concerns known. Most universities and healthcare organizations have policies and procedures about 'whistle blowing' or reporting unprofessional conduct. These include immediately making a record of what was witnessed and consulting the placement manager to ensure that the situation was not misunderstood.

If you believe you have witnessed unsafe or unprofessional practice, it is also a good idea to discuss the matter with your personal tutor, who can remind you of the normal procedure and where you can obtain additional support (e.g. the Nursing and Midwifery Council website has an advice page). Your trade union – such as the RCN Student's Association or UNISON – will provide legal advice and support should you need it. If your personal tutor considers your concerns to be legitimate, you will be advised to make a formal statement in writing, but only with the support of either a representative from your trade union or your personal tutor (or both). A special panel of senior members of clinical staff will be formed to review the evidence and make a decision about actions to be taken. They might decide to suspend the member of staff until the enquiry has been completed. If you do witness unsafe practice, you have a duty of care to the patients in the area in which you saw this practice. By not reporting it, you will be contravening your professional code of practice (see www.nmc-uk.org) as well as colluding with the person whose malpractice you observed.

Managing anger in clinical settings from patients or visitors

People's expectations of healthcare practitioners have increased enormously over the past 20 years. Without adequate management support it is often hard for practitioners to meet patients' (or their carers') high expectations. Consequently, fears and worries are sometimes expressed in angry outbursts, and even violence, projected at healthcare workers. Learning how to respond in a therapeutic manner requires great skill and training from experts. As a student, it is important to learn how to prevent such outbursts happening and be able to diffuse the anger and frustration as this second-year nursing student describes.

CASE STUDY: PROMISE

I was on duty in the Accident and Emergency Department when this relative started shouting and making a scene. I had noticed him sitting with another man and felt very frightened, because he was a big man. They had been waiting for some time. Being a Saturday afternoon we had taken several emergencies, RTAs, coronaries and a drowning.

As a result, people had been waiting a long time on the minor injuries side. We have an electronic board that notifies the waiting time, but it is waiting for repair and no-one had the chance to go and tell people. The senior nurse went up to this man and very politely asked him whether he was in pain and whether she could help him. He started swearing at her and calling her all kinds of names. She stood there very calmly and waited for him to stop and then apologized for the long wait and explained what was happening in the major injuries side. She had to do this several times as he gradually absorbed what she was saying. She seemed completely unperturbed by his violent manner, her tone of voice was very calm and almost a whisper. It was such a contrast to his manner. She offered to bring him something to drink and promised that they would be able to deal with his friend shortly (she said actually in 30 minutes). We were able to do this and to deal with the other people waiting there, as we had a quiet lull.

Accident and emergency departments and other kinds of waiting rooms are notorious for angry outbursts and assaults on staff. Often, the problem is outside the hands of the immediate staff on duty. Many NHS Trusts have successfully redesigned their waiting areas and the way they manage the through-put of patients to address the problem.

Personal ethical and professional practice

The following case study highlights the consequences that are likely to take place when a student forges the outcome of their placement.

 ### CASE STUDY: ANEKA

Aneka is second year student taking her mental-health pre-registration programme. During her 8-week placement she had 2 weeks of absence due to sickness, largely caused by an unplanned pregnancy. Aneka was desperate to complete the common foundation programme before she started maternity leave and was concerned that if she did not achieve her learning outcomes she would go down a set. In the final week of her placement, her mentor was on holiday so Aneka forged her mentor's signature on her portfolio of practice and her skills schedule and submitted it to her module leader as required, hoping it would not be noticed. The forgery was noticed and Aneka was interviewed by her personal tutor and the module leader. Initially, Aneka tried to bluff her way out of the situation, but realizing she was making it worse finally admitted what she had done. The school took the perspective that this was unprofessional conduct and that she should be dismissed from the programme. On the advice of the students' union, Aneka appealed against the decision and her appeal was heard by a panel of senior academic and clinical staff. During the appeal, Aneka was supported by an officer of the students' union who attended the hearing with her. Despite making her case as clearly and honestly as she could, the appeals committee decided against Aneka and she was discontinued from the course. She was advised that the Nursing and Midwifery Council would also be informed of her conduct and this would militate against any subsequent application to become a nurse.

Aneka made a serious mistake in trying to circumvent the requirement to have her mentor verify her progress. Perhaps she had not appreciated the importance of this verification. It constitutes the main form of quality control and by having confidence in the judgement of placement mentors the university can decide whether a student should progress through the course leading to both an academic award and a professional qualification. Academic and clinical staff are required by their professional statutory organization to protect the public and to act always in accordance with their professional code of conduct (NMC, 2008b) as are pre-registration students. Aneka admitted she had failed to do this and as a result was dismissed from the programme.

Integrating theory with practice and practice with theory

Reading and learning from case notes and drug information: keeping a notebook

Two of the most satisfying ways of learning and remembering factual information are reading patients' case notes and recording information about drugs. You may find it helpful to keep a small notebook in your uniform pocket to record any particular words or phrases that are unfamiliar, and any other new information.

By reading through case notes you will learn to see similarities and patterns in disease development. It is also helpful to look at the investigations (such as biochemistry, radiographs and so on) that have been ordered along with the reports. Again, you will begin to notice patterns and similarities, and also to learn the normal and abnormal values of the various blood tests and other investigations. If you can get an experienced staff member to explain how to read visual investigations such as X-rays and electrocardiograms, it will help you to understand the patients' symptoms and their treatment.

Another useful strategy is to attend as many different but related clinics and sessions that are relevant to your clinical placement (possibly in your own time if you cannot negotiate the time away from the placement). Sitting in on medical consultations and clinics run by other healthcare professionals (such as physiotherapists, art therapists or psychologists) provides opportunities to understand the patients' journey and to hear their accounts of their health disorder as well as to observe different treatments and therapies being delivered, thus enriching your understanding.

In your placement, you should be involved in the delivery of the different aspects of care required by your mentor's clients, as an observer, a legitimate participant or under your mentor's distant supervision. Drug administration is often one of the most ritualized and time-consuming activities, as well as being the greatest hurdle for students to address. Learning the routine of checking and delivering drugs takes practice.

Learning about the wide range of drugs used is also challenging. Taking the time to go through the drug store and test yourself on the different categories of drugs, their actions, normal dosage, side effects, symptoms of overdose and antidote is time well spent. Most of the drugs have information leaflets and the *British National Formulary* (BNF) or a good pharmacopoeia will provide this information. Making notes in your pocket notebook of these different drugs will help you to remember them. Another helpful practice is to participate in drug administration each shift, asking the registered nurse or midwife to check your knowledge on all the drugs that are being administered.

Learning to see: recognizing signs and symptoms

From the vignette about Ruth's experiences of managing a small caseload, you will know that you must always assess your patients' response to treatment, including their drug therapy. This means you should learn about their medical condition and the treatments they are receiving. When delivering care you should be constantly monitoring their condition and be alert to any side effects. Your patient is the best source of information and listening to what your patient is telling you and taking prompt action (such as reporting any changes to your mentor) can save lives.

CASE STUDY: SHOBA

Shoba is a first-year nursing student on her 4-day obstetric experience. She has been allocated to work in the busy antenatal ward. One of the mothers, a 42-year-old Bengali woman who does not speak a lot of English, is expecting her sixth child in 10 weeks time. She is on bedrest. Shoba notices that the woman is very quiet and not taking any notice of what is going on in the ward, but does not appear to be sleeping. Shoba can speak Bengali and asks her if she is alright. The woman points to her head and to her tummy. Shoba checks the woman's abdomen and discovers that it is very hard, she also notices some blood on the bottom sheet. Feeling panic stricken she nearly runs away, but decides to check the woman's blood pressure. To her horror she makes it 200 mmHg systolic over 160 mmHg diastolic. She goes to find her mentor or any of the midwives to tell them of her findings. Shoba then went back and stayed with the woman throughout the emergency and was able to tell her what was happening, thus reducing some of her anxiety. The midwives realized the woman was close to having a pre-eclamptic fit and that she might be losing her baby; they contacted the obstetrician. Without Sheba's thoughtful actions, the woman's blood pressure might have continued to rise and she could have had an eclamptic fit and died.

As you might imagine, Shoba felt quite shocked at how close she was to missing this woman's serious condition but proud that she had dealt with it so professionally. Her knowledge of the normal range of blood pressure alerted her to the possible abnormality and the need for help.

Spurred on by this experience, she read around the condition of pre-eclamptic toxaemia in pregnancy and its treatment, and kept in contact with the woman to see how she got on. As a result, Shoba learned a great deal about one of the dangers of pregnancy and was able to relate some of it to her training on how to support someone having an epileptic attack.

In another situation Ibrahim, a third-year adult nursing student, is working alongside his mentor caring for an older person with a diagnosis of 'multiple system failure' following a cardiac arrest. After they have made the patient comfortable Ibrahim has the following conversation with his mentor.

 CASE STUDY: IBRAHIM

Ibrahim: I notice that Mr Hayward has quite wheezy breathing and that his sputum is bubbly, but he has a very low output of urine. His ankles are swollen, as are his legs up to his knees, especially when he is sitting out of bed, and he is quite confused. If he has so much fluid in his system why is his urine output so low?

Mentor: Did you notice that he also has a low blood pressure and that he is prescribed Lanoxin? What could this suggest to you?

Ibrahim: Well, Lanoxin is given to strengthen the heart beat so Mr Hayward has a better cardiac output, but he still has a lot of fluid onboard.

Mentor: Yes, you're right about the action of the Lanoxin, but Mr Hayward also has some liver failure. Do you remember which of the plasma proteins that the liver produces that has a function on maintaining the fluid in the circulation?

Ibrahim: Ah, of course, if his liver's not working he will have a low serum albumin level, which means the osmotic pressure of the blood can't attract the fluid from the tissues into the circulation, and that means he won't be able to excrete the excess fluid from his kidneys, which are also failing, which is why he is also having frusemide.

Mentor: Exactly, yes well done. In fact, he is going to have two units of albumin this afternoon in an attempt to restore his osmotic pressure. Why do you think Mr Hayward is so confused?

Ibrahim: Well I suppose, if he has so much fluid on his lungs, he is probably not able to oxygenate his blood very well and this can lead to confusion. Could he also have some cerebral oedema from this albumin deficiency as well?

From this brief conversation, you will notice that Ibrahim's mentor is helping him to make connections between what he has noticed about his patient's condition and his learning, thus bringing his classroom learning and reading to life. It is often difficult to make connections between the rather generalized information in textbooks and the messiness of real life. By working with an expert, Ibrahim was able to begin to make sense of what he was seeing. If Ibrahim had not been supported by such a knowledgeable mentor he could have read the patient's notes and checked them against his textbook reading or talked to one of the other members of the healthcare team.

Summary and conclusions

In this chapter we have discussed several different approaches to learning how to deliver care knowledgeably. The two most crucial components to your success are you and your clinical supervisor.

The trouble you take to prepare yourself for the placement and your willingness to work hard and learn will influence the level of support you receive from the placement staff. Your clinical colleagues will give you their support if they see that you are interested and committed to learning from them. Most clinical staff are very stretched by their workload and receive no tangible benefits for supervising students. Yet the majority of clinical staff welcome the opportunity to support interested students.

Your willingness to engage in the everyday activities of the placement and to take responsibility for delivering care either under direct supervision or with distant supervision will provide opportunities to develop your practical knowledge and understanding of their rationale. Keeping a reflective journal will help you to record the events of your shifts, and thus to further develop your understanding of the practice and its evidence base. This chapter has provided several different approaches to recording your experiences as well as ideas about how to respond therapeutically to some of the many challenges that you might face on your journey to becoming an expert practitioner.

 CHAPTER RESOURCES

REFERENCES

Åstedt-Kurki, P. & Liukkonen, A., 1994. Humour in nursing care. Journal of Advanced Nursing 20, 183–188.

Bandura, A., 1977. Social learning. Prentice Hall, Englewood Cliffs, NJ.

Buzan, T. & Buzan, B., 1996. The Mindmap: How to use radiant thinking to maximise your brain's untapped potential. Plume, New York.

Fuhrer, U., 1993. Behaviour setting, analysis of situated learning: the case of newcomers. In: Chaiklin, S. & Lave, J. (Eds.) Understanding practice. Perspectives on activity and context. Cambridge University Press, Cambridge, pp. 179–211.

Goody, E.N. (Ed.), 1977. Questions and politeness: strategies in social interaction. Cambridge University Press, Cambridge.

Hochschild, A.R., 1983. The managed heart: The commercialisation of human feeling. University of California Press, Berkley, CA.

Jourard, S.M., 1971. The manners of helpers and healers: the bedside manners of nurses. In: Jourard, S.M. (Ed.) The transparent self. Van Nostrand Reinholdt, New York, pp. 179–207.

Lave, J. & Wenger, E., 1991. Situated learning: legitimate peripheral participation. Cambridge University Press, Cambridge.

Nicholson, N., 1987. Work role transitions: progress and outcomes. In: Warr, P. (Ed.) Psychology at work. Penguin Books, Harmondsworth, UK, pp. 160–177.

Nursing and Midwifery Council (NMC), 2008a. Standards to support learning and assessing in practice. NMC Standards for mentors, practice teachers and teachers. NMC, London.

Nursing and Midwifery Council (NMC), 2008b. Professional code of conduct. NMC, London.

Savage, J., 1995. Nursing intimacy: an ethnographic approach to nurse-patient interaction. Scutari Press, London.

Smith, P. & Lorentzen, M., 2008. The emotional labour of nursing. In: Spouse, J., Cook, M. & Cox, C. (Eds.) Common foundation studies in nursing, 4th edn. Churchill Livingstone/Elsevier, Edinburgh, pp. 67–88.

Spires, A., 2008. Learning and working as a nursing student in a multicultural world. In: Spouse, J., Cook, M. & Cox, C. (Eds.) Common foundation studies in nursing, 4th edn. Churchill Livingstone/Elsevier, Edinburgh, pp. 125–153.

Spouse, J., 1998a. Understanding learning in the professional context. Case studies of five nurses from a pre-registration degree course. Unpublished PhD thesis. University of Bath.

Spouse, J., 1998b. Learning to nurse through legitimate peripheral participation. Nurse Education Today 18, 345–351.

Spouse, J., 1999. Challenges to professional education – learning in workplace settings, 7th international improving student learning symposium 6–8 September, University of York, UK.

Spouse, J., 2003. Professional learning in nursing. Blackwell Publishing, Oxford.

Vygotsky, L. & Luria, A., 1970. Tool and symbol in child development. In: Van Der Veer, R. & Valsiner, J. (Eds.) 1994 The Vygotsky reader. Basil Blackwell, Oxford, pp. 99–174.

Vygotsky, L.S., 1978. Mind in society: the development of higher psychological processes. In: Cole, M., Steiner, V.J., Scribner, S. & Suberman, E. (Eds.) Harvard University Press, Cambridge MA.

Whaites, I., 2008. Professional standards and rules. The professional regulatory body and the nursing student. In: Spouse, J., Cook, M. & Cox, C. (Eds.) Common foundation studies in nursing, 4th edn. Churchill Livingstone/Elsevier, Edinburgh, pp. 89–124.

FURTHER READING

Smith, P. & Lorentzen, M., 2008. The emotional labour of nursing. In: Spouse, J., Cook, M. & Cox, C. (Eds.) Common foundation studies in nursing, 4th edn. Churchill Livingstone/Elsevier, Edinburgh, pp. 67–88.

Spires, A. 2008. Learning and working as a nursing student in a multicultural world In: Spouse, J., Cook, M. & Cox, C. (Eds.) Common foundation studies in nursing, 4th edn. Churchill Livingstone/Elsevier, Edinburgh, pp. 125–153.

Spouse, J. 2003. Professional learning in nursing. Blackwell Publishing, Oxford.

Reflective skills **12**

Elizabeth A. Rosser and Rebecca Hoskins

Introduction

If you are just beginning your career in nursing or midwifery, you have an exciting and fulfilling – although challenging – time ahead of you. You will be aware that the NHS is in the midst of radical change, which potentially offers you even more choice of career opportunities than ever before. In fact, change has become the one certainty that we can expect in our professional careers and the way you learn can help you to cope with the change and even harness it to your own benefit. Our regulatory body, the Nursing and Midwifery Council (NMC), acknowledges the increasing complexities of modern professional practice and requires us to be engaged in life-long learning to help us keep pace with the change and increasing expectations of our patients. The NMC (2005) has produced guidance on the principles and values of life-long learning. This can can be downloaded from (http://www.nmc-uk.org/aDisplayDocument.aspx?DocumentID=519).

Life-long learning is seen as crucial to enable you to demonstrate you are taking responsibility for your own learning throughout your career and, as a professional, you are required to articulate this through your personal professional profile (PPP). However, as the NMC acknowledges, life-long learning is more than just keeping yourself up to date. It expects you to take an enquiring approach to your practice, at both the pre-qualifying level of activity, and at the post-qualifying level, through the Post-registration Education and Practice (PREP) standards (NMC, 2008). You can download a copy of the *PREP handbook* (NMC, 2008) from the NMC website. One of the four key areas of support identified by PREP is to help you to 'think and reflect for yourself' (NMC, 2008, p. 2). Guidance on how to develop your own profile can be seen in Chapter 15.

Currently, the process of learning to think and reflect for yourself begins early in your pre-qualifying programme. You can then build on your ability to learn from the range of situations and experiences you find yourself in, up to and beyond the point of registration and throughout your career. Reflection, therefore, plays a vital role in preparing you for your professional life and for the life-long learning that is expected of you. Reflection helps you keep abreast of change as the normal expectation of professional practice. However, despite the ever-increasing body of evidence to suggest that reflective skills are crucial to the provision of holistic nursing care (Gustafsson et al., 2007), reflection is not as universal an activity as we think (Conway, 1998; Mantzoukas and Jasper, 2004).

This chapter sets out to explore what is meant by the term 'reflection' and the skills involved in undertaking it. It will also examine ways in which you can develop further the skills of reflection to help you in the study process and to gain more from the experiences you are exposed to, personally and professionally.

What is reflection?

 Jot down what you understand by the term 'reflection'.

The early work of Dewey (1933), an American educationalist, philosopher and psychologist, laid the foundation for our current concept of reflection. Dewey believed that reflection was central to human learning and professional development. More recently, a number of theorists have further developed the concept of reflection (e.g. Brookfield, 1995; Freire, 1996; Habermas, 1974; Mezirow, 1991; Schon, 1983) and helped advance our understanding of how to learn through reflection and facilitate others to learn. If you are interested in finding out more about the contribution of these different theorists, then Redmond (2004) gives a succinct overview of the literature in her first chapter.

So, how can we define reflection?

Reflection is concerned with learning by thinking, by weighing up all the aspects of the situation and making a conscious and informed decision about what to do. On a personal level, it means taking active control over what you do and how you do it. On the surface, this may seem a fairly straightforward concept; however, there is an increasing body of evidence to suggest that it is not quite as straightforward as it seems (Burns and Bulman, 2000; Moon, 1999; Taylor, 2006).

Reflection in a personal sense

We can relate reflection first to our personal lives. It is often said that we learn from the mistakes we make. Life can be seen as a series of hurdles: each time we meet new experiences, we try to fit them into our already existing understanding to make sense of them. However, not everyone does learn from their experiences. Some people are particularly self-aware and sensitive to their own response in certain circumstances, whereas others never seem to learn from their experiences and continue to make the same mistakes over and over again. Alternatively, you can learn to forget the experience – the experience can be too painful to explore or your feelings can be too strong to dissect. So, when you meet a similar situation in the future, it is easy to make the same mistakes over again. The learning has been one of forgetting.

There are two important issues here. First, feelings are an extremely important aspect of the learning process and the way you feel can dictate whether you learn from a particular experience or not. Feelings of anxiety or uncomfortable feelings can be a barrier to learning. Second, it is crucial that you do not learn to forget too many experiences. If this happens, making mistakes repeatedly may be extremely problematic for you, especially when there may be the opportunity of making life easier for yourself by responding in a different way (see the box below).

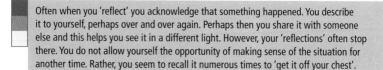

Often when you 'reflect' you acknowledge that something happened. You describe it to yourself, perhaps over and over again. Perhaps then you share it with someone else and this helps you see it in a different light. However, your 'reflections' often stop there. You do not allow yourself the opportunity of making sense of the situation for another time. Rather, you seem to recall it numerous times to 'get it off your chest'.

Merely thinking about what you did is not in itself true reflection, certainly not at a level that requires you to make sense of it and change what you do the next time.

Reflection in a professional sense

It is over 20 years since reflection and reflective practice were first introduced to nursing and midwifery in the UK, with the introduction of Project 2000 (UKCC, 1986) and the move into higher education nationally. Reflective learning has now become an essential element in both pre- and post-registration education programmes globally (Greenwood, 1998; Kember, 2001; Taylor, 2006). The belief is that reflection helps you as a nurse or midwife to learn from your practice. It helps you to make sense of how you and others deal with the complex situations you find yourselves in and it helps you to bridge the gap between the theory you learn in the classroom and your professional practice.

Prior to the introduction of reflective practice, much of the learning in practice and in the education institutions focused on rather traditional teaching styles and all assessments were written in the formal, third person academic style, with the student presenting a rather objective view of how care should be managed. The focus was more on teaching rather than learning. However, Schon (1987) believed that this rather objective, theory-driven approach to learning was inappropriate for education programmes preparing students for a professional career. He recommended that universities re-focus their activity on facilitating students, through reflective methods, to identify and address problematic issues in a more individual way (Mantzoukas, 2007; Schon, 1983, 1987). He recognized that, in dealing with human behaviour, problems in professional practice are not straightforward. They do not follow a recipe-type approach to decision making. Instead, situations in professional practice are 'messy', uncertain, complex, individual and sometimes conflicting. Rather than 'teach' theory and expect professionals to bridge the gap between the theory taught to their individual situations, Schon believed that reflective methods would enable them to analyse their unique situation and empower them to confront and address each situation in an individual and holistic way (Mantzoukas, 2007).

As a student of midwifery or nursing, you can use reflective methods to help you to deal with uncertainties and to find new solutions to dilemmas for each individual you care for. Individualized care is now a well-established way of thinking about care. The lists of textbook problems in clinical practice and, even more, the recipe-book solutions to these problems are becoming things of the past. Also, as an adult learner you will bring with you to the learning experience your own individual ways of making sense of the situations. By learning from each situation, you can build up your own portfolio of learning and be able to tailor solutions to meet the individual needs of the patients in your care.

Taylor (2006) argues that reflection encourages students to think critically. From a process of exploration, often triggered by a sense of the unexpected, reflection encourages you to make sense of an experience and learn from it to help you in the future. As already mentioned, feelings are a crucial element in terms of how they influence your learning from the experience.

 The most important aspect of reflection is learning from the experience.

To enable you to make the most of your learning, many theorists have described their own process to guide you. Before we consider different guides or 'frameworks' to help you look critically at your practice, it is worthwhile considering the relationship between reflection and expert practice.

If you look around you, you can certainly identify a number of practitioners who would fit the title of expert. But what exactly do we mean by the term 'expert'? Those 'expert' practitioners whom you have identified will have a number of different attributes, yet you have identified them all as 'experts'. Conway (1996) suggests that expertise is not definitive and in her own study she identified four different types of 'expert' as illustrated below.

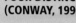

FOUR DISTINCT TYPES OF 'EXPERT' IDENTIFIED BY CONWAY (CONWAY, 1996, WITH PERMISSION)

Technologist
Characterized by wide range of knowledge, including anticipatory knowledge, diagnosis knowledge, 'know-how' knowledge and monitoring knowledge both of junior doctors and patients' conditions. Teaching by these experts was mainly didactic: images were used, as was in-depth questioning and a translator function was demonstrated. Issues arose in relation to the authority that expert nurses had vis-à-vis doctors.

Traditionalist
Characterized by the need for 'survival'. These experts were preoccupied with 'getting the work done' and managing care with scarce resources. For them, care had a medical focus and the experts operated as overseers and doctors' assistants. Management and doctors were perceived as all powerful. They did not value their own practice and saw themselves as powerless in terms of influence. They saw education as an optional extra and not as central to practice development. Value was attached to 'doing' and not to 'reflecting'. They showed that 'papering over the cracks' was what nursing was about and this others also learned to do. This dispossessed others.

Specialist
Characterized by prescribing treatment regimes, recommending medication and extending their roles. There were subdivisions within this group that reflected the traditionalists, technologists and humanistic existentialists. They had developed knowledge in terms of assessment, diagnosing, quality of life and transformative ability. Doctor–nurse relationships varied.

Humanistic existentialist
Characterized by a dynamic and strong nursing focus to care. Patients were truly viewed holistically and a humanistic philosophy was used in practice. They were passionate about nursing practice. A devolved hierarchy using primary nursing was operational. Humanistic existentialist experts were risk takers. They had supportive managers, good resources and were educationally well developed. They exerted considerable power and influence and saw themselves as creating the culture in their areas. Self-awareness and reflective abilities typified this group. They were also very aware of the influence that they had on other nurses.

Conway acknowledged that each type arose from their different 'world views'. These 'world views' were developed from the orientation of the expert to a number of issues, including:

- the resources available to them
- the amount of authority they were able to exercise

- their own goals and those of their organization
- the level and type of education (both professional and academic) that they had achieved
- their relationship with significant others, e.g. doctors and managers.

Interestingly, each group believed they were reflective although, in reality, this was not the case. Reflective ability was the hallmark of only one of the four types (the humanistic existentialists), with far less development in the other three groups. Their ways of thinking were different and the way they approached their practice was different, with those with minimal reflective abilities giving care that was limited in focus and illness orientated. In contrast, reflective practitioners gave responsive care, full of warmth and based on the needs of the individual. The different 'world views' are therefore important, as they influence the 'natural' skills individuals bring to situations, with some having more advanced critical reflective skills than others.

As Conway (1996) acknowledges, reflection in a professional sense for some, is not easy. However, as our understanding of reflective learning develops, Burns and Bulman (2000) acknowledged that, 5 years on, and through support and guidance, there was a more positive recognition by student nurses of the value of reflection and their development as curious and challenging practitioners.

More recently, however, a study (by Mantzoukas and Jasper, 2004) of sixteen nurses in four medical wards in England found that although the nurses used and acknowledged the power of reflection for developing practice, its use was devalued by those perceived as being in more 'powerful' roles; for example, doctors and managers. It was the ward culture that invalidated it as 'normal' for knowledge development and practice provision, forcing its use as a covert activity rather than an accepted and formal learning tool.

Whether you are a nurse or midwife at the beginning of your career, or returning after a break, it is important that you understand how to reflect and identify tools that will help you in the process. Using your clinical mentors or peers to support you, learning from your experience and not by any practice imposed upon you by others or by rituals or routine, will be crucial to deliver the high standards of professional practice set for us by the NMC (2005). While reflection is now accepted as a learning tool in the academic and research world, this study demonstrates that in fact there are still some barriers to its implementation in practice.

Learning from our mistakes

You will have met practitioners who have been in practice some years and have developed their practice, kept themselves up-to-date and become expert practitioners. However, you might also have had the misfortune to work with other practitioners who have been in practice for a number of years but have simply repeated their experience over time and have not learned from it.

With the drive towards more flexible career pathways and greater career opportunities from healthcare assistant to consultant, coupled with the NHS modernization agenda advocating new ways of working and better vocational training opportunities for the wider workforce (Department of Health, 1999, 2000a), the boundaries between professional work and non-professional carers have become blurred. Over 15 years ago, Dewar (1992) found that first-level nurses could not differentiate easily between their own work and that of healthcare assistants, and, with the introduction of assistant practitioners, the boundaries are likely to be less clear now. You may be quite clear in your own mind what the differences are but, if challenged, could you put them into words? Perhaps the development of reflective skills will enable the profession, as a whole, to articulate the value of the professional carer. In turn, this may allow you to distinguish between you, the professional, and your assistant, and encourage you to articulate this difference in practice.

Reflection consists of:

- Thinking about an experience
- Exploring that experience in terms of feelings and significant features
- Processing the significant features and identifying learning
- Effects on future practice

Types of reflection

As the concept of reflection has developed in relation to professional practice, a number of different types of reflection have been identified in relation to reflecting before, during or after an event.

In addition to the different types of reflection, there are different levels of reflecting. These levels are of particular importance clinically, especially when you engage in a group discussion of an incident that happened in your work. They are also important when developing your skills of reflection for academia. These are considered in more detail in Chapter 14.

Learning from practice is very important in any programme of professional development, whether pre- or post-registration. After all, the whole purpose of learning is to gain insight from our practice and to develop standards of care. Otherwise, learning and study become sterile activities.

The process of reflection

A large number of papers related to reflective practice were published during the 1990s (Hannigan, 2001) and the proliferation of papers has continued. Despite a lack of empirical evidence, reflection is seen as 'the best tool that nursing has to date for advancing its practice' (Mantzoukas and Jasper, 2004, p. 926). As a tool, therefore, different theorists have developed their own models of structured reflection to help you to follow a process to allow you to articulate your clinical decision making and learn from your experience (Boud et al., 1985; Gibbs, 1988; Johns, 2006; Rolfe et al., 2001). Jasper (2006) presents a comprehensive overview of a range of published frameworks for reflection as well as a comparison of their presentation and key questions/cues.

Reflective frameworks

One of the most popular frameworks to help you gain the most from your reflective learning is the one developed by Gibbs who uses Kolb's experiential learning cycle as a basis to help you to gain new insights into learning from your experience. Gibbs' (1988) framework is presented in Figure 12.1.

Gibbs' model helps learners work through different aspects of the learning situation and allows to break it down into different parts to make sense of it and gain new insights into how things might be done differently in the future.

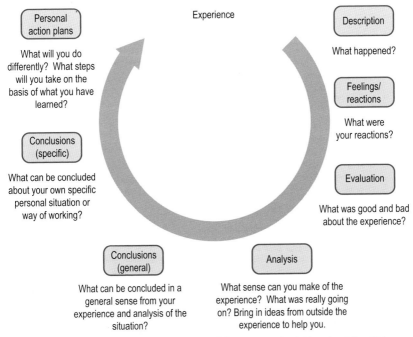

FIGURE 12.1 Gibbs' model. Debriefing sequence following experiential learning (after Gibbs, 1988).

The post-qualifying student case study below offers you a way of approaching learning through reflection, using Gibbs' tool.

CASE STUDY: JENNY

Jenny is a newly qualified Emergency Nurse Practitioner (ENP) who works in an emergency department.

Description

I attended a patient who had a cut to his dominant hand from a clean kitchen knife. Having examined him, I knew he needed referral. I bleeped the 'on call' plastics registrar and tried to make my referral over the telephone. He kept asking me questions I wasn't ready for and he became angry. In the end he told me to speak to one of my medical colleagues to make the referral. Reluctantly I did ask my colleague, who was very supportive.

Feelings/reactions

I felt mortified that I had let the patient down as well as myself. I was really anxious about making the referral and felt stupid when I couldn't seem to answer any of his straightforward questions. I have spent 6 months studying and passing exams and know I can do this role, but was so nervous about the referral. I also felt angry with the plastics registrar because I felt he undermined me.

Evaluation

The only good thing I could find was that the patient eventually received the correct treatment and that my medical colleague in the emergency department was very supportive and agreed with my clinical findings and diagnosis. The less positive aspects of the experience were that I was unprepared for the questions that I knew would be asked. I also thought I left a poor impression by making a mess of the referral. I also felt I slowed up the process for the patient who could have been transferred to the ward an hour previously.

Analysis

If I analyse the situation objectively I really wasn't prepared for making the referral. I knew the questions that I would be asked. We have covered this on my Emergency Nurse Practitioner (ENP) course and I didn't take the time to write down what I needed to say or to collect all the information I required. I also felt a bit under confident and perhaps intimidated by the plastics registrar and had a feeling of doom about the whole situation which turned out to be a self-fulfilling prophecy! When I think back over the situation and put myself in the place of the plastics registrar, it must have been very frustrating to speak to someone who was clearly nervous, didn't have the right information and sounded under confident.

Conclusions (general)

My lack of confidence didn't engender confidence in the person I was referring to. I recognize that I should not have let my emotions get in the way of the referral and also that I took the whole episode very personally when in fact it was my behaviour rather than me as a person which was the problem. I didn't need to get so upset, because it didn't help anyone, least of all the patient.

Conclusions (specific)

I recognize now that I wasn't prepared appropriately; I hadn't taken the time to prepare myself or to collect all the relevant information and I should have realized that communicating over the phone is always more challenging and I should have prepared myself for this. I recognize that I talked too much and didn't state my intention early on in the conversation so the person at the other end of the phone didn't know whether I was asking for advice, making a formal referral or had just rung for a chat!

Personal action plans

My action plan as a result of this incident is to practise making referrals to my colleagues in the team, gathering all the information needed to gain confidence and experience. I will try to rehearse the conversation in my head beforehand and ask myself what the other person would want to know. I will also practise being more succinct, stating my intention in the first sentence and being prepared for the questions, giving time for them to be asked.

You can see from this example of an experienced nurse taking over a new role that she has used Gibbs' (1988) framework to help her to analyse her situation and try to make sense of it. This abridged extract from her portfolio does show some good insight into her feelings and how she has planned to prepare for a similar situation in the future.

Think about your own practice and how Gibbs' model might help you to analyse and help you learn from a situation you have been in.

Structured reflection

A rather more detailed framework is the one described by Johns (2006). With a more comprehensive set of cues to guide your reflection than the stages offered by Gibbs (1988), Johns' framework makes it a very popular framework for those of you at the beginning of your reflective practice. Its detailed questions or cues help you begin to understand your practice in relation to the fundamental ways of knowing identified by Carper (1978). Johns' framework is continually being developed and is now in its 15th edition (Johns, 2006) since its inception in 1992. As with any tool, it can be used to help you either think or write reflectively. The written approach is considered in Table 12.1.

Johns begins by asking you to 'bring the mind home' (2006, p. 37). Here he is asking you to find your own space and focus your thoughts and feelings on a particular situation before writing a description of that experience. To reflect purposefully, it is important that you focus on a particular learning point in the situation to prevent your mind being distracted by so many different aspects that 'we [may] find ourselves scattered everywhere, in all directions, leaving nobody at home.' (Rinpoche, 1992, p. 59) He advocates meditation to bring the mind home and help create a still point within yourself to purposefully reflect (Johns, 2006, p. 37). The storytelling aspect of reflection acts as a trigger to help you tease out the issues that are important to you and with

TABLE 12.1 Johns' model of structured reflection (from Johns, 2006)

REFLECTIVE CUE	MSR MAP
1. Bring the mind home	
2. Focus on a description of an experience that seems significant in some way	Aesthetics
3. What particular issues seem significant to pay attention to?	Aesthetics
4. How were others feeling and why did they feel that way?	Aesthetics
5. How was I feeling and why did I feel that way?	Personal
6. What was I trying to achieve and did I respond effectively?	Aesthetics
7. What were the consequences of my action on the patient, others and myself?	Aesthetics
8. What factors influence the way I was/am feeling, thinking and responding to this situation?	Personal (personal, organizational professional, cultural)
9. What knowledge did or might have informed me?	Empirics
10. To what extent did I act for the best and in tune with my values?	Ethics
11. How does this situation connect with previous experiences?	Personal/reflexivity
12. Given the situation again, how might I respond differently?	Reflexivity
13. What would be the consequences of responding in new ways for the patient, others and myself?	Reflexivity
14. What factors might constrain me from responding in new ways?	Personal
15. How do I *now* feel about this experience?	Personal
16. Am I able to support myself and others better as a consequence?	Reflexivity
17. What insights have I gained? (framing perspectives)	Reflexivity
18. Am I more able to realize desirable practice?	(Being available template)
19. What have I learnt through reflecting?	

a view to learning and perhaps changing your practice, but it is only a small part of the whole process.

In Table 12.1, Johns has used Carper's (1978) four ways of knowing to help you to reflect on your clinical reasoning and action by mapping his questions and cues against these four ways of knowing. However as you can see from Table 12.1, he uses the aesthetic response as the core, influenced by ethical, empirical and the personal. These ways of knowing are as follows:

- Empirical knowledge: theoretical, scientific, accessible through the senses.
- Aesthetic knowledge: artistic and creative aspects of the situation – what is most pleasing? Knowing what to do with the moment, instantly without conscious deliberation. Producing creative and deeply moving interactions with others.

■ Personal knowledge: your personal experience, which influences the situation and also how you can manage your own concerns so they do not interfere with seeing the patients.

■ Ethical knowledge: doing the 'right' thing, doing what 'ought' to be done (Chinn and Kramer, 1995, pp. 4–11).

In addition to Carper's four ways of knowing, Johns constructed a fifth way of knowing, which he named 'reflexivity' and which helps you look back to make sense of 'the unfolding pattern' (Johns, 2006, p. 57) of events in the present situation, with a view towards the future. Johns suggests that there is a need for reflection to be guided, so the cues help you to stay as true to the meaning of the situation as you can. In this way, Johns encourages you to move away from the purely theoretical knowledge that you bring to each situation and explore other types of knowledge that help you make sense of the situation. This, of course, can be as relevant to your clinical practice as it is to your study. All aspects of knowing are important and contribute to the whole of knowing. Learning to articulate each aspect allows you to communicate and develop that knowledge to refine your understanding for practice.

It may be helpful to consider Johns' (2006) framework to guide your thoughts through a particular problem in your practice.

Take an example from your recent practice experience and follow the cues and questions Johns poses in his model (Table 12.1). This might be an example where you congratulate yourself on how well the situation turned out or it may be something that you felt unhappy about in the way you or others acted. Whatever the situation, the cues that Johns' model gives you should help you understand more fully what happened and how you might approach a similar situation in the future.

Using a guided approach, getting in touch with your feelings and responses to problems, you can learn to reflect critically and gain from your experiences. As Conway (1996) illustrated, some individuals find this easier than others. If it is not within your 'make-up' or doesn't suit your own philosophical perspective then, like any new skill, it needs practice and development, guidance and support.

As students learning the process, Holm and Stephenson (1994) present their own difficulties through their own development from a purely descriptive, storytelling approach to critical reflection. They moved on to 'find clarity and conclusion in the midst of confusion and conflict' (Holm and Stephenson, 1994, p. 62). As previously mentioned, 5 years later, these students offered a list of practical tips to help others struggling with the process of critical reflection (Burns and Bulman, 2000, p. 135).

The questioning approach

In an alternative approach to Johns' (2000) structured reflection, a very early framework is that of Borton (1970). For the more experienced reflector, its simplicity is its strength. The lack of detailed questions allows you to create your own cues around the three main questions:

- What happened? Describing the situation and identifying the focus for your learning.
- So what am I to make of this? Try to understand in a more objective way what happened and the feelings you had and the effects of what you and others did.
- Now what can I do to make the situation better? What would you do differently if you were faced with a similar situation again?

(From Rolfe et al. (2001, p. 27) after Borton (1970))

Each of these three questions can be subdivided into further questions, as shown in Table 12.2 (Rolfe et al., 2001, p. 35). Although Rolfe et al offer you a number of reflective cues under each main question, like Johns

TABLE 12.2 Borton's framework: more detail (from Rolfe et al. (2001) after Borton (1970))

WHAT...	SO WHAT...	NOW WHAT...
...is the problem/difficulty/reason for being stuck/reason for feeling bad/reason we don't get on/etc...?	...does this tell me/teach me to make things better/stop me/imply/ mean about me/my patient/others/ our relationship my patient's care/ the model of care I am better/etc...?	...do I need to do in order being stuck/improve my using/my attitudes/my patient's care/resolve the situation/feel better/get on
...was my role in the	...patient's attitudes/etc., etc.	
...was I trying to achieve?	...was going through my mind as I acted?	...broader issues need to be considered if this action is to be successful?
...actions did I take?		
...was the response of others?	...did I base my actions on?	...might be the consequences of this action?
...were the consequences: – for the patient? – for myself? – for others?	...other knowledge can I bring to the situation: – experiential? – personal? – scientific?	
...feelings did it evoke – in the patient? – in myself? – in others?	...could /should I have done to make it better?	
...is my new understanding of the situation?		
...was good/bad about the experience?		
...broader issues arise from the situation?		

(2000), once you have internalized the cues for yourself you can use your own cues to help you address the overall framework. See Table 12.1 for more detail.

More recently, Kim (1999) has developed a similar method of critical reflective inquiry for nurses to develop knowledge for nursing and to improve practice. Although originally designed as a method of research data collection, she acknowledges that it can be applied to a practice situation using reflection-on-action (Rolfe et al., 2001, p. 24). The three phases Kim refers to are:

1. The descriptive phase (examination of what happened) – 'What?'[my interpretation].
2. The reflective phase (analysis of the situation against existing theory) – 'So what?'[my interpretation].
3. The critical/emancipatory phase (demonstrating learning and a change in practice) – 'Now what?' [my interpretation].

Here she aims to develop individual practice, nursing knowledge about practice and shared learning (Kim, 1999).

 Think about something in everyday life that did not work out as well as you had hoped. Use Borton's (1970) questions to help you analyse the situation and learn from it. Does this framework help you to alter your decision making in the future?

So far, you have been concerned with decisions that have not gone according to plan. However, reflection is not just about making sense of situations when they go wrong. It is important to examine why some decisions you make are successful. You need to make sure that good decisions are repeated, rather than just changing decisions that have gone wrong. See the box below for a working example.

A WORKING EXAMPLE OF BORTON'S (1970) FRAMEWORK

A worked example of this is shown below, in which a second-year student nurse reflects on a shift in practice and the issues identified.

What? (returning to the situation)

I am currently working on a care of the elderly acute-admissions ward and spent a shift working on the general medical-admissions unit. One of the patients I was allocated was a 68-year-old woman who was admitted with acute confusion. She became very agitated and aggressive and I spent time trying to work out what the problem was; did she have a full bladder, was she in pain, was she anxious about being in a new environment? The staff nurse in charge of the shift was keen to allocate me more patients; I explained that this lady was requiring one-to-one nursing assessment and care. She became a bit short with me and I in turn felt increasingly anxious and under-confident. I came to the conclusion that the patient was probably in pain but

I did not have a way of objectively measuring this to help explain my findings at the multidisciplinary team meeting. The key issues I found were that:

- I felt anxious and inadequate by not being able to care for any more patients.
- I did not have access to the same resources as I did on the usual ward and therefore could not measure any interventions that were carried out for my patient.
- I was not assertive enough in this situation.

So what? (understanding the context)

Personal reflection: I felt frustrated in assessing and caring for my patient as I felt unsupported, I also felt under-confident in explaining why I could not safely take on any more patients, I also felt frustrated because the nurse in charge did not acknowledge that I was doing an important job and I felt glad that I helped to reduce my patient's agitated and aggressive behaviour by being able to spend time with her.

At the multidisciplinary meeting I explained about the different pain-assessment tools that were used on my usual ward and how useful they were when assessing older people who may be confused. The ward sister was interested in this and asked me to do an informal teaching session about this tool for staff. I felt pleased that my ideas had been taken seriously. She also congratulated me on assessing my patient thoroughly and appropriately.

Learning

I now feel that I should have been confident enough to have explained the consequences of me taking additional patients to the nurse in charge, because she might not have realized how dependent my patient was, and it was my responsibility to highlight this and also ask for help. It also makes me aware of some of the issues of working within teams where the members do not know each other and how important good communication is. I should also have got a copy of an appropriate pain-assessment tool from my usual ward. This would have meant I would have had to ask for help as I did not feel I could have safely left my patient alone.

Now what? (modifying future outcomes)

I now see that when I am faced with a similar issue in the future I need to take a few minutes to examine why I feel uncomfortable or anxious. This will alert me to the actions I need to carry out. I also need to realize that I work within a team and that it is acceptable to ask for help especially when dealing with a potentially difficult situation. Understanding the pressures that other people in the team are under will also help me communicate more effectively. If I had taken time to understand the pressures of the nurse in charge I would have been able to negotiate my workload more effectively. Taking time out to analyse a situation can be very helpful in contributing to the learning of the team and team members and in the future when I feel out of my depth or that things are going wrong I will spend a few minutes to identify what the problems are and how they can be addressed quickly. I think this situation and reflection will help me when I undertake the management module and undertake the shift coordinator role in a ward.

Think of a situation in your everyday life that you felt you handled particularly well. This may be the way you handled a particularly sensitive situation with a friend who sought your advice, or it may be how you mastered a skill you have recently been working on. Why do you think you handled the situation so well? What did you say/do? What other aspects were involved that made it a success?

Again, you may like to use Borton's (1970) questions to help you ana-lyse your situation in some depth. The questions should help you probe different aspects of the situation, perhaps aspects that have not readily come to mind and that at the time you felt were not significant.

This brings us on to applying what you have done so far:

- reflection as an everyday activity
- reflection applied to your study development
- reflection related to learning from your professional practice.

The three key stages in the whole reflective process can be summarized as follows as in the box below.

1. Reflection seems to be triggered by the element of surprise (when situations turn out better than you had hoped) or by an uncomfortable feeling or thought.

2. Critical analysis of the situation, involving feelings and understanding: mentally standing 'outside' yourself and using cues for guidance, ask yourself some questions about what and why you felt so uncomfortable.

3. Development of a new perspective on the situation: what have you learned from this situation that would help you in the future?

Learning practice

As you progress through your education programme, I am sure you will find there is much to learn from the theoretical side of the programme. However, learning is not just about poring over books and learning from the written text. Much of nursing and midwifery is learned in prac-tice. Theory and practice are closely linked; each supports the other and both are vital for successful patient care. Therefore, it is important to know how you can get the most out of your experiences in practice and learn from them.

Both midwifery and nursing practice are complex and uncertain. You are constantly being reminded of the need to develop holistic care, yet traditional textbooks are full of prescribed care that you should be offering patients. The complexities of midwifery and nursing are often not recognized by the very people who do it! When teaching colleagues about care activities, experienced practitioners often spend little time on the actual care aspects and much more on technical, procedural and medical treatments. Once it is mastered, it is as if professional care is self-explanatory and requires little thought. With the enormous amount that you are expected to learn in both pre- and post-registration pro-grammes, some part of your programme occurs directly in practical experiences and you need to learn from these experiences. Much can be learned and taught about both the art and science of care and you will learn a lot from the experiences you are exposed to during your pre- and post registration study programmes. To help you further, Chapter 11 is designed to give you some practical hints on how to get the most from this experience. So, to continue developing your care skills, in spite of the increasing pressures of work, consider the following questions.

- How can you make the most of your experiences in the different contexts you find yourself in?
- What is it that actually turns the experience you are getting into learning?
- Why is it that some learners appear to benefit more than others in the clinical setting?

The recent publication *Modernizing nursing careers: setting the direction* (DoH, 2006) acknowledges the radical workforce reforms across the NHS and the need for flexibility in the workforce and responsiveness to this change. Since the earlier review of nursing and midwifery (UKCC, 1999a) focusing on the pre-qualifying programme being fit for practice, the emphasis on a competency-based work system at all levels has become even more important. Additionally, life-long learning has become crucial for all practitioners to keep them up to date with all the changes (NMC, 2005). As mentioned at the beginning of this chapter, this is reinforced at the post-qualifying level through the PREP requirements and the need to maintain your professional portfolio. However, Chirema (2007) in her small study, mirrored previous research (UKCC, 1999b) that evidence from qualified practitioners of reflective practice within their personal professional portfolio was patchy. This reinforces the results of Conway's (1996) study, which found that, although all practitioners believed they did reflect, this was not the case in reality. The NMC requirements for re-registration are made quite clear in the *PREP handbook* (NMC, 2008) and this document also offers some examples from both midwifery and nursing to guide the documentation of your mandatory updating. The NMC audits compliance of this PREP (continuing professional development; CPD) standard by sampling registrants' evidence of their learning activity and its relevance to their work (NMC, 2008). The message is clear: all practitioners need to develop much stronger links between theory and practice, and encourage a positive response to the above questions for all learners of professional practice.

Your responsibilities

As you embark on your studies, you will find that current approaches to learning focus much more on your taking a more active part in the learning process. From an overuse of lectures in the past, the emphasis is now on learning rather than teaching. Techniques have been developed to help you to make real links with the world of practice and address issues that are priority areas for you. As we have already mentioned, 'learning how to learn' has become much more important than simply the acquisition of knowledge itself. Although the value of reflection has become a crucial element of this approach, reflection can be used within a number of learning strategies that you may well experience during your studies. Some examples of these techniques are problem-based learning where you will be given specific scenarios of real situations and be asked a number of questions to investigate. Other techniques include the use of action-inquiry and action-learning sets, critical-incident technique, the use of reflective diaries and journals and portfolios as well as learning the skills of contributing to an effective learning culture within the workplace. Each of these will be considered individually. What these techniques are trying to achieve is to help you to be self-aware of your own responsibilities with regard to learning, both within the classroom and in practice. Rather like Conway's (1996) traditionalist expert, it is easy to be more concerned with getting the work done than with learning from the experience and modifying your practice as you are faced with new situations.

What responsibility do you personally take to learn from the experiences you are faced with in the clinical setting? Do you expect to 'be taught' or do you 'actively seek to learn'? How can you improve on this?

Where to start

What can you do in a practical way that will help you develop your reflective skills more formally? Four main areas will be considered here:

1. the use of action-inquiry and action-learning sets
2. the use of critical-incident analysis
3. learning diaries/journals and portfolios
4. developing a learning culture within the workplace.

Action-inquiry and action-learning sets

Action inquiry and action learning have become extremely popular in both educational institutions as well as within health service organizations in recent years. Given the NHS modernization agenda and the need for service improvement and service re-design, organizations are seeking support through action learning to support their staff through major change. Moving away from didactic teaching and allowing practitioners to problem-solve organizational issues, either through individual teams or across manager groups, action-learning sets have been warmly welcomed as a way of identifying what the problems are and how they may be resolved as well as using the group for support. Much has been written about action learning and indeed, established in 2001, the Institute of Reflective Practice was set up within the UK to 'improve lives and livelihoods through reflective learning' (Institute of Reflective Practice, 2008). Additionally, from 2004, it has published a dedicated journal entitled *Action Learning: Research and Practice* to allow individuals across all types of organizations to share their experiences and engage in valuable debate. Interestingly, 2008 saw an increase in the number of publications of this journal from two per year to three, illustrating an increase in the interest of this subject area for practice.

So what do we mean by action inquiry and action learning?

There are many similarities between action inquiry and action learning particularly in relation to their theoretical assumptions and their impact on professional and management education (Pedler, 2005). Action inquiry is concerned with transforming organizations and communities to achieve greater effectiveness, trying to create a culture of collaboration and self-reflection. It has been developed as a theory as well as a life practice (Reason, 1994, p. 49) and is based on the work of Torbert, Argyris and Schon (e.g. Argyris and Schon, 1974; Argyris et al., 1985; Schon, 1983; Torbert, 1981).

Action learning, however, has its focus on learning. McGill and Beaty (2001) offer a good introduction to action learning and define it as follows:

> Action learning is a continuous process of learning and reflection, supported by colleagues, with an intention of getting things done. Through action learning individuals learn with and from each other by working on real problems and reflecting on their own experiences.
>
> (McGill and Beaty, 2001, p. 11)

By bringing together a group of people (called a set), individuals with a common purpose can work together for a specific time and be facilitated by another, often outside the initial group. As they become more confident in the approach, they may facilitate themselves. Their specific purpose is to solve problems and through their reflection be enabled into action to resolve or address those problems.

A number of government initiatives have been introduced to reduce national problems in health care such as hospital acquired infection and the Safer Patient Initiative where NHS Trusts are expected to 'integrate patient safety into hospital management, culture and across all clinical practice (The Health Foundation, 2008). To support them, NHS organizations have commissioned support from their higher-education partners to facilitate action-learning sets among senior managers to help them to find ways of addressing these problems and within their learning set, support each other through their agreed action.

The idea behind action-learning sets is that each individual member is acknowledged as being responsible for his or her own problem. Participating in the learning set, the individual seeks help in dealing with the problem but as McGill and Beaty (2001) confirm, they cannot expect anyone within the group to tell them what to do or to solve the problem. The focus is not on gaining advice from the membership but instead, for others to understand the situation better through reflection and exploration and to challenge them in their assumptions underlying the reflections to help them to identify the best way forward.

As you can see, reflection by individuals within a group and the powerful decisions they are required to take within their organizations as a result of their learning can be greatly improved by working with others (McGill and Beaty, 2001).

You may find that learning method may not be as well used at the pre-qualifying level of activity but is more widely used at the post-qualifying level. You may also find it of value as you progress through your studies in helping each other through areas of difficulty in both theory and practice.

The use of critical-incident analysis

We have seen how helpful guided reflection can be at a personal level in order to contribute to learning with the central objective of improving patient care. Reflection is also used throughout the NHS every day at an organizational level in order to examine the reasons behind the occurrence of adverse healthcare events. One million patients are safely treated in the NHS every day (Chief Medical Officer, 2005). However, it is estimated that there are more than 1.2 million safety incidents and near misses in the NHS each year (DoH, 2000b).

It is essential that a large organization like the NHS has robust systems in place for the reporting of incidents, and that the causes of adverse incidents are investigated and identified, and that learning from mistakes and lessons learned are incorporated within clinical and administrative practice in order to ensure that any clinical risk patients may be exposed to is significantly reduced (DoH, 2000b). Another important issue is that all clinical incidents are seen in an organizational context and that learning that has occurred from one incident is incorporated into practice so that critical incidents are not looked at or treated in isolation. If that was to happen then the staff working within the organization would not have the opportunity to learn lessons on a large scale.

In recent years, the NHS has focused on patient safety and has incorporated principles of good practice from other professions. The aviation industry is a high-risk area and has learnt many important lessons from aviation disasters. Research in this area indicates that errors occur most often because of failures in teamwork and coordination (Pape, 2003) and that 70% of errors involve human errors (Helmreich, 2000), such as unclear communication, poor leadership or tendencies to presume what others were doing. As a result of the learning that occurred in the aviation industry crew-resource management was developed. These principles have been further refined to develop team-resource management which is a useful concept in patient safety in the NHS (Terema, 2008).

Bradley (1992) defines critical-incident analysis as based on factual accounts of real events in which the purpose and consequences of behaviour are clear. Minghella and Benson (1995) found the technique helpful to nursing students in developing negotiation and reflective-practice skills.

While there is no one defined structured approach to critical-incident analysis several useful approaches are used within the NHS. The National Patient Safety Agency (2008) has developed a series of helpful tools to allow multidisciplinary teams seek the cause of critical incidents. A series of techniques can be employed such as:

- root-cause analysis
- nominal group technique
- brainstorming
- brainwriting
- five whys
- barrier analysis
- identifying root causes

These approaches break down components further to allow for critical analysis. For example, when looking at contributory factors, staff are asked to consider the patient, individual, task, communications, team, social, education and training, equipment, resource, working conditions, organizational and strategic issues. Each of these components is then sub-divided under sub-headings to encourage the team to analyse the issue.

More information about these techniques can be found at: http://www.npsa.nhs.uk/health/resources/root_cause_analysis

At a personal level, critical-incident analysis can be structured by using one of the reflective models discussed in this chapter in order to frame your analysis. Critical-incident analysis does not have to focus on negative events, it is important for individuals, teams and organizations to learn from situations when things went well. For example, in exceptional circumstances we can learn from situations so that the principles can be applied to the development of new processes and pathways successfully.

Think of a situation that occurred in your own practice recently. It may be a routine activity that you felt you handled particularly well or something that sticks in your mind as special in some way. Using one of the frameworks or tools identified for critical-incident analysis, identify any new knowledge you have gained from the experience and where you obtained this knowledge from.

The skill of integrating new knowledge with previous knowledge is important in all our development and helps us to individualize the care we give and to improve the standards of care overall. It is an important skill, enabling reflection to help us to adapt care in new situations and change our thinking about the way we do things.

Learning diaries/journals and portfolios

Increasingly, programmes of study encourage students to complete reflective diaries or learning journals of their learning experiences. The purpose of these is to help you understand yourself – your strengths and limitations, the opportunities that were available to you and the threats to your development (often referred to as a SWOT analysis). Diaries help you to describe your experiences, to analyse the different processes contributing to the decision making and, through learning, to develop your practice. In addition, reflective diaries or journals can help you understand your feelings during a particular clinical incident and how these feelings helped or hindered your ability to act confidently and competently.

A diary will help you to bring together the theory you have been reading and learning with the practice in clinical placements (see Chapter 2). A diary is about reflecting: thinking, analysing and learning are the key skills to a successful diary and journal. It is much more than simply telling the story. Although reflection is a skill that needs to be learned, the more you examine and explore your practice, the easier it should become to probe deeper into the complexities of your practice and begin to tease out the different issues. Knowing the 'right' questions to ask yourself is a crucial stage in this probing exercise. Reflection within your learning diary or journal will help you 'learn how to learn'.

Additionally, to help you to develop your skills of accountability, keeping a reflective diary or journal can assist you to articulate your tacit knowledge (knowing more than you can say). This can help you have a deeper understanding of your actions and help you interrogate and evaluate what you have done.

In addition to being valuable tools in themselves, the skills you are using in your learning diaries and journals can help you in the completion of your ongoing portfolio of learning. The learning you have achieved through completing a learning diary within a specific module of your programme can assist you in your personal professional portfolio both during your pre-qualifying programme and thereafter during your professional career. The NMC (2008) requirement for you to actively engage in your continuing professional development by keeping a personal professional portfolio (see Chapter 15 for more information), demonstrating you keep up to date with new developments, is being audited. You may be one of the lucky ones who is asked by the NMC to demonstrate evidence of your learning!

Nevertheless, a number of constraints to the effective implementation of reflective diaries/journals have been recognized. Among these are lack of time to complete the activity, lack of support to implement changes in practice and lack of skills of critical analysis in the documentation of this reflection (Heath, 1998). In fact, Heath offers a practical guide to keeping a reflective diary, suggesting that one side of the page is given to telling the 'story' while the other side is used for reflection and analysis notes. In this way, the points raised in the descriptive diary are addressed in some way on the other side of the page, answering your self-posed question of 'so what? – what point am I trying to make in relation to confirming my good practice or suggesting change?' Heath also recommends that you should undertake reflection without sticking to a rigid framework, rather using your own imagination and creativity to identify problems and solutions. Frameworks can then be used as a checklist after reflecting to add further dimensions and depth of thought. Alternatively, they can help get you started by offering a range of questions to ask yourself. Although there are a number of negative reports of students' indifference (Cassidy and Luxton, 1992) and complaints about having to write a journal (Holland, 1989), Chirema (2007) found in her recent study that her students were particularly positive about how writing encouraged their analysis and critical thinking. It seems from the literature that students' enthusiasm for the approach is dependent on whether the diary or journal is compulsory and the value it holds within the education programme and the promise of on-going feedback (Cunliffe, 2004; Jung and Tryssenaar, 1998; Kember et al., 1996; Kuiper, 2004).

For the purpose of your learning diary or personal professional profile, the presentation of reflective accounts of your study and practice need not be lengthy tomes but short, analytical accounts of what you gained from the experience. However, it is not until you become practised in teasing out the points for analysis in your 'stories' that you can become skilled at focusing and become more adept at identifying your learning. Moon (2006) offers a good insight into the development and use of learning journals that you might find helpful.

Finally, it is well recognized that reflection for better decision making can indeed be a painful and isolating experience:

> In the varied topography of professional practice, there is a high, hard ground where practitioners can make effective use of research-based theory and technique, and there is a swampy lowland where situations are confusing 'messes' incapable of technical solution. The difficulty is that the problems of the high ground, however great their technical interest, are often relatively unimportant to clients or to the larger society, while in the swamp are the problems of greatest human concern.
>
> (Schon, 1991, p. 42)

This difficulty needs to be recognized by us all. It is the 'messy' areas that pose the greatest challenge to us and it is crucial, therefore, to gain support in both analysing the situations and identifying possible solutions. This will be considered in more detail in the next section.

Developing a learning culture/learning community within the workplace

Clinical practice placements are seen as an essential resource in preparing pre-registration students for their professional role (McAllister, 2001). *Making a difference* (DoH, 1999) sought to strengthen UK midwifery and nurse education and training and highlighted the importance of working in a learning organization.

Seminal work in the 1980s was carried out by Orton (1981), Fretwell (1982) and Ogier (1982) with the aim of exploring the ideal clinical learning environment. All three studies identified that the ward sister was a pivotal figure in determining the quality of the learning environment in clinical areas. The leadership style of the ward sister as well as patterns of interaction were found to be important determinants of a positive learning culture.

During the last 25 years, we have seen the NHS change radically with a move from care being delivered in secondary to primary care settings. The nursing and clinical dependency of patients cared for in general ward areas has also increased dramatically. The governmental drive has been for a more accountable and responsive healthcare system which is patient centred. Alongside medical and technological advances the clinical learning environment is a very different place for pre- and post-registration students.

It is therefore understandable that for various reasons many students perceive the clinical environment as a stressful learning environment which causes them to feel anxious and vulnerable (Timmins and Kaliszer, 2002). A learning culture has been defined as one:

> ...where the nurses see their work as a source of energy and excitement and as offering opportunities for personal and professional growth: in other words, giving as much as it took and to receive constructive criticism non defensively.
> (Titchen and Binnie, 1995, p. 333)

Although this definition is 13 years old, it still captures the essence of a positive clinical learning environment at a departmental or ward level.

Think for a moment about a recent clinical placement: would you classify it as a positive learning environment? Think about issues such as: was there evidence of practice development? Was there evidence that the senior nurses displayed evidence of skills such as strategic thinking, negotiation and facilitation? Did you receive feedback which allowed you to modify your behaviour in areas in which action was required? Most importantly were the patient and their family the focus of everyone's priority?

An important characteristic of a positive learning environment is effective feedback both to students and staff. Feedback is seen as a fundamental aspect of teaching and learning (Clynes and Raftery, 2008). Rowntree (1987, p. 27) goes as far as to describe it as the 'lifeblood of learning'. Feedback in clinical practice is seen as essential for a student's growth, provides direction and helps to boost confidence, increase motivation and self-esteem (Begley and White, 2003). Weinger et al. (1998) describe the best feedback as being highly specific, and descriptive of what actually occurred. Information, including examples from practice, should be clear and the feedback offered as a measurement in terms of specific targets and standards. It is essential that feedback is objective and concentrates on behaviours and work performance and not a person's character.

What can you as a student do to benefit from a learning culture?

Various roles have been developed to meet the challenges of supporting learning in practice, such as practice educators, education facilitators, lecturer practitioners and the academic in practice. It is important that you identify the resources available to help you make the most of clinical placements as well as achieve set learning objectives.

It has been identified that students tend to rely heavily on their mentors to arrange progress meetings and offer feedback (Daelmans et al., 2006). To become an equal partner in the mentor and mentee relationship it is important that you show initiative and take responsibility for initiating the feedback process by arranging a mutually convenient time for you and your mentor to meet and being prepared for the meeting.

It has been found that the process of giving feedback is made easier for the mentor when the student identifies their practice limitations ensuring that the student is not a passive recipient of feedback (Clynes, 2008). It is important also to focus and reflect on how feedback can help you devise an action plan in order to achieve the safe and effective delivery of care. If you are unsure of what is being expected of you, ask for specific examples so you can modify behaviours. It is important, too, to reflect on positive feedback and identify why you did well so you can apply these behaviours to other situations you may encounter in your career.

Listening

One of the greatest qualities you can have to help someone in their reflections is the skill of listening. It is easy to interrupt a colleague or friend when they are exploring a situation that happened to them with a similar experience that you have had yourself. Resist the temptation and encourage your colleague to explore the situation deeply. You can provide the cues and the questioning skills to help them to do so. It can be satisfying and fulfilling to participate in another's reflective activities, as well as to share your own experiences. You can learn as much as they can from the situation from being a more objective observer of the situation. When several of you have been involved in the same situation, you should consider finding the opportunity of sharing the different perspectives of the situation together. It may surprise you to discover the different perspectives and lessons that have been learned by each of you.

Conclusion

It is important to remember that thinking about what you are doing is a natural activity that you carry out every day. Critical reflection is much more difficult. It is more analytical and encourages a more in-depth examination of your practice. It is a skill that you need to work through with support. From Conway's (1996) work we have seen that not all experts find reflection easy; we are not all natural reflectors. However, those who can develop the skill will go on to become more informed practitioners.

This chapter links closely with the previous chapters and has been designed to help you develop your understanding of how reflection can be used to help you study and, in particular, to help you gain as much as you can from both your study and your clinical practice. By attempting to make sense of both the term and the process of reflection, this chapter aims to demonstrate how meaningful reflection can help you in both a personal and professional way. A number of types of reflection, as well as a range of reflective frameworks, are available to help you understand the meaning of how and what you do, so that you can advance your work and practice and not make the same mistakes over and over. Although reflection is not easy, the practical suggestions in this chapter, e.g. critical-incident analysis and learning diaries, and the development of a learning culture/community within the workplace, will help you progress through your journey.

 ## CHAPTER RESOURCES

REFERENCES

Argyris, C. & Schon, D.A., 1974. Theory in practice: increasing professional effectiveness. Jossey Bass, San Francisco.

Argyris, C., Putman, R. & Smith, M.C., 1985. Action science: concepts, methods and skills for research and intervention. Jossey Bass, San Francisco.

Begley, C. & White, P., 2003. Irish nursing students' changing self-esteem and fear of negative evaluation during their preregistration programme. Journal of Advanced Nursing 42 (4), 390–401.

Borton, T., 1970. Reach, touch and teach. McGraw-Hill, London.

Boud, K., Keogh, R. & Walker, D. (Eds.), 1985. Reflection: turning experience into learning. Kogan Page, London.

Bradley, C.P., 1992. Turning anecdotes into data: the critical incident technique. Family Practice 9 (1), 98–103.

Brookfield, S., 1995. Becoming a critically reflective teacher. Jossey-Bass, San Francisco.

Burns, S. & Bulman, C. (Eds.), 2000. Reflective practice in nursing: the growth of the professional practitioner, 2nd edn. Blackwell Science, Oxford.

Carper, B., 1978. Fundamental patterns of knowing in nursing. Advances in Nursing Sciences 1, 13–23.

Cassidy, V.R. & Luxton, C., 1992. The use of clinical diaries by baccalaureate nursing majors. In: Unpublished paper presented at the Research in Nursing Education Tenth Anniversary Annual Meeting, February 13, San Francisco, California.

Chief Medical Officer, 2005. Medical error. Joint NHS/NPSA Publication, London.

Chinn, P. & Kramer, M., 1995. Theory and nursing: a systematic approach, 4th edn. Mosby, St Louis, MO.

Chirema, K., 2007. The use of reflective journals in the promotion of reflection and learning in post-registration nursing students. Nurse Education Today 27, 192–202.

Clynes, M., 2008. Providing feedback on clinical performance to student nurses in children's nursing: challenges facing preceptors. Journal of Children's and Young People's Nursing 2 (1), 1176–1181.

Clynes, M. & Raftery, S., 2008. Feedback: an essential element of student learning in clinical practice. Nurse Education in Practice (doi:10.1016/j.nepr.2008.02.003).

Conway, J., 1996. Nursing expertise and advanced practice. Quay Books, Salisbury, UK.

Conway, J., 1998. Evolution of the species 'expert nurse'. An examination of the practical knowledge held by expert nurses. Journal of Clinical Nursing 7 (1), 75–82.

Cunliffe, A.L., 2004. On becoming a critically reflexive practitioner. Journal of Management Education 28 (4), 407–426.

Daelmans, H.E.M., Overmeer, R.M., Hem-Stokroos, H.H., et al., 2006. In training assessment qualitative study of effects on supervision and feedback in an undergraduate clinical rotation. Medical Education 40 (1), 51–58.

Department of Health (DoH), 1999. Making a difference: strengthening the nursing, midwifery and health visiting contribution to health and healthcare. The Stationery Office, London.

Department of Health (DoH), 2000a. A health service of all the talents: developing the NHS workforce. The Stationery Office, London.

Department of Health (DoH), 2000b. An organisation with a memory. DoH, London.

Department of Health (DoH), 2006. Modernising nursing careers – setting the direction. DoH, London.

Dewar, B., 1992. Skill middle? Nursing Times 12 (88), 24–27.

Dewey, D., 1933. How we think. DC Health and Co., Boston, MA.

Freire, P., 1996. Pedagogy of hope: reliving pedagogy of the oppressed. Continuum Publishing Company, New York.

Fretwell, J.E., 1982. Ward teaching and learning. Royal College of Nursing, London.

Gibbs, G., 1988. Learning by doing. A guide to reading and learning methods. Further Education Unit, London.

Greenwood, J., 1998. The role of reflection in single and double loop learning. Journal of Advanced Nursing 27, 1048–1053.

Gustafsson, C., Asp, M. & Fagerberg, I., 2007. Reflective practice in nursing care: embedded assumptions in qualitative studies. International Journal of Nursing Practice 13, 151–160.

Habermas, J., 1974. Theory and practice [trans J Viertel]. Heinemann, London.

Hannigan, B., 2001. A discussion of the strengths and weaknesses of reflection in nursing practice and education. Journal of Clinical Nursing 10, 278–283.

Heath, H., 1998. Keeping a reflective practice diary: a practical guide. Nurse Education Today 18 (18), 592–598.

Helmreich, R.L., 2000. On error management, lessons from aviation. British Medical Journal 320 (7237), 781–785.

Holland, R.M., 1989. Anonymous journals in literature survey courses. TETYC (December), 236–241

Holm, D. & Stephenson, S., 1994. Reflection – a student's perspective. In: Palmer, A., Burns, S. & Bulman, C. (Eds.) Reflective practice in nursing: the growth of the professional practitioner. Blackwell Scientific, Oxford, pp. 53–62.

Institute of Reflective Practice. 2008. Online. Available: http://www .reflectivepractices.co.uk/index.php [accessed 27 April 2008].

Jasper, M., 2006. Professional development, reflection and decision-making. Blackwell Publishing, Oxford.

Johns, C., 2000. Becoming a reflective practitioner: a reflective and holistic approach to clinical nursing, practice development and clinical supervision. Blackwell Science, Oxford.

Johns, C., 2006. Engaging reflection in practice. A narrative approach. Blackwell Publishing, Oxford.

Jung, B. & Tryssenaar, J., 1998. Supervising students: exploring the experience through reflective journals. Occupational Therapy International 5 (1), 35–48.

Kember, D. (Ed.), 2001. Reflective teaching and learning in the health professions: action research in professional education. Blackwell Science, Oxford.

Kember, D., Jones, A. & Loke, A., et al., 1996. Developing curricula to encourage students to write reflective journals. Educational Action Research 4 (3), 329–348.

Kim, H.S., 1999. Critical reflective inquiry for knowledge development in nursing practice. Journal of Advanced Nursing 29, 1205–1212.

Kuiper, R.A., 2004. Nursing reflections from journaling during a peri-operative internship. AORN Journal 79 (1), 195–198.

Mantzoukas, S., 2007. Reflection and problem/enquiry-based learning: confluences and contradictions. Reflective Practice 8 (2), 241–253.

Mantzoukas, S. & Jasper, M., 2004. Reflective practice and daily ward reality: a covert game. Journal of Clinical Nursing 13, 925–933.

McAllister, L., 2001. An adult learning framework for clinical education. In: McAllister, L., Lincoln, M., McLeod, S. & Maloney, D. (Eds.) Facilitating learning in clinical settings. Nelson Thornes, Cheltenham, UK.

McGill, I. & Beaty, L., 2001. Action learning: a practitioner's guide, 2nd edn. Kogan Page, London.

Mezirow, J., 1991. Transformative dimensions of adult learning. Jossey-Bass, San Francisco.

Minghella, E. & Benson, A., 1995. Developing reflective practice in mental health nursing through critical incident analysis. Journal of Advanced Nursing 21, 265–273.

Moon, J.A., 1999. Reflection in learning and professional development. Kogan Page, London.

Moon, J.A., 2006. Learning journals: a handbook for reflective practice and professional development, 2nd edn. Routledge, London.

National Patient Safety Agency. 2008. RCA training and RCA toolkit. Online. Available: www.npsa.nhs.uk/health/resources/root_cause_analysis [accessed 7 April 2008].

Nursing and Midwifery Council (NMC), 2005. Supporting nurses and midwives through lifelong learning. 2 August NMC, London.

Nursing and Midwifery Council (NMC), 2008. The PREP handbook (updated). NMC, London. Accessed from http://www.nmc-org.uk/aDisplayDocument.aspx?DocumentID=4340.

Ogier, M., 1982. An ideal sister?. Royal College of Nursing, London.

Orton, H., 1981. Ward learning climate. Royal College of Nursing, London.

Pape, T.M., 2003. Applying airline safety practices to medication administration. Medical and Surgical Nursing 12 (2), 77–93.

Pedler, M., 2005. A general theory of human action. Action Learning: Research and Practice 2 (2), 127–132.

Reason, P. (Ed.), 1994. Participation in human inquiry. Sage Publications, London.

Redmond, B., 2004. Reflection in action: developing reflective practice in health and social services. Ashgate Publishing, Aldershot, UK.

Rinpoche, S., 1992. The Tibetan book of living and dying. Rider, London.

Rolfe, G., Freshwater, D. & Jasper, M., 2001. Critical reflection for nursing. Palgrave, Basingstoke, UK.

Rowntree, D., 1987. Assessing students: how shall we know them?, 2nd edn. Kogan, London.

Schon, D., 1983. The reflective practitioner – how professionals think in action. Basic Books, New York.

Schon, D., 1987. Educating the reflective practitioner. Temple Smith, London.

Schon, D., 1991. The reflective practitioner: how professionals think in action. Ashgate Avebury, UK.

Taylor, B., 2006. Reflective practice: a guide for nurses and midwives, 2nd edn. Open University Press, Maidenhead, UK.

Terema. 2008. Team resource management. Online. Available: http://www.terema.co.uk/ [accessed 7 April 2008].

The Health Foundation. 2008. Safer patients initiative. Trusts explain how they are making hospitals safer for patients. Online. Available: http://www.health.org.uk/news/blank_1_43.html [accessed 27 April 2008]

Timmins, F. & Kaliszer, M., 2002. Aspects of nurse education programmes that frequently cause stress to nursing students. Nurse Education Today 22, 203–211.

Titchen, A. & Binnie, A., 1995. The art of clinical supervision. Journal of Clinical Nursing 4, 327–334.

Torbert, W.R., 1981. Empirical, behavioural, theoretical and attentional skills necessary for collaborative inquiry. In: Reason, P. & Rowan, J. (Eds.) Human inquiry: a sourcebook of new paradigm research. Wiley, Chichester, UK.

United Kingdom Central Council for Nursing, Midwifery and Health Visiting (UKCC), 1986. Project 2000: a new preparation for practice. UKCC, London.

United Kingdom Central Council for Nursing, Midwifery and Health Visiting (UKCC), 1999a. Fitness for Practice: the UKCC commission for nursing and midwifery education. UKCC, London.

United Kingdom Central Council for Nursing, Midwifery and Health Visiting (UKCC), 1999b. UKCC PREP monitor project: summary report. UKCC, London.

Weinger, M., Pantiskas, C., Wiklund, M. & Carstensen, P., 1998. Incorporating human factors into the design of medical devices. Journal of the American Medical Association 280 (17), 1484.

WEBSITES

Action learning: http://www.ifal.org.uk

http://www.learningandteaching.info/teaching/action_learning.htm

Team resource management: http://www. terema.co.uk

National Patient Safety Association: http://www.npsa.nhs.uk/health/resources/

Life-long learning: http://www.rcm.org.uk/college/continuing-professional-development/accreditation/

http://www.lluk.org/

FURTHER READING

Jasper, M., 2006. Professional development, reflection and decision-making. Blackwell Publishing, Oxford.

Mantzoukas, S., 2007. Reflection and problem/enquiry-based learning: confluences and contradictions. Reflective Practice 8(2), 241–253.

McGill, I. & Beaty, L., 2001. Action learning: a practitioner's guide, 2nd edn. Kogan Page, London.

Moon, J.A., 2006. Learning journals: a handbook for reflective practice and professional development, 2nd edn. Routledge, London.

Redmond, B., 2004. Reflection in action: developing reflective practice in health and social services. Ashgate Publishing, Aldershot, UK.

Rolfe, G., Freshwater, D. & Jasper, M., 2001. Critical reflection for nursing. Palgrave, Basingstoke, UK.

Taylor, B., 2006. Reflective practice: a guide for nurses and midwives, 2nd edn. Open University Press, Maidenhead, UK.

13 Group work

Sian Maslin-Prothero

Introduction

Group work is frequently used as a method of learning in education and practice, and is an integral part of becoming a midwife/nurse. The aim of this chapter is to tell you about group work and how to develop your skills for working in groups so that you can get the most out of meetings, seminars and tutorials.

In health care there is increasing emphasis on student participation in learning. The belief is that through active learning students are better able to engage in the material being presented and feel more involved in the learning process. The importance of student participation in other parts of university life is important. You may be asked to become a member of a university body or committee such as a student/staff consultative committee, or represent fellow students at a meeting with the panel from the Quality Assurance Agency or Nursing and Midwifery Council (NMC) to discuss your experience of learning. Becoming a member of any group is an excellent way of developing skills that are key to your development and transferable to other situations.

If you think about it, we all belong to different groups, such as a family, a sports club, a voluntary association or a trade union. A group consists of a number of people who meet together to follow a chosen activity; being in a group is how society functions and is therefore a part of all our lives. Some groups are more personal and voluntary than others – consider the difference between a basketball team and a tutorial group.

Groups may form to achieve a specific task, and so group members are expected to work collaboratively. An effective way of learning is through interacting with other people; it not only gives us the opportunity to hear other people's ideas and thoughts but it also gives us the opportunity to try out and share our own opinions. A group will bring together a range of attitudes, knowledge and skills that would not be available if we were working alone, for example handover in your practice area or a case-based presentation. This is one of the advantages of working in a group, particularly when it involves problem solving such as problem-based learning or decision making. If all members of a group feel valued and can participate, then there is likely to be a greater commitment to, and support of, the group and the decisions made. Group discussion should help you to develop your critical thinking, and provide you with the opportunity of linking theory to practice (and vice versa).

Characteristics of groups

Groups have a number of common characteristics:

- a definable membership
- group consciousness
- a shared sense of purpose
- interdependence
- interaction
- an ability to cooperate.

Advantages of group work

If you were to reflect on your experience of working in the group, you would identify a number of advantages to working in a group, and you might include some of the following:

- enhance learning
- sharing the workload:
  - thinking
  - problem solving
  - understanding
- improve efficiency and ability to tackle complex tasks
- increased effectiveness – provide better solutions through shared dialogue and learning
- enhance satisfaction through networking and social support
- active participation
- purposeful activity.

Disadvantages of group work

There can be disadvantages to working in a group.

- Can you recall an experience of where a group activity failed?
- What do you think was the reason?
- What do you think might be some of the disadvantages of working in a group?

Jot down your thoughts.

A group might be unsuccessful for a number of reasons, some of which are listed below:

- people work at different speeds
- poor group dynamics
- lack of communication
- task set is not completed
- not all members of the group participate
- group members feel isolated
- group work does not suit your preferred learning style (see Chapter 2)
- group members compare themselves with others
- time required to set up the group
- dominance by an outspoken member.

You need to understand why groups exist, and develop strategies for ensuring they are successful. As highlighted in the advantages of groups, a group can bring together a range of skills and knowledge that an individual does not have. For the group to be successful, all the group members need to feel that they are a part of the group and that the group values their contribution.

Group dynamics

For a group to be both effective and efficient, you need to have a mix of personalities; there can be different roles assigned to members within groups – these roles are usually unconscious. The role you play in a group will depend on your personality and on the reason for the group existing. Belbin (2004) identified nine key roles for an effective group. These are:

- Coordinator: mature, confident, a good chairperson. Delegates, promotes decision making and ensures that all contributions are heard.
- Shaper: challenging, dynamic. Pushes the group and encourages them to complete the task.
- Plant: creative, imaginative, unorthodox. Solves difficult problems.
- Resource investigator: extrovert, enthusiastic, communicative. Develops contacts and explores new ideas.
- Monitor evaluator: strategic and discerning. The critic who finds the faults in arguments.
- Team worker: cooperative, perceptive, diplomatic. The individual who holds the group together and supports group members.
- Implementer: disciplined, reliable, efficient. Turns ideas into actions.
- Completer finisher: painstaking, anxious, contentious. The perfectionist who ensures that the group meets any deadlines.
- Specialist: single-minded, a self starter, dedicated. Provides knowledge and skills that are in short supply.

One person can take on more than one role in a group. It is important that there is balance between each of the roles in the group if the group is to remain effective. You might like to visit: http://www.belbin.com/ to find out more.

Having looked at the different roles in a group, which would be your preferred role?

Group life cycle

A group is dynamic and will usually have a life cycle, although they will vary according to their aim, function, size and so on; yet they will usually keep to the following phases: initial, production, consolidation and resolution.

For example, when a student midwife/nurse in practice, your time spent in an area will be limited to the length of your placement. Although you might see this as limiting, placements allow you to experience a range of different environments; in addition, you will find that you develop skills and strategies for adapting so that you can use skills learned elsewhere and apply them in a different setting (see also Chapters 10 and 11). These are referred to as transferable skills – skills learned in one context that are useful in another. Example of key skills:

- teamwork and leadership
- commercial awareness
- written communication
- interpersonal communication
- problem solving
- networking
- initiative
- planning and organisation
- adaptability and flexibility
- numeracy
- computer literacy
- time management.

Becoming a team player

Our previous experience of working in a team can affect how we approach working in a new group. In order to be effective the group may need to go through a number of stages before it becomes a functioning team. Tuckman (1965) initially identified four stages (see points 1 to 4 below), but further work identified a fifth stage (Tuckman and Jensen, 1977).

1. Forming (orientation): this is usually a positive stage when you are anticipating working with a new group of people. You might be slightly anxious at the thought of meeting people and wondering whether you will be able to successfully complete the task set.
2. Storming (dissatisfaction/conflict): at this stage you might experience some uncertainty regarding the effectiveness of the group – if the team does not seem to meet your or others' expectations. There may be disagreements as some members appear to be engaging with the group and activity more easily than you.

3. Norming (resolution/cooperation): this is where the team begins to settle down and functions more effectively, because you have addressed any conflict and negotiated how to cooperate.

4. Performing (productivity): this is where the team is working well together, where members feel that they are able to express themselves and that the task can be achieved through combined effort.

5. Adjourning (dissolution): this is when the group disbands on completion of the task.

In order for the team to develop and move forward, you may need to move through these stages; this can be facilitated by agreeing ground rules during the forming stage.

You could assess how a group is working through using the Johari window. The Johari window model was developed by American psychologists Luft and Ingham, while researching group dynamics (Luft and Ingham, 1955). This is a tool for illustrating and improving self-awareness, and mutual understanding between individuals within a group; further information about this is at the end of the chapter in the resources section.

Ground rules

Participating in group discussions allows us to learn from others, and develop our own thoughts and beliefs about a subject. For a group to be successful it is important that the group members meet and agree ground rules – these are a set of guidelines that the group acknowledges and adheres to each time it meets. Ground rules allow each member of the group to know what is expected of them.

 Imagine you are meeting in a group for the first time. Jot down the ground rules that would be important to you. Keep these and refer to them when you are asked to identify ground rules.

You might have identified some of the following as important:

- confidentiality
- being tactful, considerate and respecting others' opinions
- punctuality
- being supportive:
  - sharing knowledge
  - not 'putting down' others
- not being distracting:
  - keeping noise levels down
  - not interrupting
  - sticking to the point.
- switching off mobile phones.

The use of ground rules allows each member of the group to know what is expected of them, and they only really work when they are shared – there may need to be agreed sanctions for members who break any of the ground rules.

Managing a group

Before looking at how you can contribute to a group discussion, you need to understand about managing a group. A successful group will be purposeful, without the need for lecturer intervention. The two main factors in managing a group are:

1. group tasks
2. group maintenance.

Group tasks

The task or tasks of the group relate(s) to its purpose, structure and activities. These need to be clearly defined; for example, group composition, members' roles and responsibilities, group management, ground rules, study requirements (seminar presentations, assignments, and assessments), practice meetings, deadlines and preparation for meetings.

Group maintenance

This is all about creating a climate that encourages discussion and debate, and can be achieved through the group members being accepting of and cooperative towards each other, particularly when there are conflicts of opinion or personality clashes. Active participation makes group sessions more enjoyable, as well as producing an opportunity for learning. The amount of time spent on the maintenance of a group will vary – it is particularly important in the early stages of a group's formation.

Group meetings

For the group to be effective, everyone needs to be committed. This means attending group meetings; not turning up for a pre-arranged meeting means that you are not sharing the commitment to the group and letting your colleagues down.

The group needs to have a clear focus – a frame of reference – the subject or the task the group is going to discuss and/or achieve. For example, the lecturer facilitating your inter-professional learning group has asked you to find out about public involvement in health and social care as part of a problem-based learning activity. In order to develop your understanding you have to expand your knowledge, through thinking, brainstorming ideas, reading or discussion. Through sharing the topic with others you will be able to keep sight of the frame of reference, and move forward by using the opinions of others, as well as by cultivating your own.

Groups go through stages of development before performing success-fully (see becoming a team player above). A group that meets regularly can build on information gained at previous meetings, enabling the dialogue to become more advanced and sophisticated. The group will also change and develop over time, from its initial formation, through conflict, cooperation and task completion.

Group discussion

Many students gain support from a group – it can be a comfort to find that some students have similar thoughts to you, while others may offer a different way of looking at an issue. For example, you have been asked to read a complex article prior to an interdisciplinary case conference in practice. You read the article but you can only make sense of the abstract – the rest of the article makes no sense to you. When you arrive for the meeting, you discover that some of your colleagues were equally baffled, but some understood parts of the article. Through group discussion and debate you make sense of the article, and apply this learning to the case conference.

Groups can provide support in other ways, such as sharing skills and knowledge; remember that many skills are transferable – skills acquired through any activity (not just your studies) – and can be applied in other situations. These skills can be acquired through employment, voluntary work, hobbies and sports, almost anything.

What do you do if you don't want to participate in the discussion, possibly because you are too shy or because you are afraid that your colleagues might think what you have to say is daft? Remember that discussion is there for everyone's development, not only those who appear to have no fear of expressing their thoughts and feelings. In this situation, don't be afraid to make an observation – what appears quite simple to you might be just what another colleague needs in order to make sense of the subject. Another important point to remember is that we all feel anxious about expressing ourselves; even experienced people feel anxious about contributions they make to debates. As discussed at the beginning of the section on group dynamics, we all have different roles in a group and, so long as you participate by actively listening, you are contributing to the group discussion.

When things go wrong

There will be times when things go wrong in a group. First, it is important to remember that conflict is normal in any team – think about your relationship with friends or partner (see Cartney and Rouse, 2006). The most important thing is to maintain a climate of cooperation; this can be achieved by involving the whole group in identifying the problem and resolving it, in order that the team remains productive.

Hostile members

This can occur in small and large groups; examples include overt hostility, aggression, point scoring and inappropriate humour, all of which can hinder the success of the group. It is important to acknowledge any hostility when it occurs; if you need additional support, call on other group members to support you when you tackle hostile members.

Avoiding difficult situations

This is when members of the group avoid a specific issue by being disruptive, withdrawing from group activities or trying to change the subject. When this occurs, vocalize your thoughts – remember, communication is essential if the group is to be successful. You may find that the group relies on the same person to manage these – if this is the case, do be sure to support this person when appropriate.

Dominating members

There will be times when a member of the group dominates the conversation or prevents others from participating. If a lecturer is facilitating the group, you might see it as their responsibility to control the group; however, each member of any group has a role and responsibility for regulating the group – more so if ground rules were agreed – don't be afraid to manage unruly members. Your support will be appreciated.

Study groups

You can establish an informal self-help group to achieve specific tasks, such as revision for examinations or writing an essay (see Chapters 2 and 7). Don't wait for someone else to do this – set up the group yourself. This can be on a one-to-one basis, such as with a critical friend, or syndicated learning. There is evidence that those students who share their learning with others are more likely to complete their course successfully (Camacho Carr et al., 1996).

Active learning in groups

Experiential learning means learning by doing: you learn from experience. This refers to learning through everyday experiences in life and work – being aware of them, then thinking and reflecting on your experiences (see Chapters 12 and 14). The focus is on the learners learning.

Interactive teaching and learning methods include:

- one-to-one discussion
- buzz groups
- brainstorming
- role play.

These interactive learning methods involve active participation; the thought of participating in these different methods of learning can be quite daunting, but in reality they can be an excellent way of learning and developing other skills.

One-to-one discussions are frequently used as ice breakers. A group is divided into pairs and each pair is given a task, e.g. find out about each other and then to introduce your partner to the rest of the group. Alternatively pairs are asked a specific question, which they then have to discuss and feed back to the whole group. This also helps you to develop your listening skills.

Buzz groups are often used when there are large groups. The group is divided into sub-groups of four or five students; each sub-group is given a specific topic to discuss, which they feed back to the whole group. This is a useful way of involving the whole group and encouraging quieter members to contribute.

Brainstorming is a way of creating new ideas, solving problems, and motivating and developing teams. The group is given a problem, and a few minutes to think of possible solutions, then invited to contribute these ideas – all ideas are welcomed and recorded. The aim is to generate as many ideas as possible; once these have been recorded, then the group can use the points for discussion.

Role play is a learning technique used for developing skills such as interpersonal communication or for dealing with difficult issues. The facilitator will set the scene and explain the exercise. Students will be invited to participate by acting out specific roles, they will have their role explained, and there may even be a script. Those students observing the role play will be asked to contribute by observing what is going on in the role play and, when invited, commenting on the interactions. Don't be embarrassed – do have a go. It is important that everyone is debriefed on completion of the exercise, and that they reflect and comment on the experience.

These different methods of teaching and learning can be linked back to Chapter 2, where you identified your preferred method of learning. Even if none of these are your preferred learning style do consider that the very act of participating can allow you to learn – experiential approaches can be far more interesting and stimulating than more formal methods of teaching and learning.

Tutorials

Tutorials may occur on a one-to-one basis or with a small group of students meeting with their lecturer. The overall aim of a tutorial is to learn from a small group discussion and to develop your ability to listen, evaluate, criticize and argue. You need to be prepared for your tutorial. If you have been asked to prepare for the tutorial, i.e. to read an article or bring an outline for an assignment, then do so.

Tutorials can end up becoming mini-lectures; you might not learn much if this occurs so don't be afraid to contribute and even challenge your lecturer. As Chapter 5 highlighted, lecturers don't know everything; by contributing you will develop your argument and other critiquing skills.

Seminars

Seminars are usually recurring and focus on a particular topic. A seminar involves giving a short presentation on a chosen topic, drawing on a variety of sources, for approximately 10–15 minutes. Students may be asked to present on their own or in a small group and the presentation is followed by a general group discussion. These are sometimes assessed, either by lecturers or your peers (Elliot and Higgins, 2005).

Preparation is the key; ascertain from the facilitator exactly what they want you to cover. Do only what you were asked to do – you will be surprised how quickly the time goes. The function of your presentation is to stimulate debate among the group. You might find it helpful to have a Microsoft PowerPoint slide or a handout prepared, with the main points written down. Keep your presentation simple and be prepared to explain or illustrate certain points. Following the presentation, it may be your responsibility to engage your fellow students so that a general discussion ensues.

PREPARING A SEMINAR

- What?
  - What are you expected to present?
- How?
  - How long have you got for your seminar?
  - Is it an individual or group presentation?
  - Is it going to be assessed? If so, is it a formative or summative assessment?
- Who?
  - Who are you presenting to?
  - Who will undertake the assessment (teacher, your peers or both)?
- Finally, do you need to submit an outline of the seminar to your lecturer?

If you are presenting as a member of a group seminar, there are further points that need to be considered if it is to go well; you need to ensure that the work is shared equally and that everyone knows what they are supposed to be doing during the presentation. If there are key points to be made in the seminar, write them down on a PowerPoint, whiteboard or flip chart; these can be used to focus the discussion. As presenter, you also need to manage the group and make sure that people do not deviate too much from the topic under discussion. Finally, summarize the main points raised at the end of the seminar.

Seminars allow you to contribute to your learning by finding, collating and presenting information, and receiving feedback. The skills you develop are transferable and can be used when preparing other assignments such as essays.

Presenting

It is important that you, as a midwife or nurse, are confident about presenting – it is a part of your day-to-day activity, both in practice settings and the academy. The following are characteristics of a good presentation:

- the information is clear and relevant to your audience
- progress is logical
- there is visual as well as aural presentation
- the audience is responsive.

Again, preparation is the key, outlined in the box.

PREPARING A PRESENTATION

- Why?
  - Why are you presenting?
- Who?
  - Who is your audience? (e.g. a team meeting, a conference).
  - What is the size of the audience?
- What?
  - What format: poster or a presentation.
  - What are their requirements or, if a poster, what size?
  - What is your aim?
  - What do they already know about the subject?
  - At what level shall you pitch it?
  - What shall you include?
- How?
  - What method should you use? (e.g. poster, formal, informal).
  - What are the key points?
  - Are you there to inform, persuade or amuse?
  - How long have you got?
- Where?
  - Where will you be presenting?
  - Do you have any choice?

- Understand what you are to present (know your subject).
- Structure the presentation.
- Prepare notes to guide you.
- Identify visual aids to support your demonstration.

Structuring your presentation

You need to know your subject through researching it (see Chapter 3 on using the library and Chapters 6 and 8 on writing). Once you have the information, you need to structure your presentation; as with an essay you need an introduction, main theme and conclusion.

You should have a main theme or idea that you follow – having aims and objectives (see Chapter 1 for definitions) can help guide you and your audience. Development should be logical, your message clear and to the point. Finally, conclude by summarizing the main points, telling the audience what you have already told them, and linking it to your aims and objectives.

Delivering your presentation

This might be a face to face or poster presentation. Once again, preparation is the key. The use of motivators can attract individuals, encouraging them to attend or read your poster. This can be in the form of a question or a picture, and it will help the audience to identify the relevance of your topic to their personal experience.

Remember, you are going to be communicating with the audience using the spoken word and visually. If presenting verbally you need to decide whether you are going to present formally, with little or no interaction with the audience, or have an interactive session, where the audience engages with you. With thorough preparation, and brief notes to guide you, you can interact with your audience by maintaining eye contact and using appropriate gestures. Use the clues they provide to guide your presentation – if they look puzzled, perhaps a more detailed explanation is required.

Anyone involved in public speaking will verify that giving a presentation can be a nerve-racking experience. Ensuring that the room is ready, with the correct seating arrangements, lighting and equipment, will help make you feel much better. Finally, be enthusiastic – enthusiasm is contagious, and you will find that your audience will be eager to listen and engage with you.

Poster presentations

The poster is a visual presentation of information – use text, graphs, charts, tables and pictures. Any text should focus on the main points; it shouldn't be a copy of a written assignment or paper. And the reader should be able to read it at a distance, and understand it without any help.

Follow any guidelines given you by your lecturer or conference organiser such as:

- Give yourself plenty of time to plan, prepare, and proofread your work
- Ascertain the size of poster, and stick to this
- Content: title, introduction, methods, results, conclusion, further work and references
- Design: use text, graphs, charts, tables and pictures (appropriately)

For more excellent, detailed advice see Tham (2001).

Equipment

You can use audiovisual aids to support and enhance your presentation, for example:

- television, DVD and video recorders
- whiteboards
- flip charts
- PowerPoint, electronic whiteboards
- iPod.

Know what equipment is available, know how you are going to use it, and make sure that it works. Tables or graphs (see Chapter 4 on information technology) can act as a focus for the group participants. However, it is important not to provide too much information for your audience because this will not give them the opportunity to understand what is being said, reflect and ask appropriate questions. Use an audiovisual aid only if it can enhance your presentation, not just for the sake of it.

Audiovisual aids:

- Do be prepared
- Do have the right equipment (and make sure that it works)
- Do know how to operate the equipment
- Do use keywords
- Do use large, bold writing/print
- Don't use more than a few audiovisual aids
- Don't have too much information
- Don't obscure the view
- Don't panic: if something goes wrong, take a deep breath, find your place and continue with your presentation

Questions

As mentioned above, let your audience know at the beginning of the presentation when you are prepared to answer questions. Try to anticipate the most likely questions based on your presentation, and prepare for them.

When asked a question, be sure you have understood what you are being asked. If it is unclear, ask for the question to be repeated or re-phrased. If you are unable to answer the question, be honest and say so. You can invite other people in the audience to answer, if they have knowledge of the subject. When replying, make sure your answer is clear, relevant and to the point.

Conclusion

This chapter has looked at group work and the different types of group you might encounter when learning. It has looked at how groups are formed, how groups work, the role of different group members, how to organize group meetings, how to participate in a group and what to do if things go wrong. The last part of the chapter looked at presentations and how to prepare and present to colleagues.

Bear in mind the following:

- There is an increasing emphasis on group and team working
- Group work involves active participation
- To be successful, individuals have to adopt different roles in a team. You will probably have preferred roles
- To be successful a group must communicate and act on decisions made
- Be prepared for a group to change and develop over time

Before moving on, take some time and record in your learning diary:

- Your preferred role in a group (based on Belbin's nine key roles) and why you prefer this method of working
- Whether you have experienced conflict of opinion in a group and, if so, how this was resolved

CHAPTER RESOURCES

REFERENCES

Belbin, R.M., 2004. Management teams: why they succeed or fail, 2nd edn. Butterworth-Heinemann, London.

Camacho Carr, K., Fullerton, J.T., Severino, R. & McHugh, K.M., 1996. Barriers to completion of a nurse-midwifery distance education program. The Journal of Distance Education 11(1), 111–131. Online. Available: http://www.jofde.ca/index.php/jde/article/view/240/457 [accessed 26 September 2008].

Cartney, P. & Rouse, A., 2006. The emotional impact of learning in small groups: highlighting the impact on student progression and retention. Teaching in Higher Education 11 (1), 79–91.

Elliot, N. & Higgins, A., 2005. Self and peer assessment – does it make a difference to student group work? Nurse Education in Practice 5 (1), 40–48.

Luft, J., Ingham, H., 1955. The Johari window, a graphic model of interpersonal awareness. Proceedings of the Western Training Laboratory in group development. UCLA, Los Angeles.

Tham, M.T., 2001. Poster presentation of research work. Online. Available: http://lorien.ncl.ac.uk/ming/dept/Tips/present/posters.htm [accessed 13 January 2009].

Tuckman, B.W., 1965. Developmental sequence in small groups. Psychological Bulletin 63, 384–399.

Tuckman, B.W. & Jensen, M.A., 1977. Stages of small group development revisited. Group and Organizational Studies 2, 419–427.

WEBSITES

Belbin: the home of Belbin Team Roles. *This website has lots of different information including: team role theory, testing, games to play and many other things.* Available: http://www.belbin.com/ [accessed 26 September 2008].

Johari window model: *this is a tool for illustrating and improving self-awareness, and mutual understanding between individuals within a group. The Johari window model was developed by American psychologists Luft and Ingham in the 1950s, while researching group dynamics (Luft and Ingham, 1955).* Available: http://www.businessballs.com/johariwindowmodel.htm [accessed 13 January 2008].

Prospects: *this UK website is geared towards graduates and provides advice on careers, postgraduate study, jobs and advice. Available:* http://www.prospects.ac.uk/cms/ShowPage/Home_page/Applications__CVs_and_interviews/Job_applications/Selling_your_skills/p!eXfdpk [accessed 13 January 2009].

FURTHER READING

Forsyth, D.R., 2009. Group dynamics, international edition. Thomson Wadsworth Publishing, Belmont, CA.

Johnson. D.W. & Johnson, F.P., 2008. Joining together. Group theory and group skills. 10th edn. Merrill, Boston, MA. *Provides an overview of group dynamics and experiential learning and examines the key dimensions of group experience and the role of the leader/facilitator.*

Advanced writing skills and accreditation of experiential learning

14

Elizabeth A. Rosser and Rebecca Hoskins

KEY ISSUES

- The meaning of AEL
- The AEL process
- Types of evidence
- Presenting a claim
- Academic levels of learning
- Exemplars of writing reflectively within an academic framework

Introduction

Writing reflectively for academic credit is a well-established assessment strategy within midwifery and nursing programmes. As part of your pre-registration programme and perhaps even more so at the post-qualifying level of activity, student journals, portfolios, critical-incident analysis and assignments arising from action-learning sets are ways of integrating the theory you are learning with your practice. Each of these learning and assessment methods has been explored briefly in Chapter 12. Reflection is the approach that makes the link across each of these strategies, and by encouraging writing, encourages you to develop your analytical skills and to be critical constructively. In a small study of post-qualifying nurses, Jasper (1999) found that from initial negative views about reflective practice these nurses used their writing as a learning tool to help them to turn their thinking into action. Writing their reflections in a structured way enabled them to develop their critical and analytical skills, which, as Jasper suggests, impacts on their practice. These students recognized that writing reflectively was not a 'natural process but has to be learnt and practised (Jasper, 1999, p. 459). Additionally, they all felt that by the end of the course, the process of writing helped them to see their experiences in a new way and gave them 'a growing awareness of alternative ways of looking at the world' (Jasper, 1999, p. 459).

This chapter aims to develop your understanding of how to think and write reflectively within an academic framework. Chapter 12 explored the changing context within which nurses and midwives are working and how the way you learn can help you to cope with change and even make it work to your benefit. This chapter now explores the more formal articulation of that reflection through writing. Reflective writing is not only a tool to help you to achieve success in your study modules and influence your practice but, like the students in Jasper's study it can help you grow personally and help uncover the practice knowledge that you work from on a daily basis.

In 2006, England's chief nurse presented the changing face of nursing and health care and how it will impact on your future career (Department of Health (DoH), 2006a). The principles apply equally to midwives in terms of the need for a system of competency-based working as well as the need to develop flexibility and transferability of skills throughout your career. In relation to education, the national review of the pre-qualifying nursing and midwifery programmes advocated a more flexible approach to these programmes (UKCC, 1999a) to accommodate the changing context of health care. From this review, greater freedom to step-off and step-on the programme was advocated. Subsequently, students have been able to apply to have their previous learning recognized and they have been able to shorten their studies by up to 1 year of the total 3-year programme. More recently, through the current Nursing and Midwifery Council (NMC) consultation on the future of pre-registration nursing education, professionals are being invited to give their views on extending this recognition further (NMC, 2007). Currently, it should be possible for those with prior qualifications – National Vocational Qualifications (NVQs)/Scottish Vocational Qualifications (SVQs) and/or prior experience – to present evidence of a non-standard nature to gain entry into and/or exemption from some of the units of study within a pre-registration programme, as long as it is still relevant and current (see below). This process is called the Accreditation of (Experiential) Learning or A(E)L.

Similarly, those with prior clinical experience and qualifications within the practice area will not need to repeat work in which they are already deemed to be competent. These practitioners will be able to seek exemption from part of their programme should they wish to apply for professional preparation. Practice within the clinical area should therefore be seen much more as a continuum and development for each individual. With the possibility of further shortening the programme for those with prior learning, it is hoped that this approach will attract more recruits with a wider range of skills and abilities into the profession. It is important that you should understand what is required if you wish to make such a claim.

If you are unfamiliar with the AEL system, the box below provides a simple definition.

ACCREDITATION OF EXPERIENTIAL LEARNING (AEL)

Accreditation of experiential learning refers to the process of identification, assessment and formal acknowledgement of prior learning and achievement. 'It is the achievement of learning or the outcomes of that learning and not just the experience of the activities alone that is being accredited' (Quality Assurance Agency, 2004, p. 3).

This learning may take many forms, including professional work experience, short non-assessed courses and general life experiences. However, you need to translate this experience into evidence. This evidence needs to relate to and be comparable with an existing programme of study so that you can be exempt from that part of the programme. Most programmes of study in the UK are now modularized; that is, they are packaged up into distinct units of study. This makes the presentation of evidence a much more manageable activity for you. The modules will have clearly expressed learning outcomes or goals to be achieved and these will also be written at a particular academic level based on a typical 3-year degree programme at university.

Having this evidence accredited is only of value if you wish to follow a particular academic programme, towards a recognized award, at a particular higher-education establishment. In other words, AEL claims are only of value at the particular academic institution from which you are seeking a specific award. It is generally not possible to make a claim at one institution and have it accepted at another institution. Although there may be some locally accepted arrangements, as a rule, you must make the claim at the particular institution from which you are seeking the award. You will also see the term 'accreditation of learning' (AL). This is the gaining of academic credit for the learning that is achieved from a formally taught course that has been assessed and certificated. Some nursing and midwifery departments have produced a tariff list, which shows how much credit specific courses can attract. This is generally used when transferring actual credit from one university to another. The distinction between AL and AEL can be seen in the box below.

Accredited learning section (ALS)

In this section, you will need to identify:

- Which module or unit of the programme you are seeking exemption from on the basis of your existing credit
- Copies of any relevant certificates and any associated credit transcripts
- For non-credit-rated programmes, a copy of the associated syllabus, programme of study, length of study, number and length of assignments and assessment criteria used will need to be presented
- A copy of relevant assignments together with tutor feedback

Experiential learning section

In this section, you will need to identify:

- Which module or unit of the programme you are seeking exemption from on the basis of your experience
- The experiences you have had that have led to the learning evidenced. This must be accompanied by a written commentary to support the appropriate academic level of the unit. The learning outcomes of the matched module or unit you are interested in seeking exemption from must be presented, with the appropriate evidence alongside

In summary, AEL is a system by which you can gain non-standard access to, or exemption from, parts of a programme of study. It should be possible now to gain non-standard entry to a programme of study and exemption from parts of pre-registration programmes through the production of acceptable evidence. This may be achieved either through a system of AL (previously certificated courses) or from your past experience (through AEL). Whatever recognition you are seeking it is important to be clear that it is your prior learning that is valued and it can also contribute to and extend your learning through your on-going studies.

The AEL process

The AEL process can be divided into several distinct stages. Every institution will have its own guide or handbook for using AEL within that particular organization. Do enquire at the institution of your choice before embarking on compiling your evidence. The following is offered as a general guide only and will be considered very briefly.

Stage 1: decide on your programme of study

As someone wishing to enter or transfer into a pre-qualifying programme or a post-qualifying nurse or midwife wishing to access an undergraduate or postgraduate programme, you need to contact the programme leader of the programme you are transferring into, to find out what is required of you, and how your prior learning fits with the new programme. Always obtain as much information as you can, to make sure it is possible to make an AEL claim and what is required of you.

Stage 2: identifying and reviewing experiences

Although you may have considerable life and/or work experience, it is not the time in practice or experience that counts in AEL but evidence of the learning that has been achieved.

To present the evidence of your achievements, you need to select which prior experiences can be matched to specific learning outcomes within your chosen programme of study. To do this you need to focus clearly on experiences that have led to valuable learning. While a claim for academic credit must be current, i.e. within approximately the last 5 years, experience prior to this may be considered if you can show how you have updated older learning and applied it to your practice.

Stage 3: identifying learning achievements

When presenting your evidence against the learning outcomes of the programme, you need to consider the academic level against which you are intending to claim credit. Later on in this chapter we will offer you some guidance on this. Reflecting on your past experience and making sense of it in a critical and analytical way will help to achieve this. Chapter 12 offers you a number of analytical frameworks to help you.

These frameworks provide you with cues to help you move beyond merely telling the story towards finding meaning and learning from that experience, supported by current literature. As in any academic piece of work, organizing your work in a structured and logical manner is crucial to the achievement of a clear pass. The examiner should be able to read your work and know that you have a clear idea of its meaning in relation to the part of the programme against which you are seeking exemption.

Stage 4: matching the learning achievements against the modular learning outcomes

To be considered for accreditation, your AEL claim must contain prior learning that meets the following requirements.

- Comparability: the evidence you produce should match the learning outcomes of a specific module(s) approved by the university for the award sought. As previously suggested, not only should the type of learning match in terms of amount and range of activity, but the level of learning should also be consistent with the academic level of the learning outcomes expressed.
- Currency: as a general rule, the evidence you produce should not be more than 5 years old. Also, your reading and the literature that you present in support of your learning should be current. Do ask how much you are expected to produce; often it is the more succinct and focused work that provides the best of evidence.
- Authenticity: the evidence you produce should demonstrate that you completed the work yourself.

There may be a limit to the amount of AEL you can be exempted from in any one programme. Each institution has its own limit. Your programme leader should be able to advise you.

The evidence will be scrutinized with the same rigour required of those examining standard assignments with the institution. After all, the way candidates' work is handled within the university must be consistent across the different programmes, whether the work is produced for AEL or for standard assignment work.

Types of evidence that you may like to consider

Presentation of your learning achievements may be made in a variety of ways and you must be guided by the requirements of the institution to which you are making your claim, e.g. case studies, project work, critical-incident analysis, etc. Alternatively if you have recently completed a programme of study that has not been academically accredited, it may be appropriate to complete the actual module assignment. You may even provide a written commentary to accompany other types of learning (e.g. NVQs) to demonstrate equivalence of learning outcomes and the appropriate academic quality.

Academic portfolio

Where you need to present evidence of learning from a variety of experiences, you can do this through the development of an academic portfolio (see Chapter 15). An academic portfolio may have two distinct parts:

1. An accredited-learning section, which provides evidence of formal learning that has already been accredited and certificated by a recognized higher-education institution or assessed by recognized agencies and for which you are now seeking university credit
2. An experiential-learning section, which provides evidence of your learning from experience.

It is likely you will have some evidence in both sections.

Stage 5: summarizing the AEL claim

To help you in the submission of your AEL claim, each institution that offers this facility should have a key person, usually called an AEL coordinator, to give you advice as to how your evidence should be presented. Most institutions have a handbook or document that shows clearly how the evidence should be presented. Additionally, some institutions offer workshops or individual support for the submission of your claim and there is usually a fee required for your submission to be considered.

Once you have developed your academic portfolio and presented your evidence against a particular module or unit of study, you need to summarize your claim and submit this summary along with the main body of your claim. This acts as an aid to assessment of your AEL claim and demonstrates clearly how your learning experiences have led to a coherent learning achievement. The actual layout will vary according to the different institutions. You must be guided by your AEL adviser.

Levels of learning

Different levels of learning are expected of you at each stage of your academic development; for example, what you were expected to do at A-level is different to what is expected in the first year of your degree and different again if you move into a masters programme. It is important you understand what is expected of you at each of these stages. Various frameworks have been used to guide this learning but essentially there is a hierarchy of educational development that achievement can be measured against. Some of these frameworks are as follows.

Steinaker and Bell's (1979) experiential taxonomy of achievement in practice:

- Exposure: consciousness of an experience – having the skill demonstrated.
- Participation: deciding to become part of an experience – practice in the activity.

- Identification: union of the learner with what is to be learned – competency in achievement of the skill.
- Internalization: experience continues to influence lifestyle – mastery of the activity.
- Dissemination: attempt to influence others, e.g. through teaching.

This hierarchy can guide you to articulating different levels of practical achievement, which progress through both the doing of the practice as well as the thinking behind what you are doing. Sometimes in an academic paper it is difficult to find ways to articulate higher levels of practice when, for example, you are concerned with doing the practice safely. Translating this into academic writing may initially cause you some difficulty.

Alternatively, Bloom (1956) formulated a hierarchy of levels in each of the three areas of learning as follows:

- knowledge domain (cognitive)
- skills domain (psychomotor)
- attitudes domain (affective).

Most recently, the Southern England Consortium for Credit Accumulation and Transfer (SEEC, 2003) has adapted previous frameworks to include the practical skills and generic transferable skills as well as the cognitive skills. SEEC's (2003) credit level descriptors can be accessed at http://www.seec-office.org.uk/c+reditleveldescriptors2003.pdf. The document clearly sets out what they believe to be the expectations required from the first level of a further education programme through to undergraduate, postgraduate and doctoral study in higher education. The document is well worth considering whatever academic study you are undertaking. The credit level descriptors are of particular value when beginning your AEL claim.

Each university will have its own expectations of the different levels articulated so that you can be guided when presenting your written commentary, linked to the matched module or unit outcomes. Whatever the academic level, you must present your evidence supported by relevant and current literature. All university institutions will require you to follow a specific system of referencing; although many now advocate the Harvard system of referencing (see Chapter 9 for further information on this system).

Summary of the AEL process

In summary, therefore, AEL is a way of gaining non-standard entry to a particular programme of your choice, or exemption from some part of that programme towards the achievement of an award. Each higher education institution has its own process governed by its own rules and regulations. You must seek guidance from the AEL coordinator before embarking on this process of compiling a claim so that you are absolutely clear as to what is expected of you. We have attempted to present a general framework of the process expected from you in most institutions, the different types of evidence that you can use and the different levels of learning that can help you articulate your learning at the appropriate academic level. We believe it would be helpful at this point to present some examples of how to write reflectively for academia, especially if you have been used to producing third-person academic writing.

Writing reflectively for academia

When writing reflectively for academia, similar rules apply to both first-person reflective writing and third-person academic writing in relation to the rigour required. However, rather than write in the third person, the reflective approach encourages you to maintain a first-person reflective style of writing while at the same time supporting your thoughts and feelings with reference to the literature and research.

It is useful to think of writing in the first person as a great privilege. You need to think carefully when using this approach, so as not to use it as a chatty, letter-writing activity where it is easy to merely 'tell your story'. As you saw in Chapter 12, telling your story is only one small part of the reflective process. Jasper (2006, p. 81) presents a very useful chapter exploring in some depth the nature of reflective writing for professional development. In particular, she explores how a group of 37 nurses used reflective writing within their professional portfolios. In addition to helping them demonstrate their accountability, reflective writing helped them in four key areas, one of which was the development of their skills in critical thinking. Writing reflectively for academia helps you to make links with your reading and recognize how knowledge development and theory have influenced your practice. Conversely, reflective writing for academia helps you to see how your practice may influence theory. Early on, Argyris and Schon (1974) examined the difference between espoused theory (what we say we do) and theory-in-use (what we actually do). Through reflective writing we can begin to identify and acknowledge that in many situations there is no satisfactory off-the-shelf theory that will support or explain what we do (Schon, 1991, p. 274). By writing reflectively and analysing our theories-in-use, sharing our analysis and explanations with others, we can begin to identify new research questions and explore and even test out our theories-in-use through research. Through our research, we can build and shape new theory so that there is a constant flow of theory and practice influencing each other. Theory development will then remain alive and relevant to practice and not sterile and divorced from it. It is likely that nurses will become much more involved in research and subsequently theory making with the advent of clinical academic careers (United Kingdom Clinical Research Collaboration (UKCRC), 2007). As part of the NHS modernization agenda and the UK Department of Health's new 5-year research strategy to ensure a world-class environment for NHS research (DoH, 2006b, p. 5), a proposal for structured support for nurses to engage in a research career has been developed (UKCRC, 2007). Reflective writing can be the catalyst for nurses to engage in such a career.

In a practical way, we often ask students to look at themselves from above or outside themselves when engaging in their reflective analysis. It is almost like trying to justify and rationalize what they did and why they did it, supporting their justification with evidence from the literature. As you have probably only had experience of writing in the first person when engaging in friendly chat, e.g. letter writing, it is easy to get caught in the trap of purely descriptive passages along the lines of 'You'll never guess what happened to me the other day…'. However, as has already been explained, reflective writing for academia is about challenging your practice, analysing the situations and, by drawing on your reading, helping you towards improvement for the future. Considering it a privilege to write in the first person may allow you to use it with caution in as much as having to justify your actions.

Examples of reflective writing are becoming more evident in the literature (e.g. Burns and Bulman, 2000; Taylor, 2006; White et al., 2006) and it is important that, before writing your reflective academic assignment, you read a range of examples to give you an idea of best practice. Some of our own students and those of our colleagues have written reflective assignments to demonstrate, on reflection, how they went about planning and justifying aspects of their care. As a result of their own developments, we would like to share excerpts from their reflective writing. Mostly, these excerpts represent their first attempt at such writing and there are some insightful examples of their critical reflection.

We hope these examples will give you some idea of how to develop your reflective writing into an academic piece of work. The result offers you a truly analytical approach to your own learning. As you can see, it must be supported by current literature and, where possible, current research.

One student, Katie, undertaking a post-qualifying specialist course in intensive care explores the arguments around reflective practice for her own assignment:

 CASE STUDY: KATIE

In recent years, reflection has become popular and firmly established in nursing education; however, it is a concept that is continually debated in the literature (Girot, 2005; Hargreaves, 2003; Perry, 2000). It is important for nurses to learn from their everyday work and the development of reflective techniques encourages critical thinking in the workplace, assesses understanding and therefore facilitates the integration of theory and practice (Cotton, 2001; Girot, 2005; Gustaffson and Fagerberg, 2004). However, although many authors view reflection as an invaluable education tool

(Girot, 2005; Gustaffson and Fagerberg, 2004; Heath, 1998), other authors have argued that it may be a barrier to learning, having the potential for psychological disturbances. Rich and Parker (1995) and Cotton (2001) have considered that reflection may be painful or difficult for those who have been in vulnerable positions or experienced strong negative emotions about an experience, particularly if there are issues of confidentiality or privacy.

Here Katie is justifying to herself the importance of reflection, identifying some of the positive aspects as well as barriers to reflection. She recognizes that it is more than just telling a story and that there is a need for some structure to support the activity:

CASE STUDY: KATIE

It seems that although reflection appears to be a valid education tool, it has been suggested that nurses need guidance, support and structure to make it a positive learning experience (Cotton, 2001; Perry, 2000).

Katie moves on to critically reflect on her need to learn how to apply cricoid pressure correctly, an essential skill for nurses working in the intensive care unit (ITU).

Katie undertook a detailed review of the literature to help her improve her understanding of the skill as well as the need for education to support such activity for a range of practitioners. She concludes her reflection by being reassured that her technique was safe. However, through her reflection, she has learned to be self-aware in her clinical area and to be able to challenge and evaluate her practice. She has learned the correct application and identifies an action plan to help her own and others' development in the future.

CASE STUDY: KATIE

This may be a skill that is overlooked by other nurses, especially more junior ones. Nurses need to learn the importance of and the theory behind cricoid pressure (Matthews, 2001) and spend some time in anaesthetic rooms to gain correct training and extra practice in a controlled environment, where multiple intubations occur each day. From the literature, it seems this environment is the best equipped to train staff on cricoid pressure. This could be incorporated into the band 5 competency programme to ensure knowledge and skills of at least all junior nurses entering in the ITU.

Finally, Katie recognized the 'beliefs, frustrations, complexities and contraindications' of self-reflection (Perry, 2000, p. 139) but found the process productive, helping her learn from her experience, bridge the theory/practice divide and improve her future practice.

In addition to this example from Katie, we have a number of examples from pre-qualifying midwifery students undertaking their management module at the end of their programme. They have all chosen to use a structured model to help them. One example is that of Rebecca, who was caring for a client whose baby was presenting in the breech position. She confirms that 'the client did not want a caesarean section and wished to have a homebirth or a team delivery, with minimal intervention'. She recognized her need for good communication and advocacy skills to support her client effectively and analysed the situation, acknowledging some barriers to success, particularly during consultant appointments.

 CASE STUDY: REBECCA

For the client to feel supported and empowered, I needed good communication skills. Murray et al. (2006) makes the statement that communication skills are vital in midwifery to ensure that the client's needs are met. The verbal communication in this scenario was good, which meant that the client felt at ease. However, there were some potential barriers that could have interrupted the good verbal communication … Chant et al. (2001) found evidence that hierarchical structures could interfere with communication due to 'power gaps'. This idea is also supported by Duff (2004). Duff's idea involves the concept that if unequal relationships are present, then the client's care will be affected, as appropriate communication skills will not be practised. However, in contrast to this Randle (2004) discusses that the benefit of the midwife attending alongside the client will remove these structures and more equal relationships will be present, as seen in this scenario.

Rebecca further analyses the situation when the client went into labour, having written a birth plan confirming that she wanted midwifery-led care in hospital when in labour, without intervention.

 CASE STUDY: REBECCA

I was called as agreed when the client went into labour and my mentor and I met the client in the hospital. The registrar was informed as agreed. However, the registrar on call wanted the client to have a Venflon sited and continuous electronic fetal monitoring. This registrar was not aware of the client's previous consultations … It was my role to act as the client's advocate and put her birth plan in place, though at times this can be difficult, as I wasn't prepared for the birth plan to be challenged. I achieved this by calmly explaining to the doctor what was discussed in the antenatal period and informed the doctor of the birth plan. The Changing Childbirth report (DoH, 1993) defines an advocate as a person who acts on behalf of the client and confronts practices to meet the client's needs … In this scenario, other skills were required to be the client's advocate, these included negotiation skills and assertiveness skills … As the literature suggests at times, as I found in this scenario, it is difficult to be assertive towards a doctor and act as the client's advocate. To overcome this problem, Timmins and McCabe (2005) suggest that midwives should be offered training, as there are implications for the client if the midwife cannot be assertive.

Having evaluated the situation with reference to the literature, Rebecca identifies her own limitations and concludes by looking to the future.

CASE STUDY: REBECCA

From reflecting upon this scenario I feel that I have learned that if I am aware of my communication skills I can act as a client's advocate. However, it is also important to empower the client to self-advocate as during the antenatal consultation I often spoke on the client's behalf. If I came across a similar situation again I would use skills highlighted by Naumann and Vessey (2002) to help my client self-advocate. These skills included preparing the client as to what to expect at the consultations and provide her with any up-to-date literature surrounding the issue of breech birth, and assist the client to be assertive. This would also aid a trusting, respectful and honest relationship between the client and myself, which again is important for self-advocacy to be present (Atkinson, 1999). In relation to advocacy during childbirth, I feel that it is important to be fully prepared. In order to do this like self-advocacy I would need to be well read around breech birth and have discussed all scenarios with the client before they go into labour. It would also be appropriate to attend assertiveness training as recommended by Timmins and McCabe (2005). Then if the birth plan was challenged again I would feel more confident to advocate the birth plan to the doctor, as self-advocacy during labour may be difficult.

By using Gibbs' (1988) structured model, Rebecca has been able to recognize and critically analyse the key elements of this issue and identify what she might do if faced with a similar situation in the future. As a consequence of this process she seems more confident in her ability to manage the identified issues successfully.

Another student midwife, Sian, reflects on her own self-management by analysing her decision making, communication and autonomy in practice.

CASE STUDY: SIAN

The experience occurred on the third day postnatal visit to a breastfeeding mother whose baby was jaundiced and had lost over 10% of its birth weight. These factors, coupled with the mother having problems with feeding the baby, meant I deliberated whether to re-admit the baby to hospital.

Through her reflections, Sian articulated her thoughts and feelings as advocated by Gibbs (1988).

CASE STUDY: SIAN

I knew I had to make the decision alone; however, I was also going to be held accountable for my action, this made me feel under considerable pressure and the decision harder to make.

Following Gibbs (1988), Sian evaluated the situation, trying to make sense of her own role within it.

CASE STUDY: SIAN

The woman became upset and her partner became angry at the possibility of going back to the hospital. Decisions often call for specialist knowledge on the likely consequences or risks (Gigerenzer and Edwards, 2003); however, it is important to keep in mind that it is disrespectful and not helpful to ignore and disregard the parents (Jakobsen and Severinsson, 2006). I was aware not to dictate to the couple but to involve them in the decision I made through informing them of the possibilities of what would happen if the baby was or was not re-admitted to the hospital.

To come to an effective decision I had to negotiate, and good communication is vital to do this. Good listening can increase your negotiation power by increasing the information you have about the other side or about possible options. Once you understand the other side's feelings and concerns, you can begin to address them, to explore areas of agreement and disagreement and to develop useful ways to proceed in the future (Hall, 1993). Through listening, I understood that despite the reluctance and aggression they were showing to being re-admitted, they were extremely worried about the baby's disinterest in breastfeeding, the weight loss and by how lethargic the baby was. I then could use this information to persuade the couple of the benefits of going into hospital – the support and advice from staff and the treatment of jaundice.

Sian concluded her reflections by acknowledging the consensus that was agreed on the nature of the problem and the options available to help improve the baby's health. She then looked to develop an action plan to help her in the future.

CASE STUDY: SIAN

In future similar situations I will learn to be more aware of my body language and behaviour and how it can affect a situation. Initially, I may have been too eager to assert my decision to re-admit the baby without considering how the parents felt. Poor communication, according to Macdonald (2004), can lead to patient dissatisfaction, alienation, frustration, resentment and anger. Macdonald (2004) found research showed how the meaning in adult conversation is divided – 5% is words (i.e. what is actually said), 35% is in tone of voice and 60% is in body language and non-verbal communication. ... To control the situation I needed to ensure my body language was receptive and show I was listening to the couple.

Facial expressions can convey a range of emotions such as disapproval and encouragement. I also learnt to be aware of the tone of my voice and speech errors such as stuttering and repetitions which can show anxiety and that I had not put a lot of thought into what is being said … If this situation happened again I would remain calm and listen to the parents. I also have learnt that time management is important, although supporting and being 'with woman' should be the main aim of the care provided.

By following a structured model of reflection, Sian was able to describe the situation, explore her feelings, evaluate the situation, analyse what it meant for her, identify what else she could have done and make an action plan for the future.

One final student, Jane, used Gibbs' model to help her reflect on her own time management within the context of dealing with perinatal death. She began by presenting the context of the situation and the feelings she had at the time.

CASE STUDY: JANE

I was offered the opportunity to provide immediate postnatal care for Emma, a woman who had given birth at term to Freya, a stillborn baby 1 hour prior to the start of my shift. No attempt had been made to start the paperwork necessary following the stillbirth … I was faced with the responsibility of completing the multitude of forms and certificates, 'laying out' the baby, counselling the parents and liaising with the obstetric staff with regards to consent for post-mortem. Although I had a supportive mentor, the task ahead of me was daunting and frightening. I had never seen a dead baby or counselled a grieving family, and the mountain of paper was hugely intimidating. I realized that in order to deal with the situation, I needed to identify and prioritize the tasks in front of me and devise a plan of how I would effectively use my time over the coming hours.

Jane evaluated the situation, the conflicting demands made on her time and how she presented herself and managed to deal with the needs of the couple. In analysing her own response, Jane articulates how she managed her time.

CASE STUDY: JANE

There were times when I felt as though I wasn't coping with the amount of work I had to undertake and for a while I found myself procrastinating over my predicament rather than devising ways in which my workload could be lessened, something that is not uncommon when faced with a large quantity of equally demanding tasks (Banks, 2005). This quandary was compounded by requests made by other midwives to cover breaks. On a couple of occasions I agreed to do this, although now I realize that I was simply trying to fill my time with other tasks not related to my own (Cross, 1996; Forsyth, 2003). It soon became apparent that this would not be beneficial to Emma and Paul, and although I felt guilty at the time for refusing to help others, focusing on my own tasks took priority

(Banks, 2005; Bird, 2003). By concentrating on my own duties and asking for help with administrative tasks (Martin, 2000), I was able to spend quality time with Emma and Paul, guiding them through difficult decisions and providing opportunities for the articulation through active listening and a near constant presence (Mottram, 2004).

In conclusion, Jane recognized how she could have better managed her time and what she might do in the future if faced with a similar situation.

 ## CASE STUDY: JANE

It was a shift in which time was my most valuable resource and as such, the way in which I managed it had a significant impact on both the stress I faced and the quality of care I was able to provide (Banks, 2005; Forsyth, 2003). There were times when I felt myself falling into the trap of dithering rather than doing, and due to the difficult nature of the tasks that I was undertaking, I took longer than I should have to recognize this. I also felt guilt at declining requests to help elsewhere on the unit when I was having quiet moments. In reflecting on this experience I have been able to identify the areas in which I could have improved my time management. In particular, I am much more aware of the need to define and then place one's own priorities above others and in doing so I feel confident to be able to say no to requests for help when appropriate without feeling remorse or believing I am letting the team down. The value of devising a checklist has been cemented in my mind, although the need for flexibility in practice must be remembered, with a willingness to redefine priorities when problems arise.

As you can see, all four students used Gibbs' (1988) reflective model to make sense of their different situations. Gibbs' model is a popular one for all our students as it helps them to identify their feelings and make sense of their situation before engaging in the literature, and to identify what else they might have done in the situation before drawing up an action plan.

However, the above examples do not necessarily give you a feel for the whole picture in terms of structure. Overall, the structure of your assignment, or evidence presented for an AEL claim, will be the same as you are required to present for any third-person academic assignment; that is, it must have an introduction, main body and conclusion. In addition, the main body needs to be well structured and follow logically sequenced thoughts and arguments – all that you have learned in earlier chapters, particularly Chapter 6. However, here, you are encouraged to express your feelings, just as the major writers on reflection have identified. From the above examples, the recognition of the feelings you have experienced is a major element of the learning process. It is almost like revisiting the experience for yourself, but somehow standing outside yourself and discussing the decision-making process that you were involved in when making your decisions.

As you can see from the above examples, these students have taken time to really think about their own responsibilities to their patients in terms of acting as patient advocate, ensuring the safety of the baby while respecting the wishes of the parents and managing their time to allow for flexibility whilst constantly redefining priorities. They really thought about their own role and responsibilities, their own feelings and reactions to the different situations, their own body language and how this was being interpreted. They analysed the different situations and read around the literature and came to conclusions having reasoned through the decision-making process, discounting a number of options open to them. As in third-person academic work, it is equally important here to develop and present your analysis of the process and not merely describe the situation. It is not an easy skill to achieve. While description is a part of the process, it is only one part, and it is the development of analytical thought that will represent the hierarchy of academic levels. Like any academic assignment, it is important to identify what is expected from the different levels of academia in your particular institution, as they do vary slightly throughout the country.

In addition to the hierarchy of the cognitive domain, as identified by Bloom (1956), Mezirow (1981) offered a hierarchy of seven levels of reflectivity, ranging from a purely descriptive approach, through gaining insightful learning, to a sophisticated analytical process.

1. Reflective: becoming aware of a specific perception, meaning or behaviour of your own or the habits you have of seeing, thinking and acting.
2. Affective: becoming aware of how you feel about the way you are perceiving, thinking or acting.
3. Discriminant: assessing the efficacy of your expectations, thoughts and actions. Recognizing the reality of the contexts in which you work and identifying your relationship to the situation.
4. Judgemental: making and becoming aware of your value judgements about your perception, thought and actions, in terms of being positive or negative.
5. Conceptual: being conscious of your awareness and being critical of it (e.g. being critical of the concepts you use to evaluate a situation).
6. Psychic: recognizing in yourself the habit of making precipitant judgements about people based on limited information.
7. Theoretical: becoming aware of the influence of underlying assumptions upon your judgement.

Mezirow's levels of reflectivity have been adapted and used in a number of studies (e.g. Powell, 1989; Richardson and Maltby, 1995). Both Powell and Richardson & Maltby found that the majority of students demonstrated extensive but superficial levels of reflection with little critical and analytical thought. This was further supported by Duke and Appleton (2000) and by the UKCC's study (1999b) into the reflective activity of professional practitioners applying for re-registration. Certainly, if you wish to use your reflective practice for academic assignment work or as a contribution towards an AEL claim, these activities demand that the higher levels of reflection are used. In addition, support from the literature and research is required to justify what you have done in practice.

As previously acknowledged, critical reflection is not without its difficulties (Burns and Bulman, 2000; Duke and Appleton, 2000). However, it is clear from the examples presented in this chapter that students have gained from their experiences both in terms of academic credit, but more importantly, they have begun to articulate their deep levels of learning from practice. As shown in Chapter 12, developing a learning culture within the workplace helps the team to support each other. Gaining recognition of this learning through an AEL process also encourages you as an individual to pursue your own goals.

Conclusion

This chapter has introduced to you the notion of thinking and writing reflectively within an academic framework. It has given you an overview of the AEL process and the different levels of academic expectations. Some examples have been offered as an illustration of how to put your writing into this academic framework. Now you need to put this together with ideas from earlier chapters on the various aspects of assignment writing. Most importantly, you should recognize that, whether using a third-person academic style of writing or a first-person reflective style, the rigour required by academia is the same.

Acknowledgements

We would like to thank our four students, Katie, Rebecca, Sian and Jane, now qualified practitioners, for their enthusiasm in agreeing to contribute to our chapter.

 CHAPTER RESOURCES

REFERENCES

Argyris, C. & Schon, D.A., 1974. Theory in practice: increasing personal effectiveness. Jossey-Bass, San Francisco.

Atkinson, D., 1999. Advocacy: a review. Joseph Rowntree Foundation, Brighton, UK.

Banks, C., 2005. Using your time more effectively. Nursing Times 101 (11), 46–47.

Bird, P., 2003. Time management. Hodder Arnold, London.

Bloom, B., 1956. Taxonomy of educational objectives. Handbook 1. Cognitive domain. McKay, New York.

Burns, S. & Bulman, C. (Eds.), 2000. Reflective practice in nursing: the growth of the professional practitioner, 2nd edn. Blackwell Science, Oxford.

Chant, S., Jenkinson, T., Randle, J. & Russell, G., 2001. Communication skills: some problems in nurse education and practice. Journal of Clinical Nursing 11, 12–21.

Cotton, A.H., 2001. Private thoughts in public spheres; issues in reflection and reflective practices in nursing. Journal of Advanced Nursing 36 (4), 512–519.

Cross, R., 1996. Midwives and management: a handbook. Books for Midwives Press, Hale, UK.

Department of Health (DoH), 1993. Changing childbirth. Report of the expert maternity group (The Cumberlege report). HMSO, London.

Department of Health (DoH), 2006a. Modernising nursing careers – setting the direction. DoH, London.

Department of Health (DoH), 2006b. Best research for best health: a new national health research strategy. DoH, London.

Duff, E., 2004. No more 'quarrelling at the mother's bedside': interprofessional approaches can help stop women dying. Midwifery Digest MIDIRS 14 (1), 35–36.

Duke, S. & Appleton, J., 2000. The use of reflection in a palliative care programme: a quantitative study of the development of reflective skills over an academic year. Journal of Advanced Nursing 32 (6), 1557–1568.

Forsyth, P., 2003. Successful time management. Kogan Page, London.

Gibbs, G., 1988. Learning by doing. A guide to reading and learning methods. Further Education Unit, London.

Gigerenzer, G. & Edwards, A., 2003. Simple tools for understanding risks from innumeracy to insight. British Medical Journal 327, 741–744.

Girot, E.A., 2005. Reflective skills. In: Maslin-Prothero, S. (Ed.), Baillière's study skills for nurses and midwives, 3rd edn. Baillière Tindall, Edinburgh.

Gustaffson, C. & Fagerberg, I., 2004. Reflection: the way to professional development? Journal of Clinical Nursing 13 (3), 271–280.

Hall, L., 1993. Negotiation: strategies for mutual gain. Sage Publications, London.

Hargreaves, J., 2003. So how do you feel about that? Assessing reflective practice. Nurse Education Today 24 (3), 196–201.

Heath, H., 1998. Reflections and patterns of knowing in nursing. Journal of Advanced Nursing 27, 1054–1059.

Jakobsen, E.S. & Severinsson, E., 2006. Parents' experience of collaboration with community healthcare professionals. Journal of Psychiatric and Mental Health Nursing 13 (5), 498–505.

Jasper, M., 1999. Nurses' perceptions of the value of written reflection. Nurse Education Today 19, 452–463.

Jasper, M., 2006. Professional development, reflection and decision-making. Blackwell Publishing, Oxford.

Macdonald, E., 2004. Difficult conversations in medicine. Oxford University Press, London.

Martin, V., 2000. Managing your time. Nursing Times 96 (18), 42.

Matthews, G.A., 2001. Survey of cricoid pressure application by anaesthetists, operating department practitioners, intensive care and accident and emergency nurses. Anaesthesia 56(9), 915–917.

Mezirow, J., 1981. A critical theory for adult learning and education. Adult Education 32, 3–24.

Mottram, L., 2004. A great sadness but also a great privilege. MIDIRS Midwifery Digest 14 (3), 311–312.

Murray, K., Hamilton, S. & Martin, D., 2006. Delivering effective communication. The Practising Midwife 9 (4), 24–26.

Naumann, P. & Vessey, J., 2002. Teaching patients self-advocacy. American Journal of Nursing 102 (7), 24A–24C.

Nursing and Midwifery Council (NMC), 2007. Consultation: the future of pre-registration nursing education. NMC, London.

Perry, M.A., 2000. Reflections on intuition and expertise. Journal of Clinical Nursing 9, 137–145.

Powell, J.H., 1989. The reflective practitioner in nursing. Journal of Advanced Nursing 14, 824–832.

Quality Assurance Agency (QAA), 2004. Guidelines on the accreditation of prior learning. QAA, Mansfield. Online. Available: http://www.qaa.ac.uk/academicinfrastructure/apl/APL.pdf [accessed 27 April 2008].

Randle, S., 2004. Being an advocate for your clients in the antenatal period. Midwifery Matters 103 (winter), 4–6.

Rich, A. & Parker, D., 1995. Reflection and critical incident analysis; ethical and moral implications of their use within nursing and midwifery education. Journal of Advanced Nursing 22 (6), 1050–1057.

Richardson, G. & Maltby, H., 1995. Reflection-on-practice: enhancing student learning. Journal of Advanced Nursing 22, 235–242.

Schon, D.A., 1991. The reflective practitioner: how professionals think in action. Ashgate, Avebury, UK.

Southern England Consortium for Credit Accumulation and Transfer (SEEC). 2003. Credit level descriptors for further and higher education. SEEC, London. Online. Available: http://www.seec-office.org.uk/c+reditleveldescriptors2003.pdf

Steinaker, N. & Bell, M., 1979. The experiential taxonomy: a new approach to teaching and learning. Academic Press, New York.

Taylor, B., 2006. Reflective practice: a guide for nurses and midwives, 2nd edn. Open University Press, Maidenhead, UK.

Timmins, F. & McCabe, C., 2005. Nurses' and midwives' assertive behaviour in the workplace. Journal of Advanced Nursing 51 (1), 38–45.

United Kingdom Central Council for Nursing, Midwifery and Health Visiting (UKCC), 1999a. Fitness for practice. The UKCC Commission for Nursing and Midwifery Education (Chair: Sir Leonard Peach). UKCC, London.

United Kingdom Central Council for Nursing, Midwifery and Health Visiting (UKCC), 1999b. UKCC PREP monitor project: summary report. UKCC, London.

United Kingdom Clinical Research Collaboration (UKCRC), 2007. Developing the best research professionals: Qualified graduate nurses: recommendations for preparing and supporting clinical academic nurses of the future. UKCRC, London.

White, S., Fook, J. & Gardner, F., 2006. Critical reflection in health and social care. Open University Press, Maidenhead, UK.

WEBSITES

Higher Education Academy: this resource section has some useful information about writing reflectively: http://www.ukcle.ac.uk/resources/

Liverpool Hope University: resources include information on writing reflectively: http://www.hope.ac.uk/writing-centre/resources.html

Northampton University website: gives some further information and exercises in writing reflectively: http://pdp.northampton.ac.uk/PG_Files/pg_reflect2a.htm

Royal College of Midwives: professional resources: http://www.rcm.org.uk/home/

Royal College of Nursing: professional resources: http://www.rcn.org.uk/development/learning/learningzone

FURTHER READING

Boud, D., Keogh, R. & Walker, D. (Eds.), 1985. Reflection: turning experience into learning. Kogan Page, London. *Helpful in explaining the term 'reflection' and includes material on developing reflective learning and writing skills.*

Boulton, G., 2001. Reflective practice. Paul Chapman/Sage Publications, London.

Bulman, C. & Schutz, S. (Eds.), 2004. Reflective practice in nursing, 3rd edn. Blackwell Publishing, Oxford. *General introduction to the reflective process including writing diaries and group reflection.*

Burns, S. & Bulman, C. (Eds.), 2000. Reflective practice in nursing: the growth of the professional practitioner, 2nd edn. Blackwell Science, Oxford.

Fish, D., Twinn, S. & Purr, B., 1989. How to enable learning through professional practice. West London Press, London. *Useful for developing reflective skills for life-long learning and relevant for health care professionals.*

Jasper, M., 2006. Professional development, reflection and decision making. Blackwell Publishing, Oxford.

Johns, C., 2006. Engaging reflection in practice. A narrative approach. Blackwell Publishing, Oxford. *This book discusses the nature and application of reflective practice using many examples from professional practice.*

Rolfe, G., Freshwater, D. & Jasper, M., 2001. Critical reflection for nursing and the helping professions – a user's guide. Palgrave MacMillan, Basingstoke. *This is an in-depth look at reflection on practice which includes a useful chapter on reflective writing. It also discusses some models and theories of reflection.*

Developing a portfolio 15
Neil Gopee

KEY ISSUES

- What are portfolios and profiles? Types of portfolios
- Reasons for keeping a professional portfolio: aims and benefits
- Ways in which to develop and maintain an effective portfolio
- Assessment of portfolios and profiles

Introduction

A portfolio is more than a record of events, experiences and developments in our careers. It is a vital, 'living' document that has a secure and respected place in continuing professional development (CPD), and within mechanisms for professional regulation. It also encourages us to make sense of what we are doing and to learn through reflection. Developing a portfolio will enable you to (Palmer, 2000):

- celebrate your achievements
- target your professional development
- develop your skills of learning from professional and personal experiences
- make decisions for the future based on your knowledge of the past.

However, whilst portfolios comprise an integral aspect of contemporary learning, CPD and professional regulation (Nursing and Midwifery Council (NMC), 2008a), it does not necessarily mean that everyone feels positive about keeping one. It is important to identify and acknowledge your thoughts and feelings about this process, as you might have taken a minimalist approach to this; or you may have thrown your heart and soul into keeping a portfolio because you have always had a tendency to write about your everyday experiences as a way of understanding yourself and the world around you; or like most readers, you may be somewhere in between. As Hull et al. (2005) note, many healthcare professionals are unsure of the practical issues related to compiling a portfolio. They also tend to attach only a tenuous link between the documentation in portfolios, and portfolio learning.

This chapter offers a practical guide to portfolios through an analysis of what they are, why we need them, what the benefits of keeping them are – in particular in relation to portfolio learning, which is also associated with keeping up to date. It acknowledges the likely reservations related to portfolios, explores ways of developing and maintaining your portfolio, and how they are assessed. To assist you with your learning, as you read through this chapter, connections are made with other relevant chapters in the book.

What are portfolios and profiles?

This section defines the term portfolio, distinguishes it from profiles, and discusses two principal ways of keeping and presenting portfolios and profiles, namely as hard copies and as electronic copies (e-portfolio).

Definitions and distinctions

For healthcare professionals busy in the world of practice and for student nurses and midwives the issue of portfolios and profiles may initially appear confusing, raising such questions as 'Why do I need one?', 'What do I put in them?' and 'How often should I input items into them?'. Sensible enough questions, given the terminology and 'jargon' that tends to proliferate when new concepts about learning are introduced to the professional workplace. It is always useful to begin with the basics and to gain an understanding and appreciation of what such concepts are concerned with, and what the expectations are for both you and the profession.

A portfolio is a collection and recording of the individual's learning experiences and activities that demonstrate their personal and professional development, and achievements. Keeping a portfolio therefore allows you to document your learning and achievements, which can be done on paper or electronically. Such a record also makes it easier to explain your achievements whenever appropriate, as it is a flexible and yet comprehensive account of your professional development and how further development will be accomplished.

A profile is an extract or an adaptation of one's portfolio that contains elements that have been deliberately selected for a specific event (such as for a job interview), for supplying evidence of professional development to the professional regulatory body or for making the case for gaining credit points as part of a university course; this will take the form of Accreditation of Prior Learning (APL), or Accreditation of Prior Experiential Learning (APEL) (see Chapter 14). Your curriculum vitae (CV) that is adapted for a specific purpose is therefore also a profile.

Types of portfolio

Various forms of portfolio are available for the healthcare professional to obtain and use as they are, or to adapt to include their personal preferences. They can be kept as hard paper copy compilations and/or as electronic copy, usually referred to as e-portfolio.

Paper (hard copy) portfolios

Examples of hard paper copies of portfolios that can be purchased include *The Churchill Livingstone professional portfolio* (Kenworthy and Redfern, 2004), *A professional portfolio for dietitians* (British Dietetic Association, 2001) and various others available on the worldwide web (e.g. Health Professions Council (HPC), 2008). Some healthcare trusts also provide their employees with a portfolio to facilitate recording of continuing and mandatory professional updating. However, increasingly most healthcare professionals now tend to keep an electronic version of their portfolio that is updated whenever significant learning occurs, and it can be printed when required, and kept in a folder containing corresponding original documents such as certificates, testimonials and awards, which also constitute 'evidence' of learning.

For pre-registration nursing and midwifery students, their universities tend to provide them with a portfolio that they have to maintain as part of their pre-qualifying educational preparation programmes. The structure of these portfolios tends to be informed by research findings and guidelines from regulatory bodies (e.g. NMC, 2006). For learning from experiences, input tends to comprise a guided step-by-step process that ends with a reflective question asking the user what they have learnt from the experience. This is the most crucial component of reflective recording in portfolios, and is often followed by a further development plan.

e-portfolios

Increasingly, e-portfolios are being used particularly in profession or vocation linked courses. In some employment-related modules, students have to submit an e-profile (i.e. an extract from their e-portfolio) for summative assessments. One example of e-portfolio is Pebblepad (University of Wolverhampton, 2008), which has been in use since 2005. The publishers indicate that over 100 000 users have Pebblepad accounts, including over 40 institutions and a number of personal purchasers. Tools in e-portfolios allow for inclusion of photos (e.g. of certificates) and of videos (of presentations made by the portfolio owner) for instance.

The Pebblepad e-portfolio can, for instance, be used for recording CPD and personal development plans (PDP) and progress with them, which can be used for demonstrating conformance with standards, such as those required by professional regulatory bodies for revalidation of the individual's professional qualification.

An example of an e-profile submitted for summative assessment by Laura, a second-year BSc in Business and Human Resource Management student, is as follows. Laura had agreed to study for one short module in each of the 3 years of her course as a condition of being accepted on the course, which focuses on enhancing her chances of gaining employment straight after gaining her degree. The assessment for her second-year module, entitled *Management and teamwork in organizations*, included submitting an e-profile comprising a 600-word script documenting: a brief self-introduction, the job aimed for, reflection and evidence of use or initiative, adaptability and influence, and a SMART (specific, measurable, achievable, relevant, timed) action plan. Figure 15.1 shows parts of the e-profile that Laura submitted as one of the two assessed components for the module.

Obviously, Figure 15.1 is a profile, i.e. extracts from Laura's portfolio, that was presented for a specific purpose. As this example of e-portfolio illustrates, as with hard copies, an e-portfolio is more than a record of personal achievements because it is a 'learning system', in that it has provisions for writing up structured reflections on specific activities and experiences, and a record of aspirations and systematic forward planning.

e-portfolios also allow for certain items to be shared with selected individuals, or specific groups, or made public through the worldwide web. Other than for assessment purposes (formal or informal), over time, the e-portfolio user can store and review several 'assets' reflecting learning and achievement that can be presented for:

■ articulation: of learning from experience
■ application: for a place on a course, for funding
■ accreditation: by professional bodies
■ appraisal: by self, peer or 360 degrees feedback
■ advancement: job promotion or job transition.

Further instances of use of e-portfolios are as follows:

■ Research students can use e-portfolios to provide their supervisor with ongoing records of activities and accomplishments.
■ Art and design students keep portfolios of their designs, along with commentary from experts.
■ Students on overseas placements can confer with peers and their academic supervisors electronically with regards to validity of items for their portfolios.
■ Trainee teachers can send their lesson plans electronically to their academic supervisors, receive feedback, and document their teaching experiences.
■ Project sub-groups can share information and findings destined for their portfolios with other subgroups.

Furthermore, when students submit a profile or component of their e-portfolio for assessment, their teacher, mentor or supervisor can add feedback to the profile electronically. For summative work, moderators and external examiners can be given access to the profile for feedback and quality assurance purposes.

Research on the use of e-portfolios includes a study by Garrett and Jackson (2006), who evaluated the use of a mobile clinical e-portfolio by nursing and medical students, using wireless personal digital

Self-introduction

I am 21 years old, and in addition to being a full time student, I work at a local recruitment agency. I took a gap year after doing my A levels which is when I acquired this job. I enjoy the job, and once I have completed my degree in Business and Human Resource Management I would like to become a branch manager or a human resource manager at the same recruitment agency or at another similar large organisation.

Job aimed for: Branch manager of recruitment agency

Reflection-on-action

Initiative

An example of an objective which I have met using my initiative is when I set up my own dancing school when I was only 16. I had to arrange the insurance and licences that were required, find a suitable location, and deal with the advertising and finance myself.

I set myself the target of setting the dancing school up during the summer holidays in the year that I did my GCSE's, and ....

Adaptability

A time when things were difficult was a few weeks ago, when I was teaching dancing and we were doing a show which included stage managing approximately 150 children, and at the same time I had three 3000-word essays due in within a fortnight. As my favourite hobby, I also go camping regularly, and ....

I managed my time and had lists of everything which I needed to do, prioritized them ..... and I managed to get everything done, and it all went well – although I did feel very irritable at times.

Influence

I go camping every fortnight and organize group camping regularly, and I had to take an idea to the camping committee and prove to them that I was responsible enough to care for other people's children. In order to do this I created a leaflet with all of the information for parents, which also included a medical form and a disclaimer for injuries, which showed that I had thought of things such as health and safety. .... the committee gave the go-ahead and the camping movement is still growing after two years.

SMART action plan

One of the goals that I wish to achieve is to further develop my dancing, and my SMART action plan for this is as follows.

Goals

Specific objectives: A part-time dance teacher

Measurable: ....

Achievable: ....

Realistic: ....

Timed (Achieve by date): ....

Resources required: ....

Evidence of achievement: ....

FIGURE 15.1 Extract from Laura's 600-word e-profile submitted for summative assessment.

assistants (PDAs) with several useful functions, including helping to prevent the isolation of students whilst engaged in supervised clinical practice. The study found positive attitudes to the use of PDA based tools and portfolios.

Why do we need to keep a professional portfolio?

Why are you developing a portfolio? Is it to keep a record of your achievements, for professional development purposes, for accreditation of practice against university credit points, or because you have been told that you must do so?

Benefits and issues related to portfolios

Before we start discussing the reasons for keeping portfolios, consider and make detailed notes on what you feel are the advantages and disadvantages of keeping portfolios.

No doubt you will have noted various benefits of keeping portfolios, as well as some of the problematic aspects. The rationale for keeping a record of one's achievements and learning in portfolios (and profiles) arises from a variety of pressures in the contemporary world of work.

One major influence has been the increasing trend towards work-based vocational and professional learning, where it is necessary to keep a portfolio as evidence of what is being learnt as a continuous process. Additionally, employers expect professionals to update themselves continually and to be life-long learners who change and grow as the organization changes and grows, and record their learning.

Furthermore, in the past, nurses have not always been forthright in valuing their contribution to the healthcare team or in marketing their skills effectively. Engaging in portfolio learning can be a useful stage in doing these, developing self-awareness and building confidence and professional insights.

Another influencing factor comprises some of the more recent educational theories and approaches such as experiential learning, self-directed learning (based on 'adult education' or andragogical theories advocated by Rogers (2007) for instance), problem-based learning as well as portfolio-based learning (see Table 15.1, below, and Chapter 12). These educational theories and approaches place the healthcare professional at the centre of an active process of learning, with individuals taking responsibility for identifying and reflecting on the diverse learning opportunities that they encounter.

However, perhaps the strongest influence has emerged from professional regulatory bodies' approach that individual registered practitioners are accountable for their own updating and life-long learning (NMC, 2008a). The NMC standard is that registrants maintain a personal and professional portfolio of their learning activities as evidence of CPD and comply with requests for a relevant extract of their portfolio for audit requirements (NMC, 2006, p. 8), albeit that Snow (2007) reported that such checks are currently on hold.

The Health Professions Council (HPC) requires all healthcare professionals on its register to undertake CPD as a legal requirement (HPC, 2007). The first audit of these standards started in 2008 with a random sample of 5% of chiropodists and podiatrists being the first audited to prove they met the HPC's standards.

These influences have led to explorations and requirements to record learning and individual professional development as a meaningful process. It is generally agreed that this process should encourage further learning and facilitate professional accreditation. This accreditation is the process that offers recognition of the healthcare professional's knowledge and professional competence against professional standards, and also as credit points towards a university award.

The need to help healthcare professionals make sense of learning experiences in practice settings (experiential learning), and to make connections with planned learning (courses, in-service training, conferences or workshops) is another reason. This is all in the context of increasing professional autonomy, public accountability and quality frameworks such as clinical governance.

Furthermore, research highlights the effectiveness and various benefits of portfolios. McMullan (2008) for instance explored the use of portfolios by pre-registration students with regards to learning during practice placements and found that they helped them in their development of self-awareness and independent learning. McColgan (2008) reviewed the literature to examine the value of portfolio building by registered nurses, and found that portfolios are highly valued as long as an organizational culture of learning and support from colleagues existed.

Portfolio learning

As was discussed earlier, it should be appreciated that a portfolio contains a tangible and recognizable record of learning involving collecting, writing up and analysing significant learning experiences, including planned (or structured) and incidental learning events. Portfolio development is concerned with reflecting on your experiences and making the links between personal experiences and insights, and professional practice (see Chapters 12 and 14).

Portfolio learning is much more than good record keeping, as it is more concerned with how you engage with your thoughts and ideas. It involves working through critical incidents, collecting the evidence, and analysing such learning opportunities for yourself (see Chapter 6). Thus, a portfolio provides a safe environment, controlled by you, where you can be free to:

- acknowledge and build on your strengths
- confront your weaknesses or fears
- add perspective and depth to what you do.

Portfolio learning involves:

- focusing on your experiences
- collecting and organizing evidence
- analysing critical incidents
- having a critical dialogue with yourself (see Chapter 6)
- working with your ideas and entries
- acknowledging what you are learning and feeling
- making connections with what you are learning.

Learning opportunities include:

- exploring the everyday experiences that we have
- examining critical incidents
- learning from mistakes
- discussions with peers
- observing alternative ways of doing things through visits to other practice areas and shadowing others
- consulting mentors, preceptors and clinical supervisors.

Thus, portfolio learning can be seen as an important part of the 'educational jigsaw' that underpins the notion of the learning individual as someone committed to life-long learning. Table 15.1 details the key learning theories and approaches, and how these are integral to encouraging healthcare professionals to be continuing learning individuals. Each theory or approach has an important part to play in providing the overall 'picture' and in helping you to take responsibility for learning from your experiences and making the most of each learning opportunity that presents.

Having located portfolios within the current repertoire of learning activities it becomes easier to appreciate other advantages of keeping portfolios in the professional world of work. The NMC (2006, p. 1) suggests that the benefits of maintaining a portfolio are that it:

- Helps assess nurses' and midwives' current standards of practice.
- Helps develop nurses' and midwives' analytical skills through reflection on what they do.
- Enables review and evaluation of past experience and learning to help plan for the future.
- Demonstrates experiential learning, which may allow nurses and midwives to obtain credit towards further qualifications.
- Provides effective and current information when nurses and midwives apply for jobs or courses.

These are useful purposes that allow you to document and celebrate your achievements, and target further learning, develop your skills as a

TABLE 15.1 An overview of educational theories and approaches related to the learning individual

THEORY/APPROACH	APPLICATION
Experiential learning Concerns developing your problem-solving abilities, taking responsibility for your part in the learning process and learning from experience	Creating a desire to know more Involves thinking critically by challenging your assumptions and those of others. It includes identifying, planning and evaluating your learning opportunities
Reflective practice Concerns thinking about, mulling over and working through of ideas, issues and critical incidents	Developing abilities to integrate knowledge and find meaning within practice Involves exploring feelings and learning from practice by examining and recording actions, leading to new insights and effective practice
Professional learning support Concerns competent significant others who support and encourage us by being accessible and approachable. These are the mentors, preceptors and clinical supervisors who help us to reflect and assist our professional development	Working with critical friends Involves the building of enabling relationships that are built on mutual trust and respect to provide a supportive environment where we can consider our practice
Peer learning Refers to learning from other students on the same course, or colleagues of equal status at work	Working in formal or self-selected groups Group work, self-organized short-life self-directed study groups; learning from a buddy
Portfolio learning Concerns the regular maintenance of a portfolio that documents and draws together your experiences and provides further insights on practice	Working with your ideas and entries Writing up and engaging with the entries that allows you to demonstrate your personal and professional achievements in an organized manner, and which motivates towards further learning
Adult education/andragogy Refers to the specific ways in which adults learn, such as having clear goals about what they'd like to get out of the education programme, and seeing new learning in the context of their life experience	Having own learning plans Deciding what materials to study, when, who with and how; self-directed learning

learning individual and gain confidence in your abilities, as identified earlier by Palmer (2000). A brief example of portfolio learning is presented in Figure 15.2.

Likely reservations regarding portfolios

Despite the above-mentioned aims and benefits of portfolios, there can also be weaknesses. For instance, McMullan (2008) found that although portfolios helped students in their development of self-awareness and independent learning, the students also felt that portfolios do not sufficiently address the assessment of their clinical skills and the integration of theory and practice. Issues related to summative (i.e. pass/fail) assessment of portfolios is discussed later in this chapter.

Furthermore, there can also be barriers to utilization of e-portfolios, such as (University of Wolverhampton, 2008):

- Users being unsure and therefore reluctant to use new electronic devices.
- Some users need support to constitute their portfolios meaningfully.
- Timely access to computers, as much learning takes place outside education institutions.

Brief description of what happened

As a community nurse, I assessed a 'Return to Nursing' student administer subcutaneous medication using a Graseby syringe driver in the patient's own home. I performed this assessment with my supervisor assessing me assessing the student. The assessment was quite a long procedure, and when it was completed the two of us went to visit another patient to keep up with our schedule of work for the day.

How I felt conducting this assessment

Initially the assessment felt a little unusual. My student was nervous and appeared uncomfortable at times, but once we started and logically followed our plan and the assessment criteria, she relaxed. During the assessment I asked questions and later that morning we spent some time reflecting on both the positive and problematic aspects of the visit.

Evaluation and analysis

I am very used to working on my own, so it was a good experience taking time to assess my ability to assess a student, as indicated by the NMC (2008). During the assessment it was essential for me to be confident that the student was competent, confident and safe to practice. I was able to do this through direct observation of the student demonstrating the clinical skill and asking her questions. After the morning visits, we took 'time out' to reflect on the situation.

Learning and action plan

We both felt afterwards that reflecting on the experience is an excellent method for addressing both positive and unclear issues in a non-threatening and non-judgemental way. The student had assisted my colleagues with the skill on previous occasions, but had to wait a little while to be assessed due to my supervisor's workload. Next time I will ensure that for such a lengthy assessment, myself and the student are able to take sufficient time straight after the assessment to give feedback to the student more fully, not several hours after the procedure (Quinn & Hughes 2007).

References

Nursing and Midwifery Council (2008) Standards to Support Learning and Assessment in Practice. London, NMC.
Quinn F M, Hughes S J (2007) Quinn's Principles and Practice of Nurse Education (5th edn) Cheltenham, Nelson Thornes.

FIGURE 15.2 Extract from a student mentor's portfolio submitted for assessment.

- Different kinds of portfolios are expected by different institutions.
- Users might use an e-portfolio only when they have to.

How to develop and maintain an effective portfolio

Getting started

It is recognized that a number of nurses and midwives have trouble making a start on developing a portfolio. They often find that they are too busy, don't see the point and are unclear about what to collect or record, and what to leave out. However, as the NMC (2006) indicates, the portfolio is a personal, private and confidential document that does not belong to the NMC or to the nurse's or midwife's employer, and consequently employers and managers do not have the right to look at it. Each individual is free to present only the components that he or she wants to. Consequently, individuals should feel free to record in their portfolios whatever they feel appropriate, and the whole portfolio remains their private property.

Your portfolio is therefore your personal document, owned by you, and your own safe space where you have complete freedom to reflect on your learning encounters, be creative and decide what information and evidence you need and want to keep in your portfolio, and what these might be useful for. However, your recording needs to demonstrate that you are capable of, and therefore have the discipline, to reflect on your experiences, learn from them and document them.

One useful way of looking at portfolios is to see them as a record of significant events in your life and career (and therefore personal and professional), both being components of a journey that you are making. It is a recording of your achievements, of reflections along the way, current learning, and forward planning, which can be either timed or flexible.

Such reflections are commonly recorded in a section of the portfolio that tends to be referred to as reflective journals, diary, learning log, or learning from critical incidents. However, based on various guidelines and research findings, the following comprise useful good practice in constructing a portfolio:

- See your portfolio as your personal document, and the information should be owned by you.
- The content can be flexible and creative but it should be organized to make sense to you.
- You should be able to provide evidence to support your deliberations.
- Your learning and professional development should be related to your professional practice.
- Your portfolio should include a self-appraisal of professional development.
- Regular maintenance is essential to keep your recordings up to date and relevant.
- The contents are confidential and you need only present to others what you wish to.
- Keep your portfolio in a safe place as it may contain sensitive information about you and others.

The last two points are particularly important to allow you to engage with what you write, ask critical questions of yourself and reflect on how you are performing. The use of critical incidents can form a vital part of your portfolio development and you need to be aware that others could take incidents and events out of context. Another aspect that arises from these last two points concerns how you maintain your portfolio. It will become a living part of your practice and encourage individual learning if you consider linking parts of them to staff development discussion opportunities such as during your development and performance review.

You might choose to include the reflective elements and certain sensitive information, which is confidential to you, as you may choose to share some aspects of this section with a trusted colleague, or with your supervisor for instance as midwives are advised to do (NMC, 2008b). It is essential that information from a portfolio should not be shared or revealed without the consent (preferably written) of the owner.

Sharing some elements of your portfolio with your clinical supervisor, preceptor or mentor can also assist you in making sense of your own CPD, life-long learning and professional growth, as noted by Gopee (2008), for instance. How you do this is entirely up to you but it is preferable if you begin to make connections between your performance, professional support and any staff development openings that are available to you, or that you aspire to. This is sound advice for students on educational programmes as personal tutors, module leaders or academic supervisors are made available to assist with learning and reflecting. It is certainly worth contemplating how others can assist with the process of your portfolio learning.

The content of portfolios

What to include in your portfolio

Make a list of specific items of your own personal and professional achievement and learning that you could keep in your hard copy of your portfolio.

Having identified what portfolios are and having considered the ground rules for developing a portfolio, it is also useful to consider the precise nature of items that you are expected to keep in them. Otherwise, it may be easier to start with what you already know and any information that you have already collected about yourself. For many of us this will be factual information as a record of our academic and professional qualifications, career history and the courses or study days we have attended. Others include their CV and course certificates in their portfolio.

Next, it is a good idea to examine what is required in terms of the structure or the guidelines offered. For example when a doctor is suspected of having the tendency to use outdated practices, the General Medical Council (2008) indicates specific requirements of 'performance assessment' that the doctor needs to compile in their portfolio to demonstrate safe and effective medical practice. A wide variety of evidence of learning and achievements (outlined in the box below) can be included in portfolios.

EVIDENCE OF LEARNING AND ACHIEVEMENTS THAT CAN BE INCLUDED IN PORTFOLIOS

- Written feedback on presentations
- Reflective accounts of learning from critical incidents

- Certificates and awards
- Completed project work
- Published articles
- Testimonials
- Practice development lead
- Reviewing books/articles
- Presentation at an interest group seminar/a conference
- Feedback/written evaluation of presentations
- Approved health promotion leaflets/literature
- Organizing a significant professional event
- Planning and delivering a short course/in-service training
- National assessor for NVQ
- Representative on a committee
- Working party member
- Research/co-research report
- Involvement in design/review projects, e.g. for clinical guidelines
- Role expansion

Some of the portfolios that have been developed by publishers are organized into useful sections and are especially helpful if you are not sure of how to structure a portfolio. However, the NMC (2008a) offers flexible guidelines and suggests that there are no set procedures for building a portfolio other than three broad, inter-related steps – reviewing experience to date, self-appraisal and setting goals, and action plans. The box below identifies the likely sections of a portfolio as a possible way in which you could organize yours.

THE SECTIONS OF A PORTFOLIO

Section 1: Personal information, qualifications and awards
    1.1   Personal information
    1.2   Summary of academic qualifications, when obtained, and from which institution
    1.3   Professional and registrable qualifications
    1.4   Significant awards

Section 2: Employment history and experience
    2.1   Present full-time (and part-time) posts
    2.2   Previous post(s)
    2.3   Other associated professional roles

Section 3: Continuing professional development
    3.1   In-service training/in-house professional development courses attended
    3.2   Post-registration/post-graduate courses completed

> 3.3 Relevant research activities
> 3.4 Mapping learning against specific course outcomes (for accreditation)
>
> Section 4: Publications and other achievements
> 4.1 Publications
> 4.2 Conference presentations and teaching events/role
> 4.3 Summary of professional achievements over last 3 years
>
> Section 5: Reflections on specific significant learning experiences and critical incidents
>
> Section 6: My professional development plan
>
> Section 7: Further notes

Having started building your portfolio in this way the common concerns and issues that tend to be shared amongst nurses and midwives include 'There is too much for me to identify' and 'How do I make my records manageable?' These may become much less of an issue for some of you if you work through a prepared portfolio (the ready-made examples produced by individual Trusts and certain publishers). It is always good practice to pay attention to these but you should understand and 'own' them to help you celebrate your achievements.

However, your portfolio needs to demonstrate how you are a better practitioner as a result of keeping it. In maintaining a portfolio you need to work with and engage with what you write, making learning an integral component. Consequently, making sense of what you are recording encourages further learning, and in health care a useful way of doing this is to give structure by treating learning experiences as critical incidents (section 5 of the above box). These incidents are significant events that may be negative or positive experiences that have meaning for you or your practice, and therefore it is useful to focus on them to gain new insights.

Working with a critical incident

Identify a recent incident or experience that had significance for you, and ask yourself the following questions.

1.1 What happened?

1.2 Who was involved?

1.3 What was the outcome?

2.1 What did I feel?

2.2 What did I learn?

2.3 What would I do differently?

3.1 What have I learned from reflecting on this incident?

3.2 How will this learning impact on my practice?

In reflective write-ups related to critical incidents (see Chapters 12 and 14), the first step is to review the factual events of the incident or experience and your responses; recording them in your portfolio allows you to work with them. The second step is to engage with your feelings, which is an integral part of helping you make sense of your learning. In the third set of questions (see Figure 15.3, below) you are asked to stand back, as it were, to consider the impact of your reflection, which may result in changes to your practice.

Such inquiry requires a positive clinical culture that acknowledges that although on most occasions we do get things right and that our patients/service users are satisfied, we also encounter negative experiences, but by appreciating the experience and thinking critically about our practice, we learn from our mistakes and prevent ourselves from repeating them. Furthermore, when working with your entries:

- allow yourself adequate time
- let your ideas flow
- be honest and genuine in your recordings
- acknowledge when something is difficult
- ask yourself critical questions about what is emerging
- be creative and allow yourself to think differently
- don't confine yourself to one view
- seek help when it is required.

The process of working with your entries in your portfolio can be guided by the components illustrated in Figure 15.3, which consists of a continual cycle of:

- recording and reviewing an activity
- reflecting on and identifying the learning that has been achieved
- demonstrating the implications of this learning for practice.

The components identified in Figure 15.3 comprise a systematic approach to developing and maintaining a portfolio as they shift the balance from the relatively passive exercise of recording to reviewing your career progression, to reflecting and demonstrating portfolio learning that has facilitated personal growth and professional development based on significant experiences, and demonstrating learning that benefits your professional practice.

Support for portfolios development

As noted in the findings of the study by McMullan (2008), students feel they need ongoing support and guidance with portfolio utilization. Support with portfolio development can be obtained from various sources, such as from:

- peers: through clinical supervision and peer-reviews
- designated healthcare practitioners: such as mentors, preceptors, line managers

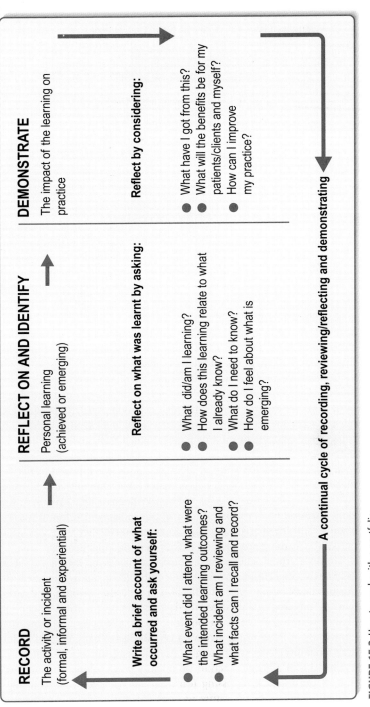

FIGURE 15.3 How to work with a portfolio.

- self-selected individuals: e.g. personal mentor, or coach
- university lecturers: e.g. personal tutor, practice education facilitators.

Moreover, if a student has any form of disability, such as dyslexia, the university's 'Student Services', Writing Support Department or Student Union can usually advise on policies on equality and diversity and the range of facilities that are available.

However, as discussed previously, as the portfolio is a confidential document, it is up to you to select information from your portfolio that you choose to share with your peers, your mentor/supervisor, in class, your line manager or for written assignments. Furthermore, it is becoming increasingly evident that nursing, midwifery and other professional courses require students to submit their portfolios for assessment.

How are portfolios and profiles assessed?

A number of professional courses, including those in healthcare, now require students to submit a portfolio by specified dates for assessment of their knowledge and competence. They form part of the coursework for the specific course or module, and students are notified as to whether they should submit them as a hard copy or as an e-portfolio. Portfolios are usually also required for assessing prior or continuing learning, with a view to accreditation and re-validation respectively. The portfolios that are required by regulatory bodies are for quality assurance purposes for instance, and are therefore audited, not assessed.

Students are provided with guidelines on the components that their portfolios are expected to include, as well as the criteria that will determine whether the portfolio is awarded a pass or fail. The pass criteria normally constitute demonstrating how specified or all learning outcomes for the course or module have been achieved, and providing evidence to support each.

Various studies have found that portfolios constitute an effective means of assessing students' levels of reflective thinking and learning (Pitts et al., 1999; Wong et al., 1995). Williams (2003) reports on a study that examined the assessment of portfolios, which found it to be a sound and transparent approach to assessments, they were viewed as part of the learning process, and encouraged life-long learning.

However, these studies also pointed to areas of inconsistency in assessment of portfolios. Wong et al. (1995) for instance identified difficulties in assessing levels of reflection in reflective writings, and problems in applying quantitative criteria to qualitative writing. Pitts et al. (1999) report that assessing portfolios is challenging and note that trained assessors can only achieve a certain degree of agreement (inter-rater reliability), even when judging portfolios against agreed criteria.

Endacott et al. (2004) report on a study that explored the effectiveness of portfolios in assessing learning and competence which highlighted the evolutionary nature of portfolio development, and a range of additional factors influencing the effectiveness of their use, including language of assessment, degree of guidance and expectations of clinical and academic staff.

Spence and El-Ansari (2004) evaluated practice teachers' experiences of portfolio assessment of specialist community nursing practitioner students in which practice teachers reported that the source of portfolio evidence supplied by students include a record of discussions during supervision, other practitioners' reports and feedback from patients. They indicate that although the practice teacher's experience of portfolios is largely positive, the quality of portfolios evidence was varied.

Another issue with assessment of portfolios relate to grading the portfolio (e.g. A, B, C, D or F) against preset criteria, which entails making judgements on the quality, or level of excellence or poorness, of the recording. This is recognized by those involved in curriculum planning for the course when identifying assessment criteria for marking portfolios. Thus, there is little doubt that assessing portfolios requires a careful approach as this exercise involves a way of objectively assessing the healthcare professional's reflective writing which includes recording of subjective personal feelings, interpretation and analysis of meaningful events, which are often less readily measurable.

Some researchers recommend a structure for portfolios that helps make assessment a more objective process. In their study, Challis et al. (1997) link portfolio learning to the completion of a learning cycle (as discussed in Chapter 2). Informants were asked to identify their learning needs and plan appropriate activities to meet these needs. The resulting portfolios included a needs analysis, an action plan and evidence that needs had been met and new learning applied to practice. Providing such a framework requires an understanding of the learning process with the identification of clear aims and learning outcomes that are linked to appropriate educational activities.

Jasper and Fulton (2005) suggest specific criteria for assessing practice-based profiles, including:

- The development of new insights which enhance and develop practice.
- Effective communication with professionals and non-professionals.
- Coherent structure that contains all required elements including use of English and referencing.

From the discussion on the approach to be taken, a key question emerges: 'What should the student include in a profile that they will submit for summative assessment?' It is clear that for portfolios to be assessed effectively, the assessment criteria need to be explicit, and include preparation of students, supervisors and assessors to ensure a common understanding of requirements. Assessors need to be clear about the specific criteria for assessment, and assessor preparation should also focus on encouraging inter-rater reliability while the students' preparation should involve strategies that encourage reflection and self-assessment. Essential components of portfolio assessment are identified in the box below.

ESSENTIAL COMPONENTS OF PORTFOLIO ASSESSMENT

- The portfolio is well organized and presented, with a contents page
- The relationship between the aims, outcomes and learning contract, and the evidence presented are explicit
- The portfolio demonstrates systematic reflection using a published model or framework
- It demonstrates connection between CPD experiences
- It shows personal or professional development in the form of action plans, and if appropriate, a PDP
- It demonstrates how new learning, including academic achievements, applies to professional practice and impact on patient or service user care
- It demonstrates links to directives and policy requirements, such as the *NHS knowledge and skills framework*, if required
- It includes documentation of self-assessment components
- The assessor provides comments on the content of the portfolio, not on the writer
- Further learning for students, and their supervisors if appropriate, is identified

---

The purpose of developing the profile should be reflected in the assessment rationale and criteria. The components identified in the box above constitute the criteria for passing/failing of the profile presented. The criteria for graded portfolios obviously need to be more detailed, but they are still at developmental stages. Furthermore, as indicated in the box, self-assessment is an important part of portfolio learning and it is therefore essential that there is a section for this to allow the individual to consider the role that they have in assessing their own work. This can also ensure that reflection continues and that they have ownership of how their work achieves the purpose required.

However, other than for summative assessment purposes, as mentioned earlier, portfolios comprise an important method of learning and facilitating learning, and therefore they do not have to be graded, and can be less structured, which in turn should encourage further learning.

Conclusion

Developing a portfolio can help you reflect and give you time to catch up with yourself in order 'to take stock, to make sense of what has happened or share other people's ideas on the experience' (Boud et al., 1985, p. 8). Working with your portfolio can also help you gain a clearer sense of knowing who you are and what you are doing – allowing you to value your uniqueness and your personal contribution to healthcare delivery.

Acknowledgement

This chapter builds on previous editions of the chapter by Liz Redfern and Anne Palmer.

CHAPTER RESOURCES

REFERENCES

Boud, D., Keogh, R. & Walker, D., 1985. Reflection: turning experience into learning. Kogan Page, London.

British Dietetic Association (BDA), 2001. A professional portfolio for dietitians. BDA, Birmingham.

Challis, M., Mathers, N.J., Howe, A.C. & Field, N.J., 1997. Portfolio-based learning: continuing medical education for general practitioners – a mid-point evaluation. Medical Education 31, 22–26.

Endacott, R., Gray, M.A. & Jasper, M.A., et al., 2004. Using portfolios in the assessment of learning and competence: the impact of four models. Nurse Education Practice 4 (4), 250–257.

Garrett, B.M. & Jackson, C., 2006. A mobile clinical e-portfolio for nursing and medical students, using wireless personal digital assistants (PDAs). Nurse Education Today 26 (8), 647–654.

General Medical Council, 2008. Doctors under investigation – performance assessments. Online. Available: www.gmc-uk.org/concerns/doctors_under_investigation/performance_assessments.asp [accessed 6 May 2008].

Gopee, N., 2008. Mentoring and supervision in healthcare. Sage Publications, London.

Health Professions Council, 2007. Countdown to CPD audits has begun… Online. Available: www.hpc-uk.org/mediaandevents/pressreleases/index.asp?id=212 [accessed 19 April 2008].

Health Professions Council, 2008. Putting your CPD profile together – CPD profile template. Online. Available: www.hpc-uk.org/registrants/cpd/profile/ [accessed 12 September 2008].

Hull, C., Redfern, L. & Shuttleworth, A., 2005. Profiles and portfolios: a guide for health and social care. Palgrave Macmillan, Basingstoke.

Jasper, M.A. & Fulton, J., 2005. Marking criteria for assessing practice-based portfolios at masters' level. Nurse Education Today 25 (5), 377–389.

Kenworthy, N. & Redfern, L., 2004. The Churchill Livingstone professional portfolio, 3rd edn. Elsevier, London.

McColgan, K., 2008. The value of portfolio building and the registered nurse. Journal of Peri-operative Practice 18 (2), 64–69.

McMullan, M., 2008. Using portfolios for clinical practice learning and assessment: The pre-registration nursing student's perspective. Nurse Education Today 28 (7), 873–879.

Nursing and Midwifery Council (NMC), 2006. Personal professional profiles: A–Z advice sheet. Online. Available: www.nmc-uk.org [accessed 26 March 2008].

Nursing and Midwifery Council (NMC), 2008a. The PREP Handbook. NMC, London.

Nursing and Midwifery Council (NMC), 2008b. Modern supervision in action: a practical guide for midwives. Online. Available: www.nmc-uk.org [accessed 26 March 2008].

Palmer, A., 2000. Freedom to learn – freedom to be: learning, reflecting and supporting in practice. In: Humphris, D. & Masterson, A. (Eds.) Developing new clinical roles: a guide for health professionals. Harcourt Health Sciences, London.

Pitts, J., Coles, C. & Thomas, P., 1999. Educational portfolios in the assessment of general practice trainers: reliability of assessors. Medical Education 33 (7), 515–520.

Rogers, J., 2007. Adults learning, 5th edn. Open University Press, Maidenhead, UK.

Snow, T., 2007. PREP compliance checks put on hold indefinitely. Nursing Standard 22 (5), 8.

Spence, J. & El-Ansari, E., 2004. Portfolio assessment: practice teachers' early experience. Nurse Education Today 24 (5), 388–401.

University of Wolverhampton, 2008. Pebblepad, not just a portfolio. Online. Available: www.pdp.coventry.ac.uk/pebblepad.aspx [accessed 2 May 2008].

Williams, M., 2003. Assessment of portfolios in professional education. Nursing Standard 18 (8), 33–37.

Wong, F.K.Y., Kember, D., Chung, L.Y.E. & Yan, L., 1995. Assessing the level of student reflection from reflective journals. Journal of Advanced Nursing 22 (1), 48–57.

WEBSITES

Centre for International ePortfolio Development at the University of Nottingham: http://www.nottingham.ac.uk/eportfolio/

General Medical Council (for *Doctors under investigation – performance assessments*): http://www.gmc-uk.org/concerns/doctors_under_investigation/performance_assessments.asp

Health Professions Council (for *Putting your CPD profile together* and a CPD profile template and the HPC guidelines on portfolios): http://www.hpc-uk.org/registrants/cpd/profile/ (and, for criteria for assessing profiles): http://www.hpc-uk.org/registrants/cpd/criteria/index.asp

Higher Education Academy (for *The e-Portfolio Project report*): http://www.heacademy.ac.uk/physsci/home/projects/jisc_del/eportfolio

Northumbria Training Programme for General Practice (The e-portfolio): http://www.gp-training.net/training/assessment/nmrcgp/eportfolio/index.htm

Nursing and Midwifery Council (for *Personal professional profiles: A–Z advice sheet*): http://www.nmc-uk.org/aFrameDisplay.aspx?DocumentID=1583

FURTHER READING

Hull, C., Redfern, L. & Shuttleworth, A., 2005. Profiles and portfolios: a guide for health and social care. Palgrave Macmillan, Basingstoke, UK.

Moon, J., 2006. Learning journals: a handbook for reflective practice and professional development, 2nd edn. Routledge, Abingdon, UK.

Timmins, F., 2008. Making sense of nursing portfolios – a guide for students. McGraw-Hill, Berkshire.

INDEX

Note: Illustrations are comprehensively referred to from the text. Therefore, significant material in illustrations and tables have only been given a page reference in the absence of their concomitant mention in the text referring to that figure.

CINAHL (Cumulative Index to Nursing and Allied Health Literature), 54, 59, 91, 166
circular argument, 136
clarity in written assignment, 125–6
client *see* patient
clinical guidelines, 99
clinical practice, 90–104, 195–337
  assessment of practice-based portfolios, 333
  information technology example in, 90–104
  learning, 32–5, 219–49
    six principles, 220–46
    of skills *see* clinical skills
  placement in *see* placement
  simulations of, 211–12
clinical questions and evidence-based healthcare, 57–8
clinical skills, 197–218
  acquisition, 200–1, 203–5
  assessment, 214–15
  feedback, 41
  for post-registration, 207–9
  for pre-registration, 205–6, 219–20
  revisiting, 212–14
  understanding, 206–7
clinical skills laboratories, 197, 198–9, 200, 202, 206
clip art, 84
Cochrane Collaboration, 175
collaborator (with supervisor/mentor/preceptor), working and learning as, 226–8
communication skills, practice setting, 225
community care, example placement in, 222, 233–6
competency stage in clinical skills acquisition, 204
complementary therapy in symptom control in cancer, 165–6
completer finisher (role in group work), 283
computers
  hardware, 78
  operating systems, 78–9
  skills using, 77
  software *see* software
conceptual level of reflectivity (Mezirow's), 311
conceptualization, abstract, 33
conclusion(s)
  in Gibbs' model of reflection, 257, 258–9

in research article, 169
in written assignment, 125
  in reports, 182
concrete experience, 33
confidence-building with clinical skills, 200
Consortium of University Research Libraries (COPAC), 69
content
  portfolios, 301, 327–30
  reports, 181–3
context and intent (reading), 112
continuing professional development (CPD), 316, 318, 322, 327
  in portfolios, 328–9
coordinator (role in group work), 283
COPAC (Consortium of University Research Libraries), 69
copying others' work *see* plagiarism
copyright, 185–6
course(s)
  online, 102–2, 103
  preparation for examination at start of and during, 144–5
  preparation in *see* preparation
CPD *see* continuing professional development
Critical Appraisal Skills Programme (CASP) website, 58
critical approach to/critical appraisal of information, 46, 109–10, 174
  articles, 64, 174
  by friend of your article, 191
Critical Care Nursing Quarterly, 172
critical-incident analysis, 269–71
  portfolios and, 329–30
critical reflection, 261, 311
  examples, 304–10
  Kim's method, 263
Cuil, 87
cultural thinking, reflection encouraging, 253
cultural values, different, 240–1
culture of learning, developing a, 273–5
Cumulative Index to Nursing and Allied Health Literature (CINAHL), 54, 59, 91, 166
currency
  of journals vs books, 51
  modular learning outcomes and learning achievements, 300
curriculum vitae (CV) on your web page, 99, 104, 106
CV on your web page, 99, 104, 106